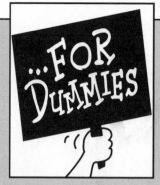

TM

References for the Rest of Us!®

BESTSELLING BOOK SERIES

Do you find that traditional reference books are overloaded with technical details and advice you'll never use? Do you postpone important life decisions because you just don't want to deal with them? Then our *For Dummies*® business and general reference book series is for you.

For Dummies business and general reference books are written for those frustrated and hard-working souls who know they aren't dumb, but find that the myriad of personal and business issues and the accompanying horror stories make them feel helpless. *For Dummies* books use a lighthearted approach, a down-to-earth style, and even cartoons and humorous icons to dispel fears and build confidence. Lighthearted but not lightweight, these books are perfect survival guides to solve your everyday personal and business problems.

> **"More than a publishing phenomenon, 'Dummies' is a sign of the times."**
>
> — The New York Times

> **"A world of detailed and authoritative information is packed into them..."**
>
> — U.S. News and World Report

> **"...you won't go wrong buying them."**
>
> — Walter Mossberg, Wall Street Journal, on For Dummies books

Already, millions of satisfied readers agree. They have made For Dummies the #1 introductory level computer book series and a best-selling business book series. They have written asking for more. So, if you're looking for the best and easiest way to learn about business and other general reference topics, look to For Dummies to give you a helping hand.

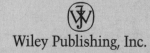

Wiley Publishing, Inc.

5/09

Pregnancy

FOR

DUMMIES®

**by Joanne Stone, MD,
Keith Eddleman, MD,
and Mary Murray**

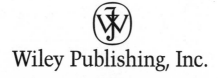

Wiley Publishing, Inc.

Pregnancy For Dummies®
Published by
Wiley Publishing, Inc.
909 Third Avenue
New York, NY 10022
www.wiley.com

For general information on our other products and services or to obtain technical support, please contact our Customer Care Department within the U.S. at 800-762-2974, outside the U.S. at 317-572-3993, or fax 317-572-4002.

Wiley also publishes its books in a variety of electronic formats. Some content that appears in print may not be available in electronic books.

Library of Congress Cataloging-in-Publication Data:

Library of Congress Control Number: 99-62376

ISBN: 0-7645-5074-8

Manufactured in the United States of America

10 9

About the Authors

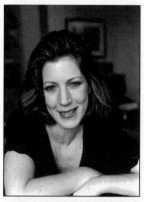

Joanne Stone, MD, is a full-time faculty member in the internationally renowned Division of Maternal-Fetal Medicine at The Mount Sinai Medical Center in New York City. She is the director of the Perinatal Ultrasound Unit and also cares for patients with problem pregnancies. She has lectured throughout the country, is widely published in medical journals, and has been interviewed frequently for television and magazines on topics related to pregnancy, with a special emphasis on the management of multifetal pregnancies. Away from the hospital she loves to spend time with her husband, George, and her two little girls, Chloe and Sabrina.

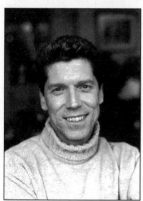

Keith Eddleman, MD, works with Joanne in the Division of Maternal-Fetal Medicine at Mount Sinai. He is also a full-time faculty member and is the director of Prenatal Diagnosis. He teaches medical students, residents, and fellows; lectures throughout the world; and appears often on television to discuss issues concerning the care of pregnant women. His areas of special expertise are ultrasound and reproductive genetics. His free time, when he has any, is split between spending time with his family at their apartment in Manhattan or at their country house in upstate New York.

Mary Murray, a former newspaper reporter, has been a magazine writer and editor since the mid-1980s. For most of that time, she has specialized in medicine and science journalism. She has written for *Discover, Allure, Reader's Digest,* and *Glamour.* She has been executive editor of *The Sciences* and a senior editor for *Vogue,* and she is currently executive editor of *Women's Sports & Fitness* magazine. She is also the mother of 9-year-old twins, Nick and Claire.

Dedication

To George, Chloe, Sabrina, Frank, Jack, Nick, and Claire for all their love and support.

Authors' Acknowledgments

Writing this book was truly a labor of love. We would like to thank everyone who played a part in the "birth" of this book, and specifically the following:

Tami Booth, Jennifer Ehrlich, Christy Beck, Elizabeth Kuball, Paula Lowell, and the other folks at Hungry Minds who conceived this idea and walked us through the whole process.

Carolyn Krupp and the folks at International Management Group for connecting us with Hungry Minds.

Dr. Jill Fishbane-Mayer for establishing the initial connection.

Drs. Lynn Friedman, Mary D'Alton, Richard Berkowitz, and Ramona Slupik for excellent comments and suggestions.

Dr. Ian Holzman for nurturing us through the newborn chapter.

Kathryn Born for taking our scrap art and turning it into terrific illustrations.

And to all our patients over the years whose inquisitive minds and need for accurate information inspired us to write this book.

Publisher's Acknowledgments

We're proud of this book; please send us your comments through our online registration form located at www.dummies.com/register.

Some of the people who helped bring this book to market include the following:

Acquisitions and Editorial

Senior Project Editor: Jennifer Ehrlich

Executive Editor: Tammerly Booth

Copy Editors: Christine Meloy Beck, Paula Lowell, Elizabeth Nededu Kuball

Technical Editors: Dr. Richard Berkowitz, Dr. Mary D'Alton, Dr. Lynn Friedman, Dr. Ramona Slupik

Editorial Manager: Mary C. Corder

Editorial Assistants: Paul E. Kuzmic, Alison Walthall

Production

Project Coordinator: Cindy L. Phipps

Layout and Graphics: Linda M. Boyer, Lisa Harrington, Angela F. Hunckler, Anna Rohrer, Brent Savage, Jacque Schneider, Mark Shirar, Rashell Smith, Michael A. Sullivan, Brian Torwelle

Special Art: Kathryn Born

Proofreaders: Kelli Botta, Betty Kish, Jennifer Mahern, Brian Massey, Nancy Price, Rebecca Senninger, Ethel M. Winslow, Janet M. Withers

Indexer: Cynthia D. Bertelsen

Publishing and Editorial for Consumer Dummies

Diane Graves Steele, Vice President and Publisher, Consumer Dummies

Joyce Pepple, Acquisitions Director, Consumer Dummies

Kristin A. Cocks, Product Development Director, Consumer Dummies

Michael Spring, Vice President and Publisher, Travel

Brice Gosnell, Publishing Director, Travel

Suzanne Jannetta, Editorial Director, Travel

Publishing for Technology Dummies

Andy Cummings, Acquisitions Director

Composition Services

Gerry Fahey, Executive Director of Production Services

Debbie Stailey, Director of Composition Services

Contents at a Glance

Cartoons at a Glance

By Rich Tennant

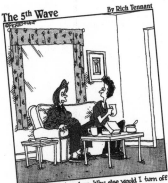

"I really think it's a boy. Why else would I turn off 'Masterpiece Theater' to hog the remote through a two-hour 'Wrestlemania?'"

page 325

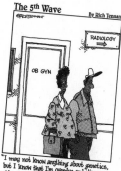

"I may not know anything about genetics, but I know that I'm overdue and it's your side of the family that's always late for family functions."

page 259

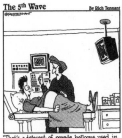

"That's a telecast of parade balloons used in Macy's Thanksgiving Day Parade. Your ultra-sound images are over here."

page 63

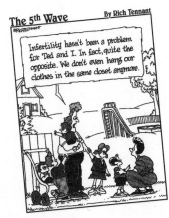

"Infertility hasn't been a problem for Ted and I. In fact, quite the opposite. We don't even hang our clothes in the same closet anymore."

page 7

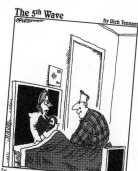

"Even the doctors were surprised at how involved you were in there. Especially right near the end when you turned on that tape of the 'William Tell Overture.'"

page 141

Cartoon Information:
Fax: 978-546-7747
E-Mail: richtennant@the5thwave.com
World Wide Web: www.the5thwave.com

Table of Contents

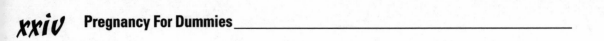

Introduction

*I*t's ironic that this book is called *Pregnancy For Dummies*, because the whole idea behind it is that couples today are *not* dummies (in the traditional sense) and are quite capable of understanding complex medical information when it's presented clearly. Our goal, in fact, has been to write a scientifically correct, comprehensive guide to what is one of the most memorable experiences in anyone's life — pregnancy. The *...For Dummies* books are known for being accurate and informative yet easy to read. That's why we found this format to be the perfect one in which to present the medical facts of pregnancy and still acknowledge, and even encourage, the humor and lightheartedness that are part of the miraculous process of having babies.

We know from our experience caring for thousands of women at Mount Sinai Medical Center in New York City that prospective parents are truly interested in and curious about everything that goes on during pregnancy. Today, you can get information about this incredible topic in so many ways — various books, magazines, and, of course, the Internet. Yet many prospective parents still have so many questions to which they have not been able to find accurate answers. In this book, we incorporate our responses to many of the commonly asked questions. Our approach to some of the more controversial ones has been to provide answers based on *real,* medically based data. We made sure to provide not just the party line answer, or the safe answer, but the response that is based on the medical literature. It took quite a bit of investigating to find data on whether it is safe to eat sushi, for example, or to dye your hair or have manicures during pregnancy. Sometimes, there are no solid data to indicate whether something is safe or unsafe, and when this is the case, we tell you. Our approach has been the same when answering questions about taking various medications during pregnancy or going scuba diving or drinking coffee.

Our experience has shown us that prospective parents also want to know about the real medical aspects of pregnancy. When is the baby's heart formed? When are fingers developed? What blood tests should be done, and why? What options are available for detecting various problems? In addressing these topics, we have attempted to write a book that is essentially a medical text on obstetrics for the layperson. We appreciate and respect each parent's desire to find out as much as possible about pregnancy, and we believe that this book is a great source of medical information — in understandable, enjoyable, and sometimes humorous form.

We are practicing obstetricians who are also board certified in the sub-specialty of maternal-fetal medicine (high-risk pregnancies), and we also teach residents, medical students, and other doctors about pregnancy and prenatal care. So we came into this project with a certain amount of exper-tise. Also, we consulted many of our colleagues in areas of medicine outside obstetrics — in pediatrics, internal medicine, and anesthesia, for example. For many topics, we conducted comprehensive searches of the medical liter-ature to make sure the information we provide is based on the most recent studies available. Working with Mary Murray on the text has been enor-mously helpful in making sure that the medical information we are providing is comprehensible to someone who is not in the medical field. In addition, as a mother of twins, Mary has been able to provide her own unique insight into various aspects of pregnancy.

Pregnancy Should Be a Joy, Not a Worry

Too often, our patients come to us incredibly worried about something they've read in another book that is either outdated, lacks any real scientific basis, or is exaggerated way out of proportion. (Guess what? You *can* eat fresh tuna when you're expecting. You can also eat the fresh fruits and veg-etables you buy at the supermarket without worrying day and night that they're overloaded with toxins.) Much of the time, information in some other pregnancy books is presented in such a way as to be alarmist, or it is not properly put into perspective. The trouble is that pregnant women are, by nature, already anxious about whether anything they do or anything they eat may hurt the baby. The guiding principle of our approach has been to put all the facts into perspective and not to create needless anxiety or fear. *Pregnancy should be a joy, not a worry.* A big part of our philosophy in writing this book is to reassure pregnant women whenever medically possible, rather than to add to the unnecessary worries they already have.

How to Use This Book

Pregnancy For Dummies is designed to be used gradually, as you enter into each stage of pregnancy. Many women are curious about what lies ahead and may want to read the whole book right off the bat. But the information is organized in such a way that you can take things one trimester at a time, if you like. You can also consult it as needed if you run into some particular question or problem.

Most of the information in this book is applicable to all pregnant women, but we also include sections dealing with atypical situations. Some couples want to read everything they possibly can about all aspects of pregnancy, find out all there is to know about the latest in medical advances, and read up on every possible pregnancy complication. Others don't want to read anything about any potential problems that don't directly relate to them. For this reason, we deal with possible complications and unusual situations either at the ends of chapters or in entirely separate chapters.

Ideally, you will pick up this book *before* you get pregnant. That way you can take advantage of our advice about how to prepare — for example, by making sure you're healthy and in reasonably good shape, by taking folic acid ahead of time, and by scheduling a preconceptual appointment with your doctor. Still, we assume that a great many expectant mothers and fathers start reading about pregnancy only *after* they've conceived. That method works, too. Most of the book covers what happens after conception.

Keep in mind that medical science advances fairly quickly. We made a great effort to ensure that all the information in this book is accurate and up to the minute as of the time of publication. But in certain ways, medical understanding of pregnancy is bound to advance. For this reason, we intend to update the book regularly.

We trust that you will use this book as a companion to regular medical care. Perhaps some of the information in it will lead you to ask your practitioner questions that you may not otherwise have thought to ask. Because there is not always just one answer or even a right answer to every question, you may find that your practitioner holds a different point of view than we do in some areas. This difference of opinion is only natural, and in fact, there are times when we disagree with each other. The bottom line is that this book provides a lot of factual information, but it is not "gospel." Remember also that many topics we discuss apply to pregnancy in general, but your particular situation may have unique aspects to it that warrant different or extra consideration.

Conventions Used in This Book

It is helpful for you to understand a few conventions that we kept in mind while writing this book.

We try to be respectful of the fact that while traditional husband-wife couples still account for the majority of expectant parents, babies are born into many different circumstances. These circumstances may involve single parents, same-sex couples, adoptive parents, or pregnancies that involve surrogacy. The bottom line is that the information we present is pertinent and useful to people in many different situations.

We also realize that obstetricians are not the only health professionals who help women through pregnancy. (See Chapter 2 for specific descriptions of the many kinds of professionals who can play a major role in helping women through pregnancy and childbirth.) That is why, in many cases, we refer to your pregnancy professional as your "practitioner." In some cases, we do specify "doctor," but usually only when we describe a situation that clearly calls for the services of a physician.

How This Book Is Organized

The parts and chapters of this book represent a logical flow of information about the pregnancy process. Check out the following sections for a more detailed overview.

Part I: The Game Plan

Sure, some women still get pregnant "accidentally." But for many women these days, pregnancy is a conscious choice. Planning ahead is a good idea — even seeing your practitioner before you conceive. Even if it's already too late to plan that far ahead, this part of the book fills you in on what's happening to your body during the first days and weeks of pregnancy. In this part, you can also find out what happens at a prenatal visit. And you can find out the general scope of what your life will be like for the next nine months.

Part II: Pregnancy: A Drama in Three Acts

Like all good narratives, pregnancy has a beginning, a middle, and an end. They're called *trimesters*. The way you feel and the kind of care you need vary with each stage. In this part, you get an idea of how each trimester unfolds.

Part III: The Big Event: Labor, Delivery, and Recovery

After you've put in your nine months, it's time for the flurry of activity that results in the birth of your baby. At this point, a lot is going on in a short time. What your experience is like depends heavily on what kind of delivery you have and how long it takes. This part covers the basic scenario of labor, delivery, and recovery — plus many possible variations on the theme.

Part IV: Special Concerns

This part is where to look for information about all kinds of special concerns that you may have as new parents — from practical challenges like how to introduce older siblings to the new baby to health problems that sometimes arise during pregnancy.

In a way, it would be nice if we didn't have to have a section about problems that come up during pregnancy. Ideally, every woman's experience would be perfectly trouble-free. On the other hand, many of the difficulties that can arise need not develop into full-blown problems if they are properly taken care of. For this reason, it's crucial that we offer information about how to deal with anything that can come up. This part is the one to consult if you think you're having any kind of difficulty, from the serious to the mundane.

Part V: The Part of Tens

The "Part of Tens" is standard in all ...*For Dummies* books. Before we began writing the book, we weren't sure how to make this part of our book useful. But in the end, we were very glad to have a place where we could put many aspects of pregnancy in a nutshell. Here, you find out more about how the baby grows and how you can view him or her on ultrasound. We also dispel some common myths and give you some good reasons to relax and enjoy your pregnancy.

Appendix

In most pregnancy books, the father of the baby is, sadly, overlooked. We think that's a shame. In this book, we throw in tidbits and tips (look for the "Just For Dads" icons) for the dad-to-be to help him be an active participant in the pregnancy process. This appendix goes a step further and gives dad an insightful overview of the entire process. Enjoy!

Icons Used in This Book

Like other ...*For Dummies* books, this one has little icons in the margins to guide you through the information and zero in on what you need to find out. The following paragraphs describe the icons and what they mean.

This icon signals that we're going to delve a little deeper than usual into a medical explanation. We don't mean to suggest the information is too difficult to understand — just a little extra detailed.

We flag certain pieces of information with this icon to let you know something is particularly worth keeping in mind.

This icon marks bits of advice we can give you about handling some of the minor discomforts and other challenges you encounter during pregnancy.

Throughout this book, we try to avoid being too alarmist, but there are some situations and actions that a pregnant woman clearly should avoid. When this is the case, we show you the Caution icon.

Many things you may feel or notice while you're pregnant will beg the question, "Is this important enough for my practitioner to know about?" When the answer is yes, you see this icon.

Dads go through pregnancy, too, we realize (though, let's face it, not nearly to the degree that moms do). And there are certain things that dads can do, or should know about, along the way. This icon points out the things that are particularly for them.

We know from experience that pregnancy can bring out the instinct to worry. It's normal and fine to feel a little anxious from time to time, but some women go overboard working themselves up over things that really aren't a problem. We use this icon — more than any other one — to point out the countless things that you really need not fret about.

Pregnancy brings about all kinds of changes in your body. Certain hormones flow more freely. You get larger (duh). We use this icon to point out the physiological changes you can anticipate.

In the interest of dispelling useless, untrue notions about pregnancy, we've mentioned a few and labeled them with the Myth icon.

Where Do I Go from Here?

If you're the particularly thorough type, start with Chapter 1 and end with the Appendix. If you just want to find specific information and then close the book, take a look at the table of contents or at the index. Dog-ear the pages that are especially interesting or relevant to you. Write little notes in the margins. Have fun and, most of all, enjoy your pregnancy!

Part I
The Game Plan

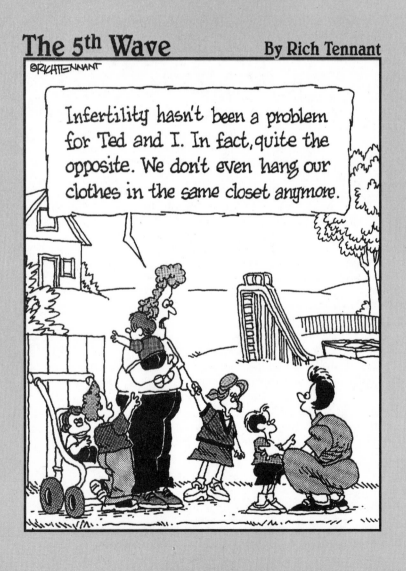

Infertility hasn't been a problem for Ted and I. In fact, quite the opposite. We don't even hang our clothes in the same closet anymore.

In this part . . .

"**I**'m not sure I'm ready for this" is a normal reaction
to finding out that you're pregnant, no matter how
long you've been thinking about having a baby and no
matter how long you've been trying to conceive.
Suddenly, you're faced with the reality that your body is
about to undergo some profound changes and a baby is
going to take shape inside you. Well, you may not *feel*
ready, but preparing is easy enough. Ideally, your preparation begins with a visit to your doctor a few months
before you conceive. But even if you're not that far ahead
of the game, this part tells you some of the many ways
you can plan ahead for the very important, very interesting next nine months (plus).

Chapter 1

From Here to Maternity

In This Chapter

▶ Discovering why it pays to think *before* you conceive

▶ Looking back at your family's health history and ethnic roots

▶ Preparing your body for pregnancy

▶ Making it happen

Congratulations! If you are already pregnant, you're about to embark upon one of the most exciting adventures of your life. The next year or so is going to be filled with tremendous changes and (we hope) unbelievable happiness. If you are thinking about getting pregnant but are not yet pregnant, you're probably excited at the prospect but also a little nervous at the same time.

In this chapter, we tell you what you can do to get ready for pregnancy — first by visiting your practitioner and going over your family and personal health history. Then you can discover whether or not you're in optimal shape to get pregnant, or if you need to take some time to gain or lose weight, improve your diet, quit smoking, or discontinue medications that could be harmful to your pregnancy. We also give you some basic advice about the easiest way to conceive, and we touch on the topic of infertility.

Before You Get Pregnant

By the time you miss your period and discover you're pregnant, the embryo, now two weeks old or more, is already undergoing dramatic changes. Believe it or not, when the embryo is only two to three weeks old, it has already developed the beginnings of its heart and brain. Because your general health and nutrition can influence the growth of those organs, having your body ready for pregnancy before you get pregnant really pays off. Scheduling what's called a *preconceptual visit* with your practitioner to be sure your body is tuned up and ready to go is your best course of action. Sometimes you can schedule this visit during a routine gynecological appointment: When you go in for your annual PAP test, mention that you're thinking about having a baby, and your practitioner will take you through the preliminaries. If you aren't due for your annual exam for several more months and you're ready to begin trying to get pregnant now, go ahead and schedule a preconceptual visit with your practitioner.

If you are already pregnant and didn't have a preconceptual visit, don't worry, because your practitioner will go over these things at your first prenatal visit, which we discuss in Chapter 5.

Going along with the mother-to-be for her preconceptual visit is a good idea, because part of the process is to go over the health background of *both* parents. In addition, you should understand what lies ahead for both of you. You can help her through the whole process better if you understand what pregnancy is all about.

Going over previous pregnancies and your gynecologic history

Information about previous pregnancies will help your practitioner decide how best to manage your future pregnancies. You'll be asked to describe any prior pregnancies, any miscarriages or premature births, twins — any situations that can happen again. It's helpful to know whether your mother ever took a medication called *DES (diethylstilbestrol)* while she was pregnant with you; if she did, you're at higher risk for having certain complications. Your gynecologic history is equally important because things like prior surgery on your uterus or cervix or a history of irregular periods also may influence your pregnancy.

Remembering your family history

Reviewing your family's medical history alerts your practitioner to conditions that may complicate your pregnancy or be passed on to the developing baby. The reason to discuss this is that, with certain disorders, such as having a family history of neural tube defects (spina bifida, for example), there are things you can do preconceptually to decrease the chance that these disorders will affect *your* pregnancy (see the sidebar "Why the sudden hype on folic acid?" later in this chapter). In Chapter 5, we discuss in more detail different genetic conditions and ways of testing for them.

For those of you considering the use of donor eggs or sperm, keep in mind that the donor's genetic history is just as important as any other biological parent's. Find out as much as you can.

Looking at your ethnic roots

Your preconceptual visit involves questions about your parents' and grand-parents' ancestry — not because your practitioner is nosy, but because some inheritable problems are concentrated in certain populations. Again, the advantage of finding out about these problems before you get pregnant is that if you and your partner are at risk for one of these problems, you have more time to become informed and to check out all of your options (see Chapter 5).

Considering your personal health

Most women contemplating pregnancy are perfectly healthy and don't have problems that can have an impact on pregnancy. Still, a preconceptual visit is very useful, because it's a time to make a game plan and to learn more about how to optimize your chances of having a healthy and uncomplicated preg-nancy. You can find out more about reaching your ideal body weight and getting started on a good exercise program, and you can begin to take prena-tal vitamins with folic acid.

Some women, however, do have medical disorders that can affect the preg-nancy. So, expect your practitioner to ask whether you have any one of a list of conditions. For example, if you have diabetes, stabilizing your blood sugar levels before you get pregnant and watching those levels during your preg-nancy are important. If you're prone to high blood pressure *(hypertension)*, your doctor will want to get that condition under control before you get pregnant. The reason is that controlling hypertension can be time-consuming and can involve changing medications more than once. If you have other problems — epilepsy, for example — checking your medications and making sure your condition is under good control are important. For a condition like systemic lupus erythematosus (SLE), your practitioner may encourage you to try to become pregnant at a time when you are having very few symptoms.

You can expect questions about whether you smoke, indulge in more than a drink or two a day, or use any recreational/illicit drugs. This isn't an interro-gation, and your practitioner is unlikely to chastise you, so be comfortable answering honestly. The point is that these habits can be harmful to a preg-nancy, and dropping them before you get pregnant is best. Your practitioner can advise you on ways to do so or refer you to help or support groups. (See Chapter 3 for more information about substance use during pregnancy.)

Why the sudden hype on folic acid?

It's something your mother never thought about when she was expecting you. But within the past decade, folic acid has become a nutritional requirement for all pregnant women. The change came in 1991, when a British medical study demonstrated that folic acid (also known as *folate,* a nutrient in the B vitamin family) reduced the recurrence of birth defects of the brain and spinal cord (also called *neural tube defects*). This reduction occurred in cases where a mother's previous child was affected — by as much as 80 percent. Subsequent studies have shown that even among women who have never had children with brain or spinal cord defects, those who consume enough folic acid can lower their baby's risk of *spina bifida* (a spinal defect) and *anencephaly* (a brain and skull defect) by 50 to 70 percent.

Today, all women who are considering pregnancy are advised to consume 0.4 milligrams of folate every day, starting at least 30 days before conception. You start early so that plenty of the nutrient is in your system at the time the neural tube is forming. If spina bifida, anencephaly, or similar conditions run in your family — especially if you have ever carried a child with these problems — you should get ten times the usual amount — 4 whole milligrams — every day.

Since 1996, the U.S. Food and Drug Administration has required that all "enriched" grains — flour, cornmeal, pasta, and rice — be fortified with folic acid. Other good sources include green leafy vegetables, beans, and liver. But to make sure that you get the full measure, take a supplement. Any good prenatal vitamin gives you at least 0.4 milligrams.

You also need to discuss any prescription or over-the-counter drugs you take regularly and your diet and exercise routines. Do you take vitamins? Do you diet frequently? Are you a vegetarian? Do you work out regularly? All of these issues should be discussed with your practitioner.

If you haven't had a recent physical exam or PAP smear, your practitioner will probably recommend that you have it done during this preconceptual visit.

Answering the Most Commonly Asked Questions

Your preconceptual visit is also a time for you to ask your practitioner questions. In this section, we answer the most common questions — about body weight, medications, vaccinations, and quitting birth control.

Getting to your ideal body weight

The last thing most women need is another reason to be concerned about weight control. But this one is important: Pregnancy goes most smoothly for women who are not too heavy and not too thin. Overweight women stand a higher-than-normal risk of developing diabetes or high blood pressure during pregnancy, and they are more likely to end up delivering their babies via cesarean section. Underweight women risk having too-small *(low birthweight)* babies.

Try to reach a healthy, normal weight *before* you get pregnant. Trying to lose weight after you conceive is not advisable, even if you are overweight. And if you're underweight to begin with, catching up on pounds when the baby is growing may be difficult. (Read more about your ideal weight and weight gain in Chapter 4.)

Reviewing your medications

Many medicines — both over-the-counter and prescription — are safe to take during pregnancy. But a few medications can cause problems for the baby's development. So let your doctor know about all the medications you take. If one of them is problematic, you can probably switch to something safer. Keep in mind that adjusting dosages and checking for side effects may take time.

Exposure to the following drugs and chemicals is considered to be safe during pregnancy:

- Acetaminophen
- Acyclovir
- Antiemetics (for example, phenothiazines and trimethobenzamide)
- Antihistamines (for example, doxylamine)
- Aspartame (brand names Nutrasweet and Equal)
- Low-dose aspirin
- Minor tranquilizers (for example, meprobamate, chlordiazepoxide, and fluoxetine)
- Penicillin, cephalexin, trimethoprim-sulfamethoxazole, erythromycin, and several others
- Zidovudine

The following are some of the common medications that women ask about before they get pregnant:

- **Birth control pills:** Women sometimes get pregnant while they're on the Pill (because they missed or were late taking a couple of pills during the month) and then worry that their babies will have birth defects. But oral contraceptives have not been shown to have any ill effects on a baby. Two to three percent of *all* babies are born with birth defects, and babies born to women on oral contraceptives are at no higher risk.

- **Ibuprofen (Motrin, Advil):** Occasional use of these and other so-called *nonsteroidal anti-inflammatory agents* during pregnancy (for pain or inflammation) is okay and has not been associated with problems in infants. However, you should avoid chronic or persistent use of these medications during pregnancy (especially during the last trimester), because they have the potential to affect platelet function and blood vessels in the baby's circulatory system.

- **Vitamin A:** This vitamin and some of its derivatives can cause miscarriage or serious birth defects if too much is present in your bloodstream when you get pregnant. The situation is complicated by the fact that vitamin A can remain in your body for several months after you consume it. Discontinuing any drugs that contain vitamin A derivatives — the most common is the anti-acne drug Accutane — at least one month before trying to conceive is important. It isn't known whether topical creams containing vitamin A derivatives — antiaging creams like Retin A and Renova, for example — are as problematic as drugs that you swallow, but you should consult your physician about them.

  Some women take supplements of vitamin A, either because they are vegetarians and don't get enough from their diet or because they suffer from vitamin A deficiency. The maximum safe dose during pregnancy is 5,000 international units (IU) daily. (You need to take twice that amount to reach the danger zone.) Multiple vitamins, including prenatal vitamins, typically contain 5,000 IU of vitamin A or less. But check the label on your vitamin bottle to be sure.

  If you're worried that your prenatal vitamin plus your diet will put you into that "danger zone" of 10,000 IU per day, rest assured that it would be extremely difficult to get that much vitamin A in your diet!

- **Blood thinners:** Women who are prone to developing blood clots or who have artificial heart valves need to take blood thinning agents every day. One type of blood thinner, *coumadin,* or its derivatives can trigger miscarriage, impair the baby's growth, or cause the baby to develop bleeding problems or structural abnormalities if taken during pregnancy. Women who take this medicine and are thinking of getting pregnant should switch to a different blood thinner. Ask your practitioner for more information.

- **Drugs for high blood pressure:** Many of these medications are considered safe to take during pregnancy. However, because a few can be problematic, you should discuss any medications to treat high blood pressure with your doctor (see Chapter 15).

✔ **Antiseizure drugs:** Some of the medicines used to prevent epileptic seizures are safer than others for use during pregnancy. If you're taking any of these drugs, discuss them with your doctor. Don't simply stop taking any antiseizure medicine, because seizures may be worse for you — and the baby — than the medications themselves (see Chapter 15).

✔ **Tetracycline:** If you take this antibiotic during the last several months of pregnancy, it may, much later on, cause your baby's teeth to be yellow.

Recognizing the importance of vaccinations and immunity

People are immune to all kinds of infections, either because they have suffered through the disease (most of us are immune to chicken pox, for example, because we had it when we were kids, causing our immune systems to make antibodies to the chicken pox virus) or because they have been vaccinated (that is, given a shot of something that causes your body to develop antibodies).

Rubella is a common example. Your practitioner checks to see whether you're immune to *rubella* (also known as *German measles*) by drawing a sample of blood and checking to see that it contains antibodies to the rubella virus. (*Antibodies* are immune system agents that protect you against infections.) It is recommended that you be vaccinated against rubella at least three months *before* becoming pregnant. If you get pregnant before the three months are over, it is highly unlikely to be a problem. The fact is that no cases have been reported of babies born with problems due to the mother having received the rubella vaccine in early pregnancy. Many vaccines, including the flu vaccine, are safe to have even while you're pregnant. See Table 1-1 for information on several vaccines.

Most people are immune to measles, mumps, poliomyelitis, and diptheria, and your practitioner is unlikely to check your immunity to all of these illnesses. Besides, these illnesses aren't usually associated with significant adverse effects for the baby. Chicken pox, on the other hand, does carry a small risk that the baby can contract the infection from her mother. If you know that you have never had chicken pox, let your practitioner know to discuss possible vaccination before you get pregnant.

Finally, if you're at risk of HIV infection, get tested before contemplating pregnancy. Some states now require that doctors discuss and offer HIV testing to *all* pregnant women.

Table 1-1	Safe and Unsafe Vaccines during Pregnancy		
Disease	*Risk of Vaccine to Baby*	*Immunization during Pregnancy?*	*Comments*
Cholera	None confirmed	Same as in nonpregnant women.	
Hepatitis B	None confirmed	OK	Used with immunoglobulins for acute exposure, newborns need vaccine.
Influenza	None confirmed	OK	
Measles	None confirmed	NO	Vaccinate postpartum.
Mumps	None confirmed	NO	Vaccinate postpartum.
Plague	None confirmed	Selected vaccination if exposed.	
Pneumococcus	None confirmed	OK, same as in nonpregnant women.	
Poliomyelitis	None confirmed	Only if exposed.	Get if traveling to endemic area.
Rubella	None confirmed	NO	Vaccinate postpartum.
Rabies	Unknown	Indication same as for nonpregnant woman.	Consider each case separately.
Tetanus-diptheria	None confirmed	OK if no primary series given or no booster in past 10 years.	
Typhoid	None confirmed	Only for close, continued exposure or travel to endemic area.	
Varicella (chicken pox)	None confirmed	Immunoglobulins recommended in exposed non-immune women and should be given to newborn if around time of delivery. Vaccine recently available but little information concerning pregnancy.	
Yellow fever	Unknown	NO	Unless exposure is unavoidable.

Quitting birth control

How soon can you get pregnant after you stop using birth control? It depends on what kind of birth control you use. The barrier methods — such as condoms, diaphragms, and spermicides — work only as long as you use them; as soon as you stop, you're fertile. Hormone-based medicines — including the Pill, Depo-Provera, and Norplant — take longer to "get out of your system." You may ovulate very shortly after stopping the Pill (weeks or days, even). On the other hand, it can take three months to one year to resume regular ovulatory cycles after stopping Depo-Provera.

There are no hard-and-fast rules about how long you should wait after stopping birth control before you start to try to conceive. In fact, you can start to try to conceive right away. If you're Fertile Myrtle, you may get pregnant on the first try. But keep in mind that if you haven't resumed regular cycles, you may not be ovulating each month, and it may be more difficult to time your intercourse to achieve conception. (At least you can have a good time trying!) If you get pregnant while your cycles are irregular, it also may be harder to tell exactly what day you conceived and, therefore, to know your due date.

If you use an intrauterine device (IUD), you can get pregnant as soon as you have it removed. Sometimes a woman conceives with her IUD in place. If this happens to you, your practitioner may choose to remove the device, if possible, because getting pregnant with your IUD in place puts you at risk of miscarriage, *ectopic pregnancy* (a pregnancy that gets stuck in the fallopian tube and never makes it to the uterus), or early delivery.

Getting pregnant with an IUD in place does not put the baby at increased risk of birth defects.

The Easiest Way to Get Pregnant

The title of this book notwithstanding, we're going to assume that you know the basics of how to get pregnant. What many people don't know, though, is how to make the process most efficient, so that you give yourself the best chance of getting pregnant as soon as you want to. To do that, you need to think a little about *ovulation* — the releasing of an egg from your ovary — which happens once each cycle (usually once per month).

After leaving the ovary, the egg spends a couple of days gliding down the fallopian tube, until it reaches the uterus (also known as the *womb*), as shown in Figure 1-1. Most often, pregnancy occurs when the egg is fertilized within

24 hours from its release from the ovary, during its passage through the tube, and the budding embryo then implants in the lining of the uterus. In order to get pregnant, your job (yours and the father-to-be's) is to get the sperm to meet up with the egg as soon as possible (ideally, within 12-24 hours) after ovulation.

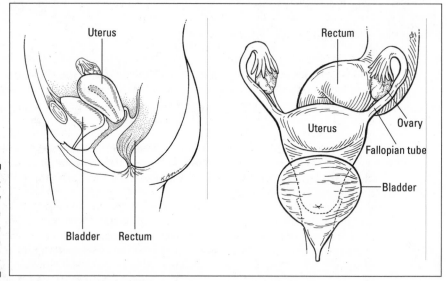

Figure 1-1:
An overview of the female reproductive system.

So when does ovulation happen? Typically, about 14 days before you get your period — which, if your menstrual cycles are 28 days long, is 14 days after the first day of your previous period. If you have a 32-day cycle, you probably ovulate on about the 18th day of your cycle. (Each cycle begins on the first day of a period.) To make sure that you get the sperm in the right place at the right time, have sex several times around the time of ovulation, starting five days before you expect to ovulate and continuing for two to three days afterward. How often? Once every two days is probably adequate, but there's no reason to resist having sex every day if your partner has a normal sperm count.

It was once thought that having sex daily would result in a lower sperm count and reduce fertility. However, later medical studies found that this is true only in men who have a lower-than-normal sperm count to start with.

The absolute prime time to have sex is 12 hours prior to ovulation. Then the sperm are in place as soon as the egg comes out. Sperm are thought to live inside a woman's body for 24 to 48 hours, although some have been known to fertilize eggs when they are as much as seven days old. No couple should count on getting pregnant on the first try. On average, you have a 15 to 25 percent chance each month. Studies have shown that roughly half of all couples trying to get pregnant conceive within four months. By six months, three-fourths of them make it; by a year, 85 percent do; and by two years, the success rate is up to 93 percent. If you have been trying unsuccessfully to conceive for a year or more, a fertility evaluation is warranted.

You can take a few steps to improve your chances of conceiving:

- ✔ If you smoke cigarettes or marijuana, quit.

- ✔ Avoid using K-Y Jelly or other commercial lubricants during sex, because they may contain spermicide. (You may want to switch to olive oil or vegetable oil.)

- ✔ Find out when you're ovulating. If you succeed in doing this, you can plan your sexual encounters at the most opportune time.

  - • Some women find that they can pinpoint their time of ovulation more easily if they keep track of their temperature, which rises close to the time of ovulation. To do this, you take your temperature (orally) each morning before you get out of bed. It typically reaches its lowest point right before your pituitary gland releases *luteinizing hormone* (LH), which triggers ovulation. (Two days after the so-called *LH surge,* your temperature rises significantly — about a half to one degree above baseline — and stays elevated until you get your period. If you get pregnant, it remains high.) You may want to invest in a special "basal body temperature" thermometer (sold in most drug stores) because it has larger gradations and is easier to read.

  Remember that a rise in your basal body temperature indicates that ovulation has already occurred. It doesn't predict when you will ovulate, but it does confirm that you're ovulating, and gives you a rough idea when ovulation occurs in your cycle.

  Reading the signals can sometimes be hard because not all women follow the same pattern. Some never see a distinct drop in temperature, and some never see a clear rise.

  - • Another way to monitor the LH surge is to use a home ovulation predictor kit, which tests the amount of LH in urine. As opposed to basal body temperatures mentioned previously, the LH surge *is* useful in predicting when ovulation will occur during any given cycle. A positive test for any cycle tells you that you're ovulating and when. In general, these kits are very accurate and effective. The main drawback is the expense. At $20 to $30 per kit, they're more expensive than taking your temperature.

In most cases, though, women are well advised to just relax and enjoy the process of trying to conceive. Don't get too anxious if it doesn't happen right off the bat. Here's one piece of advice we often give our patients: Think about stopping birth control a few months before you actually plan on getting pregnant. This way, you have some carefree months of enjoying great sex without worrying each month if you are pregnant. And if you do conceive ahead of schedule, enjoy the nice surprise!

When to see a doctor about infertility

If you're reading this book, chances are you're already pregnant, and infertility is a problem you've managed to avoid or overcome. If so, count yourself lucky, because it's a problem that is affecting more couples than ever before, as people wait longer and longer to have children. One in ten couples over the age of 30 has trouble conceiving. After age 35, the ratio is one in five. Of course, age is not a problem for everyone. Some women reportedly get pregnant even in their fifties. (*The Guinness Book of World's Records* says the world's oldest mother was 57½ when she conceived.) But let's face it: Spontaneous pregnancy in the late 40s and 50s is rare.

When should you seek a doctor's help? Generally, after you've been trying unsuccessfully to get pregnant for six months to a year. But if you have a history of miscarriages or difficulty conceiving, if you're over the age of 35, or if you already know that your partner has a low sperm count, you may want to get help before six months are up. No matter what your situation, don't despair. Reproductive technologies become more sophisticated — and more successful — with each passing year. At this point, couples can try various techniques with complicated-sounding names — ovarian stimulation with fertility medications, intrauterine insemination (with or without sperm washing), intracytoplasmic sperm injection, use of donor sperm or donor eggs, and in vitro fertilization (and its many variations) — depending on their particular cause of infertility. For a couple who has trouble conceiving right away, chances are better than ever that they will eventually become pregnant. If you're having trouble getting pregnant, and you're not sure whether it's time to see an infertility specialist, discuss it with your practitioner.

Chapter 2

I Think I'm Pregnant

So you think you may be pregnant! Or maybe you're hoping to become pregnant soon. Either way, you want to know what to look for in the early weeks of pregnancy so that you can know for sure as soon as possible. In this chapter, we take a look at some of the most common signals that your body sends you in the first weeks of pregnancy.

After you miss a period or have enough symptoms to suspect pregnancy, you'll probably want to perform a pregnancy test. We explain the various testing methods and tell you a few things about their accuracy. We also give you tips on finding the right medical professional if you don't already have one. Remember that your practitioner is an important part of your foray into parenthood.

And, of course, you want to know when your baby is due. We tell you how to calculate your due date and explain why *you* may think of pregnancy as nine months but your doctor refers to it as 40 weeks long.

Sign of the Times: Signals of Pregnancy

So let's say it has happened: A budding embryo has nestled itself into the soft lining of your womb. How and when do you find out that you're pregnant? Quite often, the first sign is a missed period. But your body gives off many other signals, sometimes even sooner than that first missed period, that typically grow more noticeable with each passing week.

Honey, I'm late!

You'll suspect that you may be pregnant if you are late for your period. By the time you notice you're late, a pregnancy test will probably yield a positive result (see the upcoming sections on pregnancy tests). Sometimes, though, you may experience one or two days of light bleeding. This is known as *implantation bleeding* because the embryo is attaching itself to the lining of the uterus.

To eat or not to eat: Cravings and aversions

What you've heard about a pregnant woman's appetite is true. You may become ravenous for pickles, pasta, and other particular foods, yet turn up your nose at things you normally love to eat. Nobody can say for certain why these changes in appetite occur. But experts suspect that these changes are, at least partly, nature's way of ensuring that you get the proper nutrients. You may find that you crave bread, potatoes, and other starchy foods, and perhaps eating those foods in the early days is actually helping you store energy for later in pregnancy, when the baby does most of its growing. You may also be very thirsty early in pregnancy, and the extra water you drink is useful for increasing your body's supply of blood and other fluids.

Breast tenderness

You'll be amazed at how early in pregnancy your breasts begin to grow. In fact, large and tender breasts are often the first symptom of pregnancy that you feel. This is because very early in pregnancy, levels of estrogen and progesterone rise, causing immediate changes in your breasts.

Joanne's story

One day a couple of years after my first daughter was born, I found myself heading to the grocery store to buy pickles and ketchup, intent on mixing them together to make a lovely, tasty, green-and-red meal. I was craving it so much that it didn't even occur to me what an odd dish it is. In fact, it wasn't until I had cleaned up the dishes that I realized that pickles and ketchup had been my only craving during the early months of my first pregnancy. I had no other reason to think I was pregnant again; I hadn't even missed a period. But the next morning I tested myself, and sure enough, it was time for round two.

Testing, Testing, 1, 2, 3

These days, you don't need to wait to get to your practitioner's office to find out whether you're pregnant. You can opt instead for self-testing. Home tests are urine tests that give simply a positive or negative result. Your practitioner, on the other hand, may perform either a urine test similar to the one you took at home or a blood test to find out whether you're pregnant.

Home tests

Suppose you've noticed some bloating or food cravings, or you've missed your period by a day or two, and you want to know whether you're pregnant, but you aren't ready to go to a doctor yet. The easiest, fastest way is to go to the drugstore and pick up a home pregnancy test. These tests are basically simplified chemistry sets, designed to check for the presence of *human chorionic gonadotropin* (hCG, the hormone produced by the developing placenta) in your urine. While these kits are not as precise as laboratory tests that look for hCG in blood, in many cases they can provide positive results very quickly — by the day you miss your period, or about two weeks after conception.

The results of home pregnancy tests aren't a sure thing. If your test comes out negative but you still think you're pregnant, retest in another week or make an appointment with your doctor.

Urine tests

Even if you had a positive home pregnancy test, most practitioners want to confirm this test in their office before beginning the rest of your prenatal care. Your practitioner may decide to simply repeat a urine pregnancy test or to use a blood pregnancy test instead (discussed next).

Blood tests

A blood pregnancy test checks for hCG in your blood. This test can be either qualitative (a simple positive or negative result) or quantitative (an actual measurement of the amount of hCG in your blood). The test your practitioner chooses depends in part upon your history and your current symptoms and in part on his or her own individual preference. Blood tests can be positive even when urine tests are negative.

Choosing a Practitioner Who's Right for You

Midwives, obstetricians, maternal-fetal specialists — many kinds of professionals can help you through pregnancy and delivery. Be sure to choose a practitioner with whom you feel most comfortable. Here is a list of the basic four:

- **Obstetrician/gynecologist:** This physician has four years of special training in pregnancy, delivery, and women's health. He or she should be *board certified* (or be in the process of becoming board certified) by the American Board of Obstetrics and Gynecology (or an equivalent program if you're from a country other than the United States).

- **Maternal-fetal medicine specialist (also known as a *perinatologist* or *high-risk obstetrician*):** This type of doctor has completed a two-to-three-year fellowship in the care of high-risk pregnancies, on top of the standard obstetrics residency, to become board certified in maternal-fetal medicine. Some maternal-fetal medicine specialists act as consultants, and some also deliver babies.

- **Family practice physician:** This doctor provides general medical care for whole families — men, women, and children. He or she is board certified in family practice medicine. This kind of doctor is likely to refer you to an obstetrician or maternal-fetal medicine specialist if complications arise during your pregnancy.

- **Nurse-midwife:** A nurse-midwife is a registered nurse who is certified in the care of pregnant women and is also licensed to perform deliveries. A certified nurse-midwife typically practices in conjunction with a physician and refers patients to a specialist when complications occur.

When you're deciding on a practitioner, be sure to ask yourself the following key questions:

- **Am I comfortable with and do I have confidence in this person?** You should trust and feel at ease not only with your practitioner but also with the whole constellation of people who work in the practice. Would you feel free to ask questions or express your anxieties to them? Another point to keep in mind is how your general personality fits in with the philosophy of the practice. Some women prefer a low-key, low-tech approach to prenatal care, while others want to have every possible diagnostic test under the sun. Your past medical and obstetrical history will also influence the approach you take to your pregnancy.

✔ **How many practitioners are involved in the practice?** You may end up choosing between a practitioner who works with one or more partners and one who is in solo practice. In a group practice, you usually rotate through appointments with each of the doctors, getting to know them all so that you feel comfortable having any one of them deliver your baby. Practically speaking, you're likely to bond more with one or two people in the practice than with others. This is natural, given that most women and most practitioners have many varied personalities. A practitioner who practices alone should tell you who handles deliveries when he or she is ill, off duty, or out of town.

Be sure to ask your practitioner about his or her policy for after-hours problems or emergencies — including questions you may need to ask by telephone on evenings or weekends.

✔ **What's the hospital like?** If your pregnancy is uncomplicated, any good hospital or birthing center will be fine for you. If you're at risk of some complications, you may want to ask whether your hospital has a labor and delivery suite and a nursery equipped to handle any problems that may arise if, for example, the baby is born early. You may also want to ask

- Is an anesthesiologist on site 24 hours a day, or can your doctor call in an anesthesiologist quickly in case of an emergency?

- Can the hospital provide you with *epidural* anesthesia (a form of pain control during labor)? If epidural anesthesia is not readily available, or you're not interested in this form of pain relief, you should find out what other options are available for pain management.

- Are you allowed to *room in* — that is, keep the baby in your room as much as possible — after delivery? Also, are accommodations available for your partner to stay with you during your postpartum hospitalization?

✔ **Are specialists close by?** Consider whether you may end up needing the services of a maternal-fetal medicine specialist or a *neonatologist,* a physician who specializes in the care of infants who are born early or who have other medical problems. Ideally, your practitioner can refer you to someone quickly if anything comes up.

✔ **Will my insurance plan cover the costs of this doctor?** Now that managed care has become an important part of the health insurance industry, it may be important to you to know whether your practitioner of choice is covered by your plan. Some places allow you to select physicians from "outside the network" if you pay part of the cost yourself.

TIP

Am I at high risk?

The question of whether you and your pregnancy are at high risk has no black-and-white answer, especially at the beginning. But it helps to be aware of the kinds of situations (which you may either have or develop) that can put a pregnancy at high risk:

✔ Diabetes

✔ High blood pressure

✔ Lupus

✔ Blood disorders

✔ Heart, kidney, or liver disorders

✔ Twins, triplets, or other multiple fetuses

✔ A premature delivery in a prior pregnancy

✔ A previous child with birth defects

✔ A history of miscarriage

✔ An abnormally shaped uterus

✔ Epilepsy

✔ Some infections

✔ Bleeding

Calculating Your Due Date

The average pregnancy lasts 280 days — 40 weeks — counting from the first day of the last menstrual period. Your due date — what doctors once referred to as the *EDC,* for *estimated date of confinement* (in the old days, women were actually "confined" to the hospital around the time of their delivery) — can be calculated by starting with the date on which your last menstrual period (LMP) started. If your cycles are 28 days long, you can subtract three months from your LMP and add seven days. If your last period started on June 3, for example, your due date would be March (subtract three months) 10 (add seven days).

DON'T WORRY

If your periods didn't follow 28-day cycles, don't worry. You can establish your due date in other ways.

If you can pinpoint the date of conception, coming up with an accurate date is especially easy. If not, you can get an ultrasound exam during the first three months to get a good idea of your due date. Pinpointing the due date as precisely as possible is important in order to ensure that the tests you need along the way are performed at the right time. Knowing how far along you are also makes it easier for your doctor to see that the baby is growing properly. A first trimester ultrasound predicts your due date more accurately than a second or third trimester one.

Only 1 in 20 women delivers *on* her due date. Most women deliver anywhere from three weeks early to two weeks late.

If you're wondering how far along you are at this moment (and you happen to have an elephant's memory), you can just keep track of the number of days that have passed since your last period. An alternative to this system is to use a *pregnancy wheel* to calculate. To use this handy tool, line up the arrow to the date of your last menstrual period and then look for today's date. Just below the date you see the number of weeks and days that have gone by. You can see what a pregnancy wheel looks like in Figure 2-1.

If you know the date of conception, rather than your last period, you can follow the same procedure and then subtract two weeks.

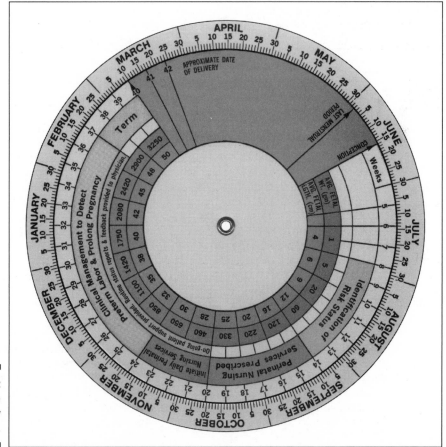

Figure 2-1:
A sample pregnancy wheel.

Weeks versus months

Most of us think of pregnancy as lasting nine months. But face it — 40 weeks is a little longer than nine times four weeks. It's closer to ten lunar months (in Japan, they actually speak of pregnancy as lasting ten months) and a bit longer than nine 30-to-31-day calendar months. That's why your doctor is more likely to talk in terms of weeks.

Because you start counting from the date of the LMP, you actually start the count a couple of weeks *before* you conceive. So when your doctor says you're 12 weeks pregnant, the fetus is really only ten weeks old!

Chapter 3

Preparing for Life during Pregnancy

*E*ven though you're pregnant and your body is already undergoing miraculous changes, your day-to-day life goes on. If you're like most pregnant women, you want to find out what you need to change in your lifestyle in order to make your pregnancy go as smoothly as possible. But you also want to know what things in your life you don't need to change, or what things need to be modified only slightly. You have a lot to consider: your job, the general level of stress in your life, what medications you take, whether you smoke or drink alcohol regularly, and what to do about routine things like going to the dentist or hairdresser. If you're like most normally healthy women, you'll probably find that for the most part, your life can go on largely as usual.

All the issues we mention are subjects for discussion with your practitioner. But in this chapter and the next, we offer a general outline for how to plan your life during pregnancy. If you consider from the beginning how your daily habits and health practices interact with your pregnancy, you're likely to have a smoother time getting used to your new state of being. The earlier you get started on the right diet, exercise, and overall health program, the better (see Chapter 4 for more).

Prenatal Visits

After you finish celebrating the results of your positive pregnancy test, it's time to get down to business and think about what lies ahead. After you decide who your practitioner will be, give the office a call to find out how next to proceed. Some practices want you to come in for a visit with the office nurse to give a medical history and confirm your good news with either a blood or urine test, while others schedule a first visit with the practitioner. How soon your first visit will be scheduled depends in part on your past or current history. If you didn't have a preconceptual visit (see Chapter 1) beforehand and you haven't been on prenatal vitamins or other folic-acid containing vitamins, let the office know. The office will be able to call in a prescription for prenatal vitamins so you can start taking them even before your first prenatal visit.

Some things are consistent from trimester to trimester — like checking your blood pressure, urine, and the baby's heartbeat — so we cover these topics in this chapter. In Chapters 5, 6, and 7, we go over the specifics of what happens during prenatal visits for each trimester. But just to give you an overview, here's a typical schedule for prenatal visits and what happens at each visit.

Stage of Pregnancy	*Frequency of Doctor Visits*
First visit to 28 weeks	Every four weeks
28 to 36 weeks	Every two to three weeks
36 weeks to delivery	Weekly

If you develop problems during pregnancy or if your pregnancy is considered "high risk" (see the risk factors we describe in Chapter 2), your practitioner may suggest that you come in more frequently.

This schedule of prenatal visits is not set in stone. If you're planning a vacation or need to miss a prenatal visit, let your practitioners know and reschedule your appointment. If your pregnancy is going smoothly, rescheduling is usually not a big deal. However, because some prenatal tests have to be performed at specific times during pregnancy, just make sure that missing an appointment won't affect any of these tests.

Prenatal visits vary a bit according to each woman's personal needs and each practitioner's style. Some women need particular laboratory tests or physical examinations. But a few things are standard during your prenatal visits.

✔ **A nurse checks your weight and blood pressure.** For more information on how much weight you should be gaining and when, see Chapter 4.

✔ **You give a urine sample (usually an easy job for most pregnant women!).** Your practitioner checks for the presence of protein or glucose to look for any signs of preeclampsia or diabetes (see Chapters 14 and 15). Some urine tests also enable your doctor to look for any signs that you have a urinary tract infection.

✔ **Starting sometime after 14 to 16 weeks, a nurse or doctor measures your fundal height.** This procedure is when a nurse or doctor uses a tape measure or her hands to measure your uterus to get a rough idea about how the baby is growing and whether you have an adequate amount of amniotic fluid (see Figure 3-1). Technically speaking, she is measuring the *fundal height* — the distance from the top of the pubic bone to the top of the uterus (the fundus). By 20 weeks, the fundus usually reaches the level of the naval. After 20 weeks, the height in centimeters roughly equals the number of weeks pregnant you are. *Note:* The fundal height measurement may not be useful in women who are expecting twins or more, or in women who have large fibroids or who are very obese.

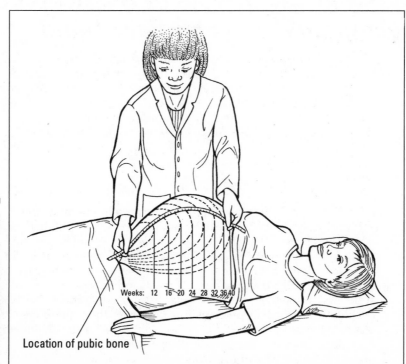

Figure 3-1: Your practitioner may measure your fundal height to check that your baby is growing properly.

Weeks: 12 16 20 24 28 32 36 40

Location of pubic bone

✔ **A nurse or doctor listens for and counts the baby's heartbeat.**
Typically, the heartbeat ranges between 120 and 160 beats per minute.
Most offices use an electronic Doppler device to check the baby's heartbeat. With this method, the baby's heartbeat sounds sort of like horses
galloping inside the womb. Sometimes, you can hear the heartbeat using
this method as early as 8 or 9 weeks, but often it isn't clearly discernible
until 10 to 12 weeks. Prior to the availability of Doppler, a special stetho-
scope called a *fetoscope* was used to hear the baby's heartbeat. Using
this method, the heartbeat can first be heard around 20 weeks. A third
way of checking the baby's heartbeat is by seeing it on ultrasound. The
heart can usually be seen at around six weeks.

In some practices, a medical assistant or nurse performs tasks such as checking your blood pressure; in other practices a doctor may perform this task.
No matter who performs the technical components of the prenatal visit, you
should always have the opportunity to ask your practitioner questions before
leaving the office.

Looking at the Effects of Medications, Alcohol, and Drugs on Your Baby

Alcohol, "recreational" drugs, and some medications that you take into your
body can cross the placenta and get into the baby's circulation. Some of
these substances are completely harmless, whereas others can cause problems. Knowing which substances you can safely use and which to avoid is
crucial to the health of your child. The following sections outline which substances you can safely use and which you should steer clear of.

Taking medications

During your pregnancy, you'll probably experience at least a headache or two
and an occasional case of heartburn. The question of whether you can safely
take pain relievers, antacids, and other over-the-counter medicines is bound
to come up. Many women are afraid to take any medicine at all, for fear of
somehow harming their babies. But most nonprescription drugs — and even
many prescription drugs — are safe during pregnancy. It's a good idea, even
at the first prenatal visit, to go over with your practitioner what medications
are okay to take during pregnancy — both over-the-counter medications and
medications prescribed to you by another physician. If you're being treated
by another physician for a medical condition, let him or her know that you're
pregnant, in case any adjustments need to be made.

Don't stop taking a prescription medication or change the dosage on your own without talking to your doctor first.

Many medications are labeled "Do not take during pregnancy" because they have not been adequately studied in pregnant women. However, this does not necessarily mean that adverse effects have been reported, or that you can't use them. Whenever you have a question about a particular medication, ask the advice of your practitioner. Don't be surprised if opinions vary between practitioners, because there is not always only one right answer.

Certain medical problems, such as high blood pressure, pose more risk to the growing fetus than the medication you would take to treat it does. Even a common headache, if it's bad enough to cause you to miss a traffic signal when you're behind the wheel, could be more dangerous than a little aceta-minophen (Tylenol), which actually isn't dangerous at all when taken in therapeutic doses. The fact is, we find many pregnant women suffer need-lessly with common symptoms that could be treated with medications that are safe for the baby.

In Chapter 1, we list many of the drugs/chemicals that are safe for most preg-nant women to take. We also discuss some of the drugs that are known to have *teratogenic* effects, which means they have the potential to cause birth defects or problems with growth and development.

If you took any teratogenic medications before you knew you were pregnant — or before you knew that the drugs could pose a problem — don't panic. In many cases, the drugs do no harm, depending on when during pregnancy they were taken and in what quantities. Some medications can cause problems in the first trimester, but are totally safe in the third trimester, and vice versa. In fact, relatively few substances are proven to be teratogenic to humans, and even those that are don't cause birth defects every time they are used. It's important to discuss with your practitioner what medications you've been taking, and what tests are available to check on your baby's growth and development.

You can also call any one of a number of telephone services, including those in the following list, for more information about teratogenic substances. These services get their information from medical databases (also listed), so if the information you get over the phone is overly technical, ask your practi-tioner to interpret for you.

- ✔ Micromedex, Inc., REPRODISK (REPROTEXT, REPROTOX, Shepard's Catalog of Teratogenic Agents and TERIS), Englewood, CO; 800-525-9083.

- ✔ National Library of Medicine, MEDLARS Service Desk GRATEFUL MED (TOXLINE, TOXNET, and MEDLINE), Bethesda, MD; 800-638-8480.

- ✔ Reproductive Toxicology Center, REPROTOX, Columbia Hospital for Women Medical Center, Washington, D.C.; 202-293-5137.

> ✔ Shepard's Catalog of Teratogenic Agents, University of Washington, Seattle, WA; 206-543-3373.
>
> ✔ Teratogen Information System, TERIS and Shepard's Catalog of Teratogenic Agents, Seattle, WA; 206-543-2465.

Smoking

Unless you have been living on Mars for the past ten years, you no doubt are aware that smoking is a health risk for you. When you smoke, you run the risk of developing lung cancer, emphysema, and heart disease, among other illnesses. During pregnancy, however, smoking poses risks to your baby as well.

The carbon monoxide in cigarette smoke decreases the amount of oxygen that is delivered to a growing baby, and nicotine cuts back on blood flow to the fetus. Consequently, women who smoke stand an increased chance of delivering babies with low birthweight. In fact, babies born to smokers are expected to weigh a half pound less, on average, than those born to non-smokers. The exact difference in birthweight depends upon how much the mother smokes.

If you quit smoking during the first three months you're pregnant, give yourself a pat on the back and be reassured that your baby is likely to be born at a normal weight.

In addition to low birthweight, smoking during pregnancy is associated with a greater risk of preterm delivery, miscarriage, placenta previa (see Chapter 14), placental abruption (see Chapter 14), preterm rupture of the amniotic membranes, and even sudden infant death syndrome after the baby is born.

Quitting smoking can be extremely difficult. But keep in mind that even cutting back on the number of cigarettes you smoke is a benefit to your baby.

Some women use nicotine patches or gum to help them kick the habit. The nicotine from these products is still absorbed into the bloodstream and can still reach the fetus, but at least the carbon monoxide and other toxins in cigarette smoke are eliminated.

Drinking alcohol

This topic is one we feel really needs to be put into perspective. Clearly, pregnant women who abuse alcohol put their babies at risk of *fetal alcohol syndrome,* which encompasses a wide variety of birth defects (including growth problems, heart defects, mental retardation, or abnormalities of the face or limbs). The controversy arises because medical science hasn't been able to define an absolute safe level of alcohol intake during pregnancy.

Scientific data shows that daily drinking or heavy binge drinking can lead to serious complications, but no studies indicate that an occasional glass of wine or an occasional drink will cause harm to your baby. Moderation and common sense should be your guidelines. Some practitioners advise their patients to avoid alcohol during the first trimester, when the baby's organ systems are forming, and after that to limit their alcohol consumption to one to two drinks per week.

If you think you may have a drinking problem, be sure to inform your practitioner. A T-ACE questionnaire helps to identify patients whose drinking is excessive enough to pose a risk to the fetus. If you think you may have a problem, discussing this questionnaire with your practitioner is crucial to your baby's health — and to yours.

Using recreational or illicit drugs

Many studies have been conducted to evaluate the effects of drug use during pregnancy. But the studies can be confusing because they tend to lump all kinds of "users" together, regardless of which drugs they use and how much they use them. The mother's lifestyle also influences the degree of risk to the baby, which complicates the information even more. For example, women who abuse drugs are more likely to be malnourished than other women, they

---

Our patients want to know . . .

Questions about alcohol consumption during pregnancy are very common. So we've gathered some of the most frequently asked questions and provided the answers you need.

Q: "On my Caribbean vacation, I enjoyed many piña coladas on the beach. I didn't find out I was pregnant until a few weeks later. Will my baby have birth defects?"

A: There's no evidence that a single episode of binge drinking has any adverse effects on pregnancy. Now that you know you're pregnant, an occasional drink is thought to be safe, but large amounts of alcohol, even over short periods, may be problematic.

Q: "Is hard liquor worse for the baby than wine or beer?"

A: Not necessarily. A can of beer, a glass of wine, and a mixed drink containing one ounce of hard liquor contain roughly the same amounts of alcohol. No one choice is worse than another.

Q: "My doctor suggested I have a glass of wine on the evening after my amniocentesis. Is this okay?"

A: Yes. Alcohol is a *tocolytic,* which basically means that it relaxes the uterus. After amniocentesis, many women feel a little uterine cramping. The alcohol in a glass of wine minimizes that discomfort without hurting the baby.

are typically of lower socioeconomic status, and they suffer a higher incidence of sexually transmitted diseases. All of these factors, independent of drug use, can cause problems for your pregnancy and for your baby.

The following list tells the basics about the use of various recreational drugs and their effects on unborn babies:

- **Marijuana:** This is the illicit drug most frequently used during pregnancy. The data on marijuana use are controversial, but they do suggest that women who use marijuana when they're pregnant stand a higher-than-average risk of delivering their babies early or at low birthweight.

- **Cocaine and crack cocaine:** In a pregnant woman, the use of cocaine or crack can lead to severe high blood pressure, stroke, heart attack, and even sudden death. What's more, cocaine use raises the risk of problems with the baby's growth, preterm delivery, placental abruption (see Chapter 14), and fetal stroke. Women who use cocaine early in pregnancy put their babies at higher risk of developing a variety of birth defects. Also, infants born to women who use cocaine during pregnancy are more likely to have behavioral and neurological problems, seizures, and sudden infant death syndrome (SIDS).

- **Narcotics and opiates (including heroin, methadone, codeine, Demerol, and morphine):** Narcotic addiction alone puts both the mother and the baby at a greater risk. It is associated with fetal growth problems, preterm delivery, fetal death, and small head size. Perhaps even more important, narcotic addiction places the newborn at a high risk of complications (including death) due to withdrawal from the drug. If you are addicted to narcotics or opiates, beginning a treatment program during your pregnancy can minimize the effects of the drugs on your baby.

  We don't mean to imply that occasional short-term use of medications containing narcotics in therapeutic doses causes any problems. If you're undergoing a surgical or painful dental procedure during your pregnancy, for example, using such medications for short-term pain control is perfectly acceptable.

- **Amphetamines and other uppers (including crystal methamphetamine and blue ice):** Because these substances historically have not been used as widely as narcotics and cocaine, we have less information about their side effects during pregnancy. We do know that they decrease the user's appetite, which, in turn, could lead to poor fetal growth. Also, evidence shows that the drugs themselves can increase the risk of fetal growth problems (including small head size), placental abruption (see Chapter 14), and fetal stroke or death.

Figuring Out How Your Lifestyle Will Change during Pregnancy

Your lifestyle will inevitably change during the nine months of your pregnancy. You may wonder whether it's still okay to do some of the things you may have been used to doing on a regular basis before you were pregnant. This section provides information on things like whether you can safely color your hair while you're pregnant, whether you can go into saunas and hot tubs, whether you can travel and when, and whether you can continue working.

Pampering yourself with beauty treatments

When your friends and relatives hear that you're pregnant, they'll probably tell you how beautiful you look or what a lovely maternal glow you have. And you may feel more beautiful, too, although some women feel the exact opposite. You may find that you're not happy with the physical changes that are happening to your body. Either way, if you're like most of our patients, you may wonder whether your customary beauty habits are safe to follow during pregnancy. In this section, we go over them one by one and let you know if there are any risks at all.

Is it safe to continue using wrinkle creams?

The two most common antiwrinkle creams used today are Retin-A and Renova. Both of these preparations contain vitamin A derivatives. Substantial data exists to suggest that oral medications containing vitamin A derivatives (for example, Accutane) can cause birth defects, but the information that's available on topical preparations such as Retin-A and Renova doesn't indicate that these are a problem. Due to the significant effects of oral preparations, however, many practitioners are reluctant to recommend any medications containing these compounds — oral or topical — to their patients.

Are chemical peels okay?

Alpha-hydroxy acids are the main ingredients in chemical peels. The chemicals work topically, but small amounts are absorbed into your system. We have been unable to find any data on whether chemical peels are safe during pregnancy. They're probably okay, but if you want to, discuss it first with your practitioner.

Can I have my legs waxed or a bikini wax?

Waxing legs or the bikini line involves applying a heated wax preparation topically and then removing it along with the hair. There is nothing in the wax preparations that can lead to problems for the baby. So it's okay to keep doing it while you're pregnant to help you remain carefree and hair-free.

Can I have my hair dyed?

One of the first questions some of our patients bring up is, "Can I have my hair dyed?" or "Can I have my hair highlighted?" (Others wait until their roots have grown halfway down their heads and then plead for permission.) Most women worry about hair dyes because they've read in a magazine or heard from their friends that hair dye can be toxic and can cause problems for the baby. Practitioners tend to disagree on this issue. Your practitioner may tell you to stick to vegetable hair dyes during pregnancy. But your friend, on the other hand, may have been told by her practitioner that dyeing her hair is fine.

The bottom line is that using hair dyes during pregnancy is probably fine. No evidence suggests that hair dyes cause birth defects or miscarriage. Years ago, some of them contained formaldehyde and other potentially dangerous chemicals that could harm a baby. But the newer dyes don't contain these chemicals.

Can I keep perming my hair?

There is also no scientific evidence suggesting that the chemicals in hair permanents are harmful to the developing baby. These preparations usually do contain significant amounts of ammonia, however, and for your own safety they should be used in well-ventilated areas.

Should I stop having my nails done?

Another frequently asked question is: "Can I have a manicure/pedicure or have nail tips or acrylic nails placed while I'm pregnant?" Again, the answer is that it's okay. Common sense suggests that if you go to a reputable salon where the equipment is properly cleaned and the area is well ventilated, the risk is nil.

Are facials and massages still okay?

You may notice that your complexion has changed over the past few months, because sometimes pregnancy hormones can wreak havoc on your skin. Facials may or may not help. But go ahead and have one anyway, if only to enjoy the time it will give you to sit back and relax! (See earlier comments about chemical peels.)

Likewise, massages are fine too. Many massage therapists offer special pregnancy massages aimed at accommodating your pregnant belly. Some use special tables with the center cut out so that you are able to comfortably lie face down, especially in the latter part of the pregnancy.

Going into hot tubs, whirlpools, saunas, or steam rooms

Using hot tubs, whirlpools, saunas, or steam rooms when you're pregnant can be risky because of the high temperatures involved. In laboratory animals, exposure to high levels of heat during pregnancy has been known to cause birth defects or miscarriage. Studies involving humans suggest that pregnant women whose core body temperatures rise significantly during the early weeks of pregnancy stand an increased risk of miscarriage or having babies with neural tube defects (spina bifida, for example).

However, it is generally accepted that problems occur only if the mother's core temperature rises above 102 degrees Fahrenheit (or about 39 degrees Celsius) for more than ten minutes during the first seven weeks of her pregnancy.

In general, soaking in a warm, soothing bath is fine during pregnancy. Just make sure that the water temperature is not too high, for the reasons just mentioned.

Common sense would suggest that occasional use of hot tubs, saunas, and steam rooms for less than ten minutes, and after the first trimester, is probably okay. However, remember to drink plenty of fluids to avoid getting dehydrated.

Traveling

The main potential problem with traveling during pregnancy is that it puts distance between you and your prenatal care provider. If you're close to your due date or if your pregnancy is considered high-risk, you probably shouldn't travel far from home. This, of course, depends on what the risk factors actually are. If you have diabetes but it's well controlled, it's probably okay to go on a trip. But if you have triplets, it's probably not a good idea to travel to Timbuktu. If your pregnancy is uncomplicated, travel during the first, second, and early third trimesters is usually okay.

Traveling by car poses no special risk, aside from requiring that you sit in one place for a long time. On long trips, stop every couple of hours to get out and walk around a bit. Wear your seat belt and shoulder strap; they keep you safe, and they won't hurt the baby, even if you're in an accident. The amniotic fluid surrounding the fetus serves as a cushion against any constriction from the lap belt. *Not* wearing restraints clearly poses a greater risk; studies show that the leading cause of fetal death in auto accidents is death of the mother.

Wear your seat belt below your abdomen, not above it, and keep the shoulder strap in its usual position.

Most airlines allow women to fly if they're less than 36 weeks pregnant, but you may want to carry a note from your practitioner indicating that he or she sees no medical reason why you shouldn't fly. Flying is perfectly safe, especially if you take a couple of precautions:

✔ **Get up from your seat occasionally during longer flights and walk around the plane.** Prolonged periods of sitting can cause blood to pool in your legs. Walking around keeps your circulation going.

✔ **Carry a water bottle with you and drink water frequently.** Airplane air is always very dry. (A pilot once told us that the relative humidity in airplanes is typically lower than it is in the Sahara Desert. Planes can't carry enough water to keep the humidity up, because the extra water would add too much cargo weight.) Because airplane air is so dry, you can easily become dehydrated during long flights.

Drinking extra water also ensures that you get up frequently to go to the restroom, which keeps the blood from pooling in your legs.

You don't need to worry about airport metal detectors — or any other metal detectors — because they don't use ionizing radiation. (The conveyor belt that carries your luggage after you check it in does use ionizing radiation, however, so we don't recommend that you climb onto the counter and send yourself through that machine.)

If you're prone to air sickness and have found Dramamine helpful in the past, using it in normal doses while you're pregnant is okay.

If you plan to visit tropical countries, where some diseases are particularly prevalent, you may want to be vaccinated before you go. But check with your doctor to see whether any vaccines you're considering are safe to have during pregnancy. (For more information on vaccines, see Chapter 1.)

Considering occupational hazards

Maybe your job requires minimal standing or walking, allows you to work regular hours, and never stresses you out. If that's the case, and if you have no previous medical problems, you may just as well skip this section (and let us know what your job is!). But if you're like the rest of us, read on.

Should you continue working during your pregnancy? Unfortunately, this question doesn't have a simple answer, because jobs are too diverse, and individual pregnancies are so different. Stress-free, sedentary jobs are perfectly safe. On the other hand, occupations that are physically very demanding can be problematic. Most jobs fall somewhere in between, but even then the amount of stress varies according to the individual. If your pregnancy proceeds without complications, there is no reason you can't continue to work right up until it's time for you to deliver. However, some complications may arise during pregnancy that make reducing your workload or stopping work altogether advisable. For example, if you develop preterm labor, your practitioner will most likely advise you to stop working so that your physical activity is limited. Other conditions that may warrant a reduction in physical activity are hypertension or problems with the baby's growth.

If you work at a computer terminal, you may wonder whether you're being exposed to anything harmful. But you have no need to worry — there is no evidence to suggest that the electromagnetic fields that computer terminals emit is a problem.

No matter what type of work you do, it's a good idea to discuss your working conditions with your doctor.

Getting dental care

Most people see their dentist for routine cleanings every 6 to 12 months, which means you'll probably need to visit your dentist at least once during your pregnancy. Pregnancy itself should not affect your dental health. Neglected cavities can become infected, which is all the more reason to see your dentist when you're pregnant.

Pregnancy causes an increase in blood flow to the gums. In fact, about half of all pregnant women develop a condition called *pregnancy gingivitis,* which is simply a reddening of the gums caused by this increased blood flow. In this condition, gums have a tendency to bleed easily. So try to be gentle when you brush and floss your teeth.

If you need routine dental work — cavities filled, teeth pulled, crowns placed — don't worry. Local anesthesia and most pain medications are safe. Some dentists also recommend antibiotics during dental procedures. Most antibiotics that dentists recommend are also safe during pregnancy, but you should check with your prenatal care provider to make sure. Even dental X-rays pose no significant problem for the fetus, as long as a lead "apron" is placed over the abdomen.

Remember, if you plan on having extensive dental work that requires general anesthesia, make sure your anesthesiologist knows that you're pregnant and has experience in giving anesthesia to pregnant women.

Having sex

For most couples, having sex during pregnancy is perfectly safe. In fact, some couples find that sex during pregnancy is even better than before. There are other issues to consider, however.

In the first half of pregnancy, because your body hasn't changed that noticeably, sex can usually continue as before. You may notice that your breasts are particularly sensitive to the touch, or even tender. Later, as the uterus grows, some sexual positions become more difficult. You and your partner may find that you have to be a little creative in making things work. If you find that intercourse is too uncomfortable, other forms of sexual gratification may work better for you and your partner.

A lot of women ask us if it's still okay to have sex at the end of pregnancy, even if the cervix is a little bit dilated. It is perfectly fine as long as your membranes haven't ruptured (your water hasn't broken).

There are a couple of circumstances in which intercourse should be avoided: If you are at a high risk for preterm labor, most practitioners suggest refraining from intercourse because of the concern that intercourse could introduce an infection into the uterus and because semen contains substances that are known to make the uterus contract. There is some controversy about whether orgasm itself can set off preterm labor. Several studies conducted in the 1960s and 1970s showed that in patients at high risk for preterm labor (see Chapter 14), orgasm was associated with an increase in preterm delivery. But more recently, studies have shown that in low-risk women, the frequency of intercourse and orgasm was not associated with a higher risk for preterm delivery. If you have placenta previa in the third trimester, you should also avoid intercourse.

Another important aspect to consider is how each of you feel psychologically about having sex during pregnancy. Like some women, you may find that your libido or sex drive has increased. Often, you may find that you have vivid sexual dreams and that orgasm itself is heightened. On the other hand, you may find that your interest in sex is less than it was before you got pregnant. You may feel less attractive because of the physical changes that have taken place. This is perfectly normal. Your partner may also experience changes in his desire for sex due to the excitement and normal apprehension that goes along with being a father and due to (unfounded) fears that intercourse will hurt the baby or that the baby will somehow know what mom and dad are up to.

Preparing for Physical Changes

When you're pregnant, your body is constantly changing. Some of the things you can expect to experience — mood swings, leg cramps, and stress — you've probably experienced before, just not with such intensity. The following sections cover these and other problems and let you know what you may be in for. Have your family and friends read these sections, too — then tell them to consider themselves warned.

Dealing with mood swings

Hormonal shifts affect mood, as most women, especially those who suffer from PMS (premenstrual syndrome), already know. The hormonal fluctuations that support pregnancy are perhaps the most dramatic a woman experiences in her lifetime, so it's hardly surprising that emotional ups and downs are commonplace. And these ups and downs can easily be made more severe by the fatigue that also goes along with pregnancy. Add to this biochemical mix the normal anxieties that the average expectant mother has about whether the baby will be healthy and whether she'll be a good mother, and you have plenty of fuel to produce good, old-fashioned mood swings.

You're not alone. Moodiness is a normal part of pregnancy, and you're not the first or only woman to experience it. So don't blame yourself. Your family and friends will understand.

Your moodiness may be especially pronounced during the first trimester, as your body adjusts to its new condition. You may find yourself overreacting to little things. A silly, mushy television commercial, for example, may leave you in tears. Misplacing your appointment book may send you into a panic. A grocery store clerk who accidentally smashes your loaf of bread may draw you into a teeth-clenching rage. Don't worry — you're just pregnant. Take a few deep breaths, go out for a walk, or just close your eyes and take a few seconds' break. These feelings often pass as quickly as they arise.

Remember dad, it may be difficult to deal with her sudden and unexpected mood swings, but try to be patient. Consider all the changes her body is going through and be as understanding as possible.

Living through leg cramps

Leg cramps are a common annoyance of pregnancy, and they're likely to become more frequent as the months go along.

The fact is that doctors aren't quite sure what really causes leg cramps. Because some think it may be related to low levels of calcium or magnesium, supplementing with calcium or magnesium tablets has been suggested. However, the medical benefit of doing so has never been medically proven. Some doctors believe that leg cramps may be related to a decrease in circulation, which gets worse when you are sedentary. This may be why leg cramps are more common at night. You may find that stretching and extending your legs and feet helps diminish the cramping.

Sometimes walking helps ease the pain of leg cramps. A foot or leg massage can also be useful — and leg cramps are a great excuse for getting frequent massages!

Noticing vaginal discharge

During pregnancy, your vaginal discharge normally increases substantially. Some women find that they need to wear thin panty liners every day. The discharge tends to be thin, white, and virtually odorless. Vaginal douches are not a good idea because they may alter a woman's natural ability to fight off vaginal infections.

If your vaginal discharge takes on a brown, yellow, or green color, or if it develops a noxious odor, let your practitioner know. (Be sure to use your judgment about how much of an emergency this is — it is not the sort of problem that requires a 3 a.m. phone call to his or her office.)

Pregnancy doesn't prevent you from getting a vaginal infection, and because of the high levels of estrogen in your blood, you may be predisposed to developing a yeast infection. A yeast infection usually produces a thick, white-yellow discharge, and it may in some cases cause itchiness or redness. Topical vaginal creams should solve the problem, and they pose no risk to the fetus. Most over-the -counter preparations come in 1-, 3-, and 7-day preparations and are completely safe for the baby.

Putting up with backaches

Backaches are a common complaint or symptom that many women experience during pregnancy. They typically occur in the latter part of pregnancy, although they can occur earlier. The shift in your center of gravity can be one cause. Another can be the change in the curvature of your spine as the baby grows and the uterus enlarges. You may get some relief by getting off of your feet when you can, by applying mild local heat, and by taking acetaminophen (Tylenol). Our patients often ask us about using a specially designed pregnancy girdle that they've seen advertised or heard about. While some find this helps, others do not.

Some women experience pain extending from their lower back to their buttocks and down one leg or the other. This pain, or less commonly, numbness, is known as *sciatica*. It is due to pressure on the sciatic nerve, a major nerve that branches from your back, through your pelvis, to your hips and down your legs. Mild cases of sciatica can be relieved by bed rest, warm baths, or heating pads. If you develop a severe case, you may need prolonged bed rest or special exercises.

Occasionally, preterm labor can present itself as low back pain. However, when it is preterm labor, the pain is more crampy, and it comes and goes, rather than being continuous.

Handling stress

Many women wonder whether stress has any effect on pregnancy. But that question is difficult to answer because stress is such an elusive concept. We all know what it is, but each of us seems to handle it in her own way, and no one can really measure its intensity. We do know that chronic stress — day after day and unrelieved — can increase the levels of stress hormones circulating in the bloodstream. Many doctors think that such elevated levels of stress hormones can promote preterm labor or blood pressure problems during pregnancy, but few studies have been able to prove this idea.

While you're pregnant, paying attention to your own personal comfort and happiness is especially important. Everyone has her own way of relaxing — whether it's by getting a massage, going to a movie, having dinner with friends, taking a hot shower or bubble bath, or just sitting back and putting her feet up. Take the time you need to be good to yourself.

Chapter 4

Diet and Exercise for the Expectant Mother

. . . .

In This Chapter

▶ Thinking about what — and how much — you eat

▶ Staying active during pregnancy

. . . .

*T*hrough the ages, women have received all kinds of advice about what, and how much, to eat while they're expecting. Cultural traditions, religious beliefs, and even scientific thinking all have had their influence. As recently as a generation ago, women were told to limit how much they ate and drank and thus keep their weight gain to a minimum. At other times, they were encouraged to eat lots of fatty foods — that the greater the weight gain, the healthier the child. These days, your practitioner's advice is likely to depend on your particular health habits and your size when your pregnancy begins. Also, if you are carrying more than one baby, you're expected to gain more than the average number of pounds. This chapter provides you with the information you need in order to properly nourish yourself and your baby.

Sneak preview: In general, you need to eat a balanced, healthy diet and gain a moderate amount of weight. For women of average size — that is, not underweight or overweight — and with only one baby on the way, this translates into about 25 to 35 pounds (11.5 to 16 kilograms).

Choosing the Proper Diet

If your diet is balanced and not too heavy in sugar or fat, you don't need to modify the way you eat dramatically. During pregnancy, you should take in roughly 300 *extra* calories a day, on average. That means that if you're at a healthy weight and you're taking in 2,100 calories per day, while pregnant you should take in an average of 2,400 calories per day (perhaps a little less during your first trimester and a little more during your third trimester).

The need to increase your caloric intake to this degree doesn't mean that you should eat a hot fudge sundae every day, though. It is obviously important that you fill these additional requirements with nutritious foods. Your practitioner will likely advise you to take some supplemental vitamins and minerals, too. The most important components of prenatal vitamins are the iron, folic acid, and calcium, because these are the minerals that tend to get depleted and the ones that most women tend not to consume in adequate amounts. We discuss more about these components later in this chapter.

Your growing body

Starting pregnancy at a healthy weight and gaining weight at a moderate pace throughout pregnancy can help ensure that your baby grows and develops normally, and that you stay healthy as well.

The best way to figure out your ideal weight — and weight gain — is to look at a measurement that's known as *body mass index,* a number that takes into account both height and weight. Here's the formula for figuring your body mass index:

Body mass index = weight (in kilograms) ÷ height (in meters) squared

Or

Body mass index = weight (in pounds) ÷ height (in inches) squared, and then multiplied by 700.

For example, if you are 5 feet tall and weigh 110 pounds, your formula would be 110 ÷ (60 x 60) x 700 = 21.4. According to the chart in Figure 4-1, this would fall into the normal weight range, and the weight gain should be 25 to 35 pounds (11.5 to 16 kilograms).

Or

Skip the calculations and just find your body mass index by looking up your measurements on the chart in Figure 4-1. To find your body mass index, locate your weight on the vertical line on the left-hand side of the chart and your height on the horizontal (bottom) line. (Alternatively, use the metric measurements on the top and right-hand side.) The place where those two points intersect on the chart is your body mass index (follow the diagonal lines until you find the BMI number).

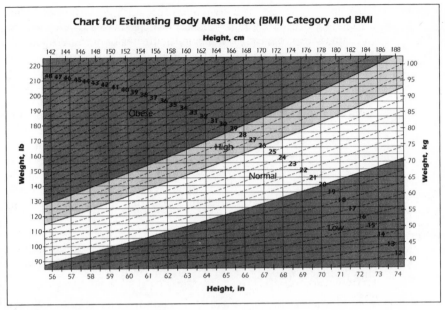

Figure 4-1:
The body
mass index
chart.

Source: *Nutrition During Pregnancy and Lactation,* National Academy Press, 1992

After you know your body mass index, you can figure out your ideal weight gain during pregnancy by consulting the following table. (But don't forget, this refers to women carrying only one baby!)

Body Mass Index	Recommended Weight Gain
Less than 19.8 (underweight)	28 to 40 pounds (12.5 to 18 kilograms)
19.9 to 26 (normal weight)	25 to 35 pounds (11.5 to 16 kilograms)
26 to 29 (overweight)	15 to 25 pounds (7 to 11.5 kilograms)
29 or more (obese)	15 pounds (6 kilograms) or less

These numbers refer to total weight gain during the entire pregnancy, so you won't know whether you hit the target until delivery day.

Unfortunately, far less is known about the optimal pattern of weight gain throughout pregnancy. Some research suggests that gaining very little weight early on (when you are, perhaps, in the throes of morning sickness) has less effect on fetal growth than does poor weight gain in the late second or third trimesters. Some women gain weight very inconsistently, putting on a large number of pounds early and then much less later on. Nothing is necessarily unhealthy about this pattern. For the most part, you should use the charts of optimal weight gain as a guide, but try not to become fanatical about how much you weigh. Even if the amount you gain is somewhat off course, if your doctor says that the baby is growing normally, you have nothing to worry about. Women who gain more than average can still have healthy babies, and so can women who gain very little. If your weight gain is way too high or way too low, your doctor can check the baby's growth by measuring the fundal height (see Chapter 3) or scheduling you for a sonogram if he or she is at all concerned.

The bottom line is that you want to do all you can to improve your baby's chances of optimal growth and development, but not at the expense of driving yourself crazy.

If you deviate significantly from the recommended weight gain, your doctor will probably want to evaluate your diet. He or she may refer you to a nutritionist or dietitian who can give you specific advice about what and how much to eat.

Sticking to a well-balanced and low-fat, high-fiber diet is also important not only for your baby but for your own health. It is important that you consume adequate protein, because protein is important for carrying out many of the body's functions. The fiber in your diet helps to prevent or reduce constipation and hemorrhoids. By not consuming too much fat, you help keep your heart healthy, and also avoid putting on a lot of extra pounds that may be difficult to get rid of. By avoiding excessive weight gain, you also decrease the chances of developing stretch marks. To read more about stretch marks, see Chapter 7.

Choosing the best foods

Where are you going to get the extra 300 calories a day you need during pregnancy? You could stop off for a double cheeseburger and fries (actually, that would put you well over 300). Or you could opt for low-fat yogurt or cottage cheese. It's easy to see which choice is wiser. The key is to make sure that your extra calories are packed with nutrients, protein, and carbohydrates.

Where does the weight go?

The good news is, the weight you gain during pregnancy doesn't all go to your thighs. Then again, it doesn't all go to the baby. A pregnant woman typically adds a little to her own body fat. It's a myth, however, that you can tell by a woman's pattern of weight gain — more in the hips or more in the belly — whether she's going to have a boy or a girl. (See Chapter 18 for some other myths regarding determining your baby's sex.)

Here's a realistic view of what you're gaining — assuming a total weight gain of 27 pounds, which is fairly average:

Baby	7 pounds (3,180 grams)
Placenta	1 pound (455 grams)
Amniotic fluid	2 pounds (910 grams)
Uterus	2 pounds (910 grams)
Breasts	1 pound (455 grams)
Fat stores	7 pounds (3,180 grams)
Body water	4 pounds (1,820 grams)
Extra blood	3 pounds (1,360 grams)

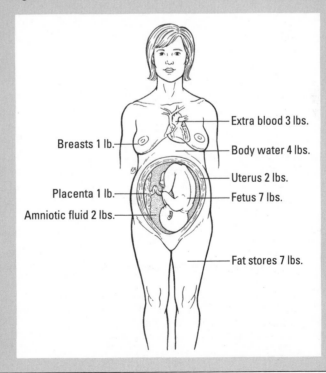

Breasts 1 lb.
Placenta 1 lb.
Amniotic fluid 2 lbs.
Extra blood 3 lbs.
Body water 4 lbs.
Uterus 2 lbs.
Fetus 7 lbs.
Fat stores 7 lbs.

It is very common for women to experience morning sickness during the first trimester (see Chapter 2). If you are experiencing this nausea and are unable to eat a well-balanced diet, you may wonder whether or not you are getting enough nutrition for you and the baby. The fact is, you can go for several weeks not eating an optimal diet without any ill effects on the baby. You may find that the only foods you can tolerate are foods heavy in starch or carbohydrates. If all you feel like eating are potatoes, bread, and pasta, go right ahead. It is more important that you keep something down rather than starve.

No single food can satisfy all of your important nutritional needs. The food pyramid from the USDA (shown in Figure 4-2) is a general guideline that illustrates how much food from each group you should eat. An important underlying concept in the food pyramid is that the most important food groups are grain products, fruits, and vegetables. These should be complemented by low-fat foods from the other groups (protein and dairy products) as well. While fats, oils, and sweets are also included in the pyramid, these groups should constitute only a small part of your diet. The food pyramid shows you the relative proportions of servings you should eat in each group.

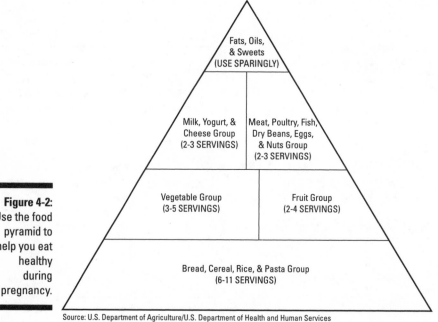

Figure 4-2:
Use the food pyramid to help you eat healthy during pregnancy.

Fats, Oils, & Sweets (USE SPARINGLY)

Milk, Yogurt, & Cheese Group (2-3 SERVINGS)

Meat, Poultry, Fish, Dry Beans, Eggs, & Nuts Group (2-3 SERVINGS)

Vegetable Group (3-5 SERVINGS)

Fruit Group (2-4 SERVINGS)

Bread, Cereal, Rice, & Pasta Group (6-11 SERVINGS)

Source: U.S. Department of Agriculture/U.S. Department of Health and Human Services

✔ The tip of the pyramid includes fats, oils, and sweets. Foods containing these yummy but less nutritional substances include candy, many desserts, butter, mayonnaise, and salad dressings. You can look for low-fat varieties of these foods in the supermarket, but remember that even though they may be lower in fat, they often still contain lots of calories.

✔ The second level of the pyramid contains food rich in protein and calcium: meat, chicken, fish, nuts, beans, eggs, and milk products such as cheese, yogurt, and, of course, milk. You want to eat 2 to 4 servings of protein, and 3 or 4 servings of dairy a day. A single serving of chicken, turkey, lean meat, or fish is about 2 to 3 ounces. Two tablespoons of peanut butter or one egg is equal to 1 ounce of meat.

✔ The next-to-the-bottom level on the food pyramid is the fruit and vegetable group. You need to eat about 3 or 4 servings of each of these. Fruits and vegetables are not only a good source of vitamins and minerals, they also provide fiber, which is very important during pregnancy to help reduce constipation. Vegetables are high in vitamins A, C, and folate, as well as iron. Fruits, too, contain healthy amounts of vitamins A and C, as well as potassium.

✔ The bottom tier on the pyramid is the broadest and largest, comprising such foods as bread, cereal, pasta, rice, and other grains. This group is important because it provides complex carbohydrates, which are long-lasting energy sources. In addition, grains are a good source of vitamins, minerals, and fiber. On average, you need to try to eat about 8 to 10 servings from this group each day. While this may seem like quite a lot of food, satisfying this requirement is easier than you think. One slice of bread, a few crackers, or half a cup of pasta each make up only a single serving. If you are like most of us, when you sit down to order some pasta primavera or shrimp marinara, you usually eat more than ½ cup.

Water

As your pregnancy progresses, your body needs a lot of extra fluid. Early on, some women who don't drink enough liquid feel weak or faint. Later in pregnancy, dehydration can lead to premature contractions.

Make a point of drinking plenty of water — or milk or juice — about 6 to 8 glasses a day.

Vitamins

If your diet is healthy and balanced, you get most of the vitamins and minerals you need naturally — with the exception of iron, folic acid, and calcium. To make sure that you get enough of these nutrients and as insurance against inadequate eating habits, your practitioner is likely to recommend prenatal vitamins. In the case of vitamins, more isn't necessarily better; take only the prescribed number of pills each day.

Is caffeine safe during pregnancy?

While some women think that the only food that contains caffeine is a strong cup of coffee, caffeine is actually found in many of the things you eat and drink on a daily basis: tea, many sodas, cocoa, chocolate, and of course, coffee. There is no evidence that caffeine causes birth defects. However, if you consume caffeine in large enough amounts, it can raise the risk of low birthweight and miscarriage.

Most studies suggest that it takes more than 300 milligrams of caffeine a day to affect the fetus. The average cup of coffee has between 100 and 150 milligrams of caffeine (remember, this is an *average* cup — not the super-mondo size or an espresso or cappuccino!). So drinking up to two average-sized cups of coffee (or the equivalent caffeine content in other foods or beverages) per day is usually okay during pregnancy.

Remember too, though, that consuming caffeine often increases the already frequent trips to the bathroom, so if you are already bothered by frequent urination, you may want to cut your caffeine intake further. Also, many women find that, especially in the last trimester, it is difficult to get a full night's rest, not only because of needing to go to the bathroom so often but also because it's difficult to find a comfortable position to sleep in. Drinking coffee or tea at nighttime may only aggravate your inability to get some rest!

If you miss taking a vitamin, don't worry. Nothing bad is going to happen. During the early months, if your vitamins make you nauseous, skipping them until you're feeling better is perfectly safe for the baby. Remember that the baby is still very small, without large nutritional requirements. If you are very early in your pregnancy (4 to 7 weeks), it's a good idea to take a folic acid supplement only, which is sometimes easier to tolerate, until you can handle the complete prenatal vitamin pill. If later on in the pregnancy, you get a stomach virus and can't tolerate vitamins for some time, it is also not a problem. The growing baby is able to get what it needs, even at the expense of the mom (a theme that continues throughout life!).

Iron

You need more iron when you're expecting, because both you and the baby are making new red blood cells every day. On average, you need 30 milligrams of extra iron every day of your pregnancy, which is what most prenatal vitamins contain. Blood counts can easily drop during pregnancy, as your body gradually makes more and more blood *plasma* (fluid) and *relatively* fewer red blood cells (what is called a *dilutional anemia*). If you do develop an anemia, you may need to take an extra iron supplement.

Foods rich in iron include chicken, fish, red meat, green leafy vegetables, and enriched or whole-grain breads and cereals. You can raise the iron content of foods by cooking them in cast-iron pots and skillets.

Sodium

In the old days, doctors told pregnant women to minimize their salt intake. But it turns out that sodium doesn't really cause any problems. Now, experts pretty much agree that if you're healthy and your blood pressure is normal, you don't need to restrict your salt intake. If you find that you are prone to retaining lots of fluid, then lowering your salt intake may be helpful. Also, if you have underlying hypertension, a lower sodium diet also is a good idea.

Foods heavy on salt include some cheeses, canned soup, canned vegetables, and some deli meats.

Calcium

You need about 1,200 milligrams of calcium every day while you're pregnant. As a matter of fact, the U.S. Recommended Daily Allowance (USRDA) of calcium for *all* women is about 1,000 milligrams. Most women actually get much less than this, which is why so much effort is currently aimed at educating women and enriching foods with calcium. If you are already starting out somewhat calcium deficient, the calcium requirements of the developing baby will only make matters worse for you. A fetus is able to extract enough calcium from its mother, even if it means getting it at the expense of the mother's bones. So the extra calcium needed during pregnancy is really aimed at protecting you and your health.

Prenatal vitamins contain only about 200 to 300 mg of calcium (only about one-quarter of the USRDA), so you need to get it from other sources as well.

Getting enough calcium from your diet alone is possible if you really pay attention. You can get it from three to four servings of calcium-rich foods — such as milk, yogurt, cheese, green leafy vegetables, and canned fish with bones (if your stomach can take it). Supermarkets also stock special lactose-free foods that are high in calcium. The following list indicates portions of foods that qualify as one serving (300 mg of calcium):

- ✔ 1 8-ounce glass of milk (*Tip:* choose low fat or skim milk)
- ✔ 4 ounces of cooked broccoli
- ✔ 4–5 ounces of canned salmon with bones
- ✔ 1¹⁄₂–2 ounces of cheese (*Tip:* cottage cheese has less calcium than many other cheeses)
- ✔ 8 ounces of yogurt

If your diet is low in calcium, take a supplement. Tums and some other antacids contain quite a bit of calcium and, at the same time, they help relieve any pregnancy heartburn you may have. (A single Tums tablet has the equivalent calcium content of an 8-ounce glass of milk.)

Special considerations

Try as you might to follow all the rules of healthy nutrition, you may encounter certain problems with digestion — such as constipation or heartburn. Or you may find that you need to tailor the rules to fit your particular eating habits — for example, if you are a vegetarian. In this section, we address some of the issues that arise for women with special nutritional considerations and for all women who might experience any digestive problems.

Vegetarians

If you're a vegetarian, rest assured that you can produce a healthy baby without eating steak. But you do have to plan your diet more carefully. Vegetables, whole grains, and legumes (peas and beans) are rich in protein, but most do

---

Foods pregnant women ask about most often

When our patients ask us about nutrition and which foods they may want to avoid, certain items come up again and again. Here are some of the foods we're most often asked about:

Sushi: Raw fish carries a small risk of a parasitic infection, whether you're pregnant or not. Pregnancy doesn't increase the danger, and your fetus is unlikely to suffer any harm from such an infection. It is very important, however, that the fish comes from a reliable source.

Smoked meats or fish: Many pregnant women worry about eating smoked meats and fish because they've heard that these foods are high in nitrites or nitrates. But while these foods do contain these substances, they won't hurt your baby if eaten in moderation.

Cheeses: Processed and pasteurized cheeses are not only safe, but they're also a great source of both protein and calcium. Cheeses made from *un*pasteurized milk, on the other hand, may contain *listeria monocytogenes* bacteria, which can cause infection or even miscarriage or premature labor.

Listeria is sometimes found in other foods — some patés, for example, or prepackaged salads that have been contaminated with soil that contains listeria. If you inadvertently eat any of these foods, however, don't panic; your actual risk of infection is still quite low. The problem is relatively uncommon.

Raw or very rare meat: Steak tartare or very rare beef or pork may contain bacteria, such as listeria, or parasites, such as toxoplasma. Adequate cooking kills both bacteria and parasites. In other words, you want your food to be cooked medium-well to well done.

Aspartame (Equal or Nutrasweet): Aspartame (a common component of low-calorie foods and beverages) is a type of amino acid, a kind of substance the body is used to because it is what all proteins are made of. There is no medical evidence to show that aspartame causes any problems for the growing baby.

not have complete proteins — that is, they don't contain all the essential amino acids that your body can't produce by itself. To get all your protein, you can combine whole grains with legumes or nuts — rice with kidney beans, for example, or even peanut butter with whole-grain bread. The combination doesn't have to occur at the same meal, only on the same day.

If you don't eat any animal products, including milk and cheese, your diet may not provide enough of six other important nutrients: vitamin B12, calcium, riboflavin, iron, zinc, and vitamin D. Bring up the topic with your doctor, and you may want to discuss your diet with a nutritionist.

Pica

In certain cultures, or under such conditions as malnourishment, pregnant women have demonstrated cravings for nonfood substances such as clay and laundry starch. This syndrome is known as *pica*. Sometimes these cravings may be indicative of an underlying nutritional deficiency. For example, the desire to eat clay may indicate that the woman has iron deficiency. If you have any such cravings, do not give in to them; instead, discuss them with your practitioner. Besides the risk of poisoning, eating nonfoods can interfere with your body's absorption of nutrients.

Constipation

Progesterone, a hormone that circulates freely through your body during pregnancy, can slow down your digestive system and thus cause constipation. The extra iron from your prenatal vitamin only makes matters worse. Women who are on bed rest because of pregnancy complications are at particular risk of constipation because they are so inactive.

You can counteract constipation by drinking plenty of fluids, by eating adequate fiber (in the form of fruits, vegetables, beans, bran, and other whole grains), and, if possible, by getting exercise every day. Keep in mind, however, that some women experience abdominal discomfort, bloating, or gas from eating too much of very high-fiber foods. You may have to use a little trial and error to see which fiber-rich foods you tolerate best. If constipation bothers you, your practitioner may recommend a stool softener.

Diabetes and other diseases

If you are diabetic or if you develop diabetes during pregnancy, you must adjust your diet so that it includes specific quantities of proteins, fats, and carbohydrates — to ensure that you maintain a normal level of blood glucose (sugar). We discuss this more in Chapter 14.

Getting Enough Exercise

The great fitness movement has not left pregnant women behind. You see them jogging in the parks, working out in gyms, or stretching their limbs in yoga classes. During pregnancy, exercise helps your body in two ways: It keeps your heart strong and your muscles in shape, and it relieves the basic discomforts of pregnancy — from morning sickness to constipation to achy legs and backs. Studies show that the earlier in pregnancy a woman gets regular exercise, the more comfortable she is likely to feel throughout the nine months. Some evidence shows that regular exercise makes for shorter labor, too. It can even help alleviate the symptoms of diabetes. So if you're in good health and not at risk for obstetrical or medical complications, by all means go ahead and continue with your exercise program — unless your program calls for climbing Mount Fuji, entering a professional boxing match, or some other super-strenuous activity. It's a good idea to go over your exercise program with your practitioner, so he or she knows what you are doing, and so that you can ask any other questions you have.

Adapting to changes in your body

Even if you work out in moderation, keep in mind that pregnancy causes your body to undergo real physical changes, which can affect your strength, stamina, and performance. The following list details some of those changes:

- **Cardiovascular changes:** When you're pregnant, the amount of blood that your heart pumps through your body increases. That increase in blood volume usually has no effect on your workout. But if you lie flat on your back, especially after about 16 weeks of pregnancy, you may find yourself feeling dizzy or faint — or even nauseous. Known as the *supine hypotension syndrome,* this dizziness sometimes happens when the enlarging uterus presses down on major blood vessels that return blood to the heart, thus decreasing the heart's output. It happens even more readily if you're carrying twins or more and your uterus is that much heavier.

  If you are doing any exercises that require you to lie on your back (and also if you're accustomed to sleeping on your back), put a small pillow or foam wedge under the right side of your back or your right hip. This tilts you slightly sidewise and effectively lifts your uterus off the blood vessels.

- **Respiratory changes:** Your body is using more oxygen than usual to support the growing baby. At the same time, breathing is more work than it used to be because the enlarging uterus presses upward against the diaphragm. For some women, this difficulty makes performing aerobic exercise a little harder.

✔ **Structural changes:** As your body shape changes — bigger abdomen, larger breasts — your center of gravity shifts, which can affect your balance. You notice it especially if you dance, bicycle, ski, surf, ride horses, or do anything else (walk tightropes, maybe?) where balance is important. In addition, pregnancy hormones cause some laxness in your joints, which also can make balance more difficult and may increase your risk of injury.

✔ **Metabolic changes:** Pregnant women use up carbohydrates faster than nonpregnant women do, which means that they are at a higher risk of developing *hypoglycemia* (or *low blood sugar*). Exercise can be very useful in helping lower and control blood sugar levels, but it also increases the body's need for carbohydrates. So if you exercise, make extra sure that you're eating an adequate amount of starch.

✔ **Effects on the uterus:** One study of women at *term* (far enough along to deliver) showed that their contractions increased after moderate aerobic exercise. Another study indicated that exercise is associated with a lower risk of early labor. But most studies have shown that exercise has no effect either way, and exercise does not pose a risk of preterm labor in healthy pregnant women.

✔ **Effect on birthweight:** Some studies have shown that women who work out strenuously (at high intensity) during pregnancy have lighter-weight babies. The same effect appears to occur in women who perform heavy physical work in a standing position while they're pregnant. But this decrease in birthweight seems to be due mainly to a decrease in the newborn's subcutaneous fat. In other words, more exercise has no effect on the fetus's normal growth.

Reasons not to exercise

As good as exercise is for most pregnant women, it's not advisable for everyone. If you have any of the following conditions (discussed in detail in Chapter 14), you may be better off not working out — at least not until you discuss the situation with your doctor:

✔ Bleeding

✔ Incompetent cervix

✔ Intrauterine growth restriction

✔ Low volume of amniotic fluid

✔ Placenta previa (late in pregnancy)

✔ Pregnancy-induced hypertension

✔ Premature labor or preterm rupture of the membranes

✔ Triplets or more

Workout guide

No matter what your particular exercise regimen may be, keep in mind the basic rules for working out during pregnancy. The following is a list of things to consider when keeping up activities as your baby grows larger and larger.

✔ If you have a moderate exercise routine, keep it up. If you've been pretty sedentary, don't suddenly plunge into a strenuous program; ease in slowly.

Keeping up a regular schedule of moderate activity is better than engaging in infrequent spurts of intense exercise.

✔ Avoid overheating, especially during the first six weeks of pregnancy.

✔ Avoid exercising flat on your back for long periods of time; doing so may reduce blood flow to your heart.

✔ Try not to beat yourself up if you find that pregnancy makes it harder to continue the workout routine you're accustomed to. Modify your program according to what you can reasonably tolerate. Listen to your body. If weight-lifting suddenly hurts your back, lighten up. You may find it easier to perform nonweight-bearing exercises like swimming or bicycling.

✔ Watch how your center of gravity shifts. You probably should avoid surfing, horseback riding, skiing, or any other sport that can cause injury if you're out of balance. Also avoid anything that puts you at risk of being hurt in the abdomen, and high-impact, bouncy exercises that can tax your loosening joints.

✔ Carry a bottle of water to every exercise session and stay well hydrated.

✔ Eat a well-balanced diet that includes an adequate supply of carbohydrates (see "Choosing the best foods" earlier in this chapter).

✔ Talk to your practitioner about what your peak exercise heart rate should be. (Many practitioners suggest 140 beats per minute as the upper limit.) Then regularly measure your heart rate at the peak of your workout to make sure that it's at a safe level.

✔ Stop exercising — and talk to your doctor — if you experience any of these symptoms:

- Shortness of breath out of proportion to the exercise you are doing

- Vaginal bleeding

- Rapid heartbeat (that is, more than 140 beats per minute)

- Dizziness or feeling faint

- Any significant pain

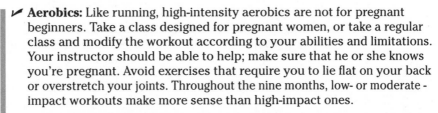

Here's a more specific look at how pregnancy affects the most common kinds of exercise:

✔ **Aerobics:** Like running, high-intensity aerobics are not for pregnant beginners. Take a class designed for pregnant women, or take a regular class and modify the workout according to your abilities and limitations. Your instructor should be able to help; make sure that he or she knows you're pregnant. Avoid exercises that require you to lie flat on your back or overstretch your joints. Throughout the nine months, low- or moderate - impact workouts make more sense than high-impact ones.

During the third trimester, you may have difficulty keeping your balance all the way through an aerobics class or tape.

✔ **Bicycling:** Bike riding is nonweight-bearing — the bicycle supports your weight — and that makes it good for pregnant women. Still, biking entails some risks. As your center of gravity shifts, you may be more likely to fall. Your heavier abdomen can also put stress on your back as you lean toward the handlebars.

Stationary bicycles are ideal because they pose very little risk of falling. In fact, stationary bike riding is an exercise that even the most sedentary woman can begin after she gets pregnant, because she can start slowly and gradually increase riding time as she gets in better shape.

✔ **Downhill skiing, water skiing, horseback riding:** All of these activities put you at risk of falling with significant impact, which could injure you or your baby. While they may be fine early in pregnancy, talk to your doctor before doing any of these sports in your second or third trimester. Cross-country skiing is less risky, especially if you're experienced.

✔ **Golf and bowling:** Joanne's favorite exercises — maybe not so great for your muscles or conditioning, but you don't have to sweat! They're per- fectly okay, but be careful not to overextend or overheat.

✔ **Running/jogging:** If you're a runner, you can keep on running. Competitive runners often maintain their training during pregnancy. But if you haven't been running for a while, starting up during pregnancy doesn't make sense. You put yourself at risk of *musculoskeletal* injuries — knee and hip problems and the like — especially after the body's center of gravity shifts significantly in the third trimester. Better to try brisk walking, 30 to 60 minutes a day, which can also raise your heart rate to fitness range. Many runners find that later in pregnancy, fatigue keeps them from going their usual distance.

Try not to overheat or become dehydrated, and if you feel fatigued, dizzy, faint, or nauseous, by all means stop. On very hot or humid days, don't exercise outdoors.

✔ **Stair-climbing machines:** Stair climbing *is* weight-bearing, but most machines help lighten the load so that it isn't as weight-bearing as aerobics or running. And the stationary machines pose little risk of falling. As your stomach grows, you put more stress on your back muscles. But all things considered, stair climbing is an excellent form of exercise for pregnant women, especially if the room you're in gets plenty of fresh air.

✔ **Stretching and body sculpting:** These are fine as long as you don't do them flat on your back or overextend. You don't get any cardiac benefit, but stretching does help you maintain muscle tone and flexibility, which can come in handy during labor and delivery. Kegel exercises (see Chapter 11), which involve targeting and contracting the muscles of the pelvic floor (around the opening of your bladder and vagina), may not help so much during pregnancy. But afterward, they can make it easier for your pelvic muscles to return to normal, and they may prevent problems with urinary incontinence later in life.

✔ **Swimming:** If you swam before you got pregnant, keep swimming now. In fact, swimming is one of the best exercises a pregnant woman can do because it puts no stress on your joints and poses little risk of overheating or losing your balance and falling. However, most doctors advise that you avoid scuba diving because the dramatic pressure changes could have adverse effects on the baby.

✔ **Tennis and other racquet sports:** Tennis may be continued during pregnancy. But be aware of how your center of gravity is shifting so that you don't lose balance. Try to avoid very bouncy or jerky movements, and don't get overheated.

✔ **Weight lifting:** Weight-lifting machines may be preferable to using free weights, because you know you won't drop the weights onto your abdomen. Use free weights only with caution, preferably with the help of a trainer or a skilled friend. A trainer can also show the proper way to exhale and inhale during lifting. Breathing well is important because it lessens the chance that you might *bear down* (otherwise known as *valsava,* or increase your abdominal pressure), which can reduce blood flow, raise your blood pressure, and stress your heart.

Avoid using very heavy weights, which can cause injury to your joints and ligaments.

✔ **Yoga:** Most forms of yoga are fine during pregnancy and may even relieve some of your stress. Many yoga teachers offer special pregnancy classes, but regular classes are also fine. Just avoid lying flat on your back or overstretching.

Part II

Pregnancy: A Drama in Three Acts

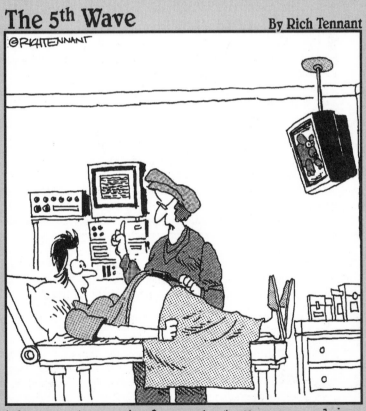

The 5th Wave

By Rich Tennant

"That's a telecast of parade balloons used in Macy's Thanksgiving Day Parade. Your ultra-sound images are over here."

In this part . . .

*I*f you're like most women, you're likely to become a bit calendar-conscious during pregnancy. It's 40 weeks. It's nine months (plus). But perhaps the most useful way to think of pregnancy is to divide it, as doctors always have divided it, into three trimesters. They do it this way because the baby's growth, as well as the changes that occur in your own body, happen in these three fairly distinct stages. In this part, we let you know what's likely to happen — how the baby develops, how you're likely to feel, and how your practitioner takes care of you — in each trimester.

Chapter 5

The First Trimester

. . . .

In This Chapter

▶ Understanding the way your baby develops from conception through the first trimester

▶ Being prepared for physical changes as your pregnancy begins

▶ Anticipating tests and questions at your prenatal visits

▶ Understanding when certain diagnostic tests are necessary

▶ Recognizing some of the signs that things may not be going smoothly

. . . .

The first trimester of your pregnancy is an exciting time, full of many changes for both you and your baby. In this chapter, we cover everything from the development of your fetus over the course of the first three months (or 13 weeks) to the changes that you see in your body at the same time. In the following pages, you find out what happens at your first prenatal visit and at the visits that follow. We provide information on diagnostic tests that may be performed during the first trimester and let you know the reasons to consider them as well as the risks involved. Finally, we let you know when you have reason to be concerned and tell you when you should call your practitioner — and when you can take a deep breath and relax. We cover everything that you — and your baby — experience during your first trimester in the following pages. So read on!

A New Life Takes Shape

Pregnancy begins when the egg and sperm meet, which happens in the fallopian tube. At this stage, the egg and sperm together form what we refer to as the *zygote* — a single cell. The single-celled zygote divides many times into multiple cells called a *blastocyst*. The blastocyst travels down the fallopian tube and into the *uterus* (also called the *womb*), shown in Figure 5-1. When it reaches the uterus, both you and your baby begin to experience major changes.

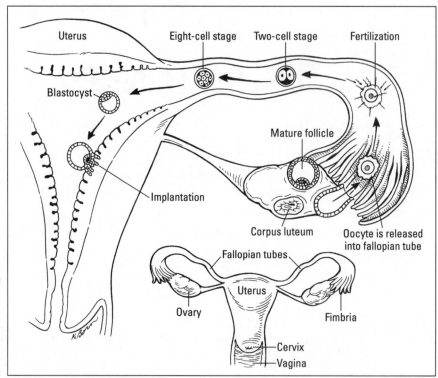

Figure 5-1:
The female
reproductive
system in
action.

On or about the fifth day of development, the blastocyst attaches to the blood-rich lining of the uterus (called *implantation*). Part of the blastocyst grows to become the *embryo* (the baby in the first eight weeks of development), and the other part becomes the *placenta*.

Your baby grows within the *amniotic sac* in the uterus. Try to imagine a baby developing inside a balloon (the amniotic sac), but instead of the balloon being filled with air, it's full of clear fluid, known as the *amniotic fluid*. The balloon itself is actually two thin layers of membrane, called the *chorion* and *amnion* (which are together known as the *membranes*). When people talk about "breaking the bag of water," they are referring to rupturing the membranes. These membranes line the inner walls of the uterus. The baby "swims" in this fluid and is attached to the placenta by the umbilical cord. Figure 5-2 shows a diagram of an early pregnancy, including a developing fetus and the *cervix,* which is the opening to the uterus. The cervix is what opens up, or *dilates,* when you are in labor.

The placenta begins to form very early on — soon after the embryo implants in the uterus. Maternal and fetal blood vessels lie very close to one another inside the placenta, which allows various substances (such as nutrients, oxygen, and waste) to transfer back and forth. The mother's blood and the baby's blood are in close contact, but they don't actually mix.

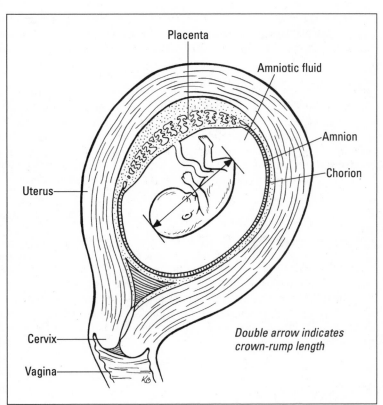

Placenta

Amniotic fluid

Amnion

Chorion

Uterus

Cervix

Vagina

Double arrow indicates crown-rump length

Figure 5-2: An early pregnancy.

Like a tree, the placenta forms large branches that in turn divide into smaller and smaller ones. The tiniest buds of the placenta are called the *chorionic villi,* and it is within these *villi,* or branches, that small fetal blood vessels form. About three weeks after fertilization, these blood vessels join to form the baby's circulatory system, and the heart begins to beat.

After eight weeks into your pregnancy, the developing embryo is referred to as a *fetus.* Amazingly, by this time almost all of the baby's major organs and structures are already formed. The remaining 32 weeks allow the fetus's structures to grow and mature. On the other hand, the brain, although also formed very early, continues to develop as well as grow throughout the pregnancy (and even into early childhood).

When we refer to weeks, we mean menstrual weeks, which means weeks from the last menstrual period, not weeks from conception. So at eight weeks, the baby is really six weeks from conception.

By the end of the second month, arms, legs, fingers, and toes begin to form. In fact, the embryo begins to perform small, spontaneous movements. If you have an ultrasound examination performed in the first trimester, you can see these spontaneous movements on the screen. The brain enlarges rapidly, and ears and eyes appear. The external genitalia also emerge and can be differentiated as male or female genitalia by the end of the second month, although sex differences are not yet detectable by ultrasound.

By the end of the third month, the fetus is about 4 inches long and weighs about 1 ounce. The head looks large and round, and the eyelids are fused shut. The intestines, which protruded slightly into the umbilical cord at about week 10, are by this time well inside the abdomen. Fingernails appear, and hair begins to grow on the baby's head. The kidneys start working during the third month. Between 9 and 12 weeks, the fetus begins to produce urine, which can be seen within the small fetal bladder on ultrasound.

Your Body Adapts to Pregnancy

Your baby isn't the only one growing and changing during your pregnancy (not that we have to remind you of that!). Your own body also has to adjust, and the adjustments it makes are not always the most pleasant and comfortable for you. Being prepared for what lies ahead can help ease your mind. So in the following sections, we let you know what is in store for you during the first trimester.

Breast changes

One of the earliest and most amazing changes in your body happens to your breasts. Even during the first month of pregnancy, most women notice that their breasts grow considerably larger and feel very tender. The nipples and *areolae* (the circular areas around the nipples) also grow bigger and may begin to darken. Breast changes are caused by the large amounts of estrogen and progesterone your body produces during pregnancy. These hormones cause the glands inside your breasts to grow and branch out, in preparation for milk production and breast-feeding after the baby is born. Blood supply to the breasts also increases markedly. You may notice large, bluish blood vessels coursing along your breasts.

Plan to go through several bra sizes while you're pregnant — and don't skimp on buying new bras. Good support helps reduce stretching and sagging later on. Although some women like the way they look with larger breasts, others feel more self-conscious. Whichever way you feel, we guarantee that other pregnant women feel the same way, and it's nothing to feel embarrassed about.

Fatigue

During the first trimester, you're likely to feel overwhelming fatigue. This fatigue may be a side effect of all the physical changes your body is experiencing, including the dramatic rise in hormone levels. Rest assured that your exhaustion will probably go away somewhere around the 12th to 14th week of your pregnancy. As your fatigue lessens, you'll probably feel more energetic and almost normal, until about 30 to 34 weeks into your pregnancy, when you may tire out again. In the meantime, remember that fatigue is nature's way of telling you to get more rest. If you can, try to catch a short nap during the day and go to bed earlier than usual at night.

Dad, by all means, help the mother-to-be as much as possible during this time — without making a big stink about it.

Any-time-of-day sickness

For some women, the nausea that can strike during the first trimester is worse in the mornings, maybe because the stomach is empty at that time of day. But ask anyone who's had morning sickness, and she'll tell you: It can hit any time it wants. It often starts during the 5th or 6th week (that is, three to four weeks after you miss your period — we describe how doctors calculate the timing of pregnancy in Chapter 2) and goes away, or at least becomes much less severe, by the end of the 11th or 12th week. It can last longer, though, particularly in women who are expecting twins or more, because multiple placentas release more hCG.

The cause of morning sickness is not absolutely clear, but it appears to be related to the rise in *hCG* (human chorionic gonadotropin), a hormone released by the placenta.

You may hear some women say that morning sickness is a sign that you're experiencing a "normal" pregnancy, but that claim is a myth — and so is the reverse. If you're not having morning sickness, or if it suddenly disappears, don't worry that your pregnancy isn't normal; just enjoy your good fortune. Similarly, you may hear that the severity of your queasiness indicates whether you're having a girl or a boy. But that's a myth, too, so don't buy those pink or blue outfits just yet (and turn to Chapter 18 for even more myths about determining the sex of your bundle of joy).

If you *are* experiencing nausea, we sympathize. Even when nausea doesn't actually cause you to vomit, it can be extremely uncomfortable and truly debilitating. Certain odors — from foods, perfumes, or musty places — can make it worse. Look in the nearby sidebar called "Tips for keeping nausea at bay," for recommendations on how to minimize morning sickness.

Tips for keeping nausea at bay

Unfortunately, we can't tell you how to make your nausea totally disappear. But you can try a few things to make it better. Here are a few suggestions:

✔ Eat small, frequent meals, so that your stomach is never empty.

✔ Don't worry too much about adhering to a balanced diet; just eat whatever appeals to you during this relatively short period of time.

✔ Avoid perfume counters, active kitchens, smelly taxi cabs, barnyards, or other places where odors may be strong.

✔ If your prenatal vitamins make the symptoms worse, try taking them at night just before you go to bed. If you find that they are still causing a problem, skipping them for a few days is okay.

✔ Keep crackers by your bedside — some women find that eating them before getting out of bed in the morning helps to decrease the nausea.

✔ Ginger (in the form of tea or tablets, for example) may help some women.

✔ You may notice that your nausea worsens when you brush your teeth. Switching toothpaste brands may help.

✔ Try eating dry toast, saltines, whole wheat crackers, potatoes, and other bland, easy-to-digest carbohydrates.

✔ If you are bothered by the accumulation of saliva in your mouth, sucking on lemon drop candies may be helpful.

✔ Accupressure wrist bands, sold in drug stores and health food stores, give some women relief.

✔ Relaxation exercises and even hypnosis work for some women.

✔ Try vitamin B6. Some evidence suggests that 25 milligrams of this nutrient three times a day can reduce queasiness. But talk to your doctor before starting on a B6 regimen.

✔ For extreme nausea, talk to your doctor about prescription medicines or other over-the-counter medicines that may help.

✔ Above all, don't compound the problem by worrying about it. The nausea is harmless — to you and the baby. Your optimal weight gain for the first three months is only 2 pounds. Even losing weight probably isn't a big problem.

Occasionally, the nausea and vomiting are so severe that you develop a condition called *hyperemesis gravidarum*. The symptoms include dehydration and weight loss. If you develop hyperemesis gravidarum, you may need to be given fluids intravenously.

If your queasiness gets out of control — if you experience weight loss, if you find that you can't keep down food or liquids, or if you feel dizzy or faint — call your doctor.

If you're less than six weeks pregnant, you can take folic acid alone instead of your prenatal vitamin. Folic acid is the main supplement that you need early in your pregnancy, and it's much less likely to upset your stomach than the multivitamin you normally take during pregnancy.

Bloating

Well before the baby is big enough to stretch out your stomach, your belt may begin to feel uncomfortable and your belly may look bloated and distended. This side effect of the hormone shift starts happening as soon as you conceive. *Progesterone,* one of the two key pregnancy hormones, causes you to retain water. Plus, it slows down the bowels, causing them to enlarge and thus increase the size of the abdomen. *Estrogen,* the other key pregnancy hormone, causes your uterus to enlarge, which also makes your abdomen feel bigger. This effect is often more pronounced in second or third pregnancies because the first pregnancy caused your abdominal muscles to relax to a greater degree.

Frequent urination

From early on in your pregnancy, you may feel as if you're spending your whole life in the restroom. There's no question about it — during pregnancy, you need to urinate more frequently for a variety of reasons. At the beginning of your pregnancy, your uterus is inside your pelvis. But toward the end of your first trimester (at around 12 weeks), your uterus expands enough to rise up into your abdominal cavity. Your enlarging uterus may compress your bladder, which both decreases its capacity and increases the feeling that you need to urinate. Also, your blood volume rises markedly during pregnancy, and that means the rate at which your kidneys produce urine also increases.

You can't do much about your need to urinate frequently, except use common sense. Before going out for long (or even short) trips, empty your bladder so that you don't find yourself needing facilities when none are available. Be sure to drink plenty of fluids during pregnancy to avoid dehydration, but try to drink more during the day and less in the evening, so that you aren't up all night going to the restroom. Coffee and tea contain caffeine (a *diuretic,* which increases the flow of urine) and may aggravate the situation, so try decreasing the amount of caffeine you consume. (For more information about caffeine, see Chapter 4.)

If you find yourself urinating even more than your pregnancy norm or if you feel any discomfort or burning or notice blood during urination, talk to your practitioner. When you're pregnant, bacteria in your urine are more likely than usual to cause a urinary tract infection (see Chapter 15).

Headaches

Many pregnant women notice that they get headaches more often than they used to. This may be the result of nausea, fatigue, hunger, the normal physiologic decrease in blood pressure that starts to occur at this time, tension, or even depression. Acetaminophen (for example, Tylenol), in recommended doses, is perfectly fine to take for occasional headache relief. Some women find that a little caffeine can also alleviate symptoms of a headache. In fact, some women find relief from occasional headaches by taking a combination of acetaminophen and caffeine (Aspirin-free Excedrin). Although this combination is fine to take once in a while, it should not be used on a regular basis.

Food and rest can usually cure headaches that are caused by nausea, fatigue, or hunger. So try eating and getting some extra sleep. If neither of those tactics work, your headache is probably being caused by something else.

Simple pain relievers like acetaminophen (Tylenol) or ibuprofen (such as Motrin) are often the best treatment for headaches, including migraines. If over-the-counter medications don't relieve your headache, talk with your practitioner about taking a mild tranquilizer or anti-migraine medication.

Base your decision on whether to use migraine medications on the severity of your problem. If your headaches are chronic or recurrent, you may need to take medications, despite their effects on your fetus. As always, be sure to consult with your practitioner before taking these medications.

Avoid taking regular doses of aspirin, because adult doses of aspirin can affect platelet function (important in blood clotting).

If your headaches are severe and unremitting, you may need a thorough medical evaluation or you may need to be referred to a neurologist. Later on in pregnancy, a headache may signal the onset of a condition called preeclampsia (which is covered in more detail in Chapter 14). In that case, your headache may be accompanied by swelling of your hands and feet and by high blood pressure. If you suffer a severe headache in the late second or third trimester, call you practitioner.

Constipation

About half of all pregnant women complain of constipation. When you are pregnant, you may become constipated because the large amount of progesterone circulating in your bloodstream slows the activity of your digestive tract. The iron in prenatal vitamins may make matters worse. Here are a few suggestions for dealing with the problem:

✔ **Eat plenty of high-fiber foods.** Bran cereals, fruits, and vegetables all are good sources of fiber. Some women find it helpful to eat some popcorn, but choose the low-fat kind, without all the butter and added oil. Check the fiber content on package labels and choose foods with a higher fiber content.

✔ **Drink plenty of water.** Staying well hydrated helps keep food and waste moving through the digestive tract. Some juices (especially prune juice) may help, while others (such as apple juice) may only exacerbate the problem.

✔ **Take stool softeners.** A stool softener, such as Colace (docusate sodium), is not a laxative — it just keeps the stool soft. Stool softeners are safe during pregnancy, and you may take them two to three times a day. It is better to avoid laxatives, because they can cause abdominal cramping and, occasionally, uterine contractions. For any person, pregnant or not, chronic laxative use should be avoided. If you are extremely constipated, though, and are not at risk for preterm labor, you may want to talk to your practitioner about the short-term use of a very mild laxative, like a glycerin suppository.

✔ **Exercise as regularly as you can.** Exercise is known to help constipation, so enjoy some safe exercise (even if it's only walking).

Cramps

You may feel a vague, menstrual-like cramping sensation during the first trimester. This is a very common symptom and nothing that should cause you concern. It is probably related to the uterus growing and enlarging.

If, however, you experience cramping along with vaginal bleeding, give your practitioner a call. Although the majority of women who experience bleeding and cramping go on to have perfectly normal pregnancies, sometimes these two symptoms together are associated with miscarriage. Cramping alone, without bleeding, is unlikely to be a problem.

Prenatal Visits

Visits to your practitioner should be a regular part of your pregnancy, not only to ensure your health, but to ensure the health of your baby. Prenatal visits differ from your typical yearly exams, and you may be wondering what they are like. So in the following sections we've highlighted exactly what you need to know to feel prepared when you visit your practitioner's office throughout your first trimester.

Your first prenatal visit

After the at-home pregnancy test reveals the news, you should set up an appointment with a practitioner. Your first prenatal visit may be your first meeting with the practitioner who will guide you through your pregnancy. (If you don't already have a practitioner selected, see Chapter 2 for information on the kinds of care available and tips for choosing a health care provider.) Or you may have a long-standing relationship with an ob/gyn or family-practice doctor, with whom you have already discussed many of the topics that are typically covered at an initial prenatal visit. Whatever your particular situation, you're moving into new territory. The following sections describe the usual parts of your first prenatal visit.

Consultation

During your first visit, your practitioner discusses with you your medical and obstetrical history. He or she asks about various aspects of your physical health, as well as elements of your lifestyle that may affect your pregnancy.

Lifestyle

Your practitioner asks about your occupation to find out whether your job is sedentary or active, if you spend your days standing or lifting heavy objects, or whether you work nights or long shifts. You are also asked about your general lifestyle — for example, smoking, heavy alcohol use, dietary restrictions, and exercise patterns.

Date of your last menstrual period

You are asked the start date of your last menstrual period to determine your due date. (For more information on calculating your due date, see Chapter 2.) If you don't know exactly the date that your last period began, try to remember the exact date of conception. If you are unsure about either of these dates, your practitioner may want to check on how far along you are by scheduling an ultrasound exam.

Obstetrical and gynecological history

If you have not already seen your practitioner for a *preconceptual visit* (covered in more detail in Chapter 1), you are asked about your obstetrical and gynecological history, including any prior pregnancies and any experiences with fibroid tumors, vaginal infections, and other gynecological problems. Your past history can help determine how best to manage this pregnancy. For example, if you have a history of preterm labor (see Chapter 14) or gestational diabetes (Chapter 15), knowing that history prepares your practitioner for the possibility that it may happen again.

Medical problems

Your practitioner also asks you about any medical problems you have had and any surgeries you have undergone, including problems that aren't gynecological in nature. Certain medical conditions may affect pregnancy, and others don't. You are also asked about any allergies to medications you may have. It's important that your practitioner knows everything he or she can about you and your health.

Family medical histories

The family medical histories of both you and the baby's father are important for two reasons. First, to identify pregnancy-related conditions that can recur from generation to generation, like having twins or exceptionally large babies. The other reason is to identify serious problems within your family that can be inherited by your baby. Some of these problems can be screened for by blood tests — cystic fibrosis, for example.

Ethnic roots

Even if your and your partner's family history is free of any known genetic disorders, your ethnic backgrounds are important because some genetic disorders occur more frequently in one ethnicity than others. Jewish people of Eastern European descent, for example, are ten times more likely than others to carry the rare gene for *Tay-Sachs,* a disease of the nervous system that is usually fatal in early childhood. French Canadians and Cajuns (from Louisiana) also have a higher-than-normal risk of carrying this gene. Most of the time, a simple blood test can determine whether you're a carrier of this disease.

This condition is inherited in what's known as a "recessive" manner, which means that both parents would need to be carriers to place the baby at risk for having the disease. Being a carrier doesn't mean that you *have* Tay-Sachs, only that you carry a gene for it. Most genetic counselors recommend that both members of a couple undergo the blood tests for carrier status, because it often takes several weeks to find out the results. If one member of a couple is tested only after the other is found to be a carrier, the whole process can take a long time, perhaps even too long to leave time for certain prenatal diagnostic tests (like CVS or amniocentesis, described later in this chapter and in Chapter 6).

Although Tay-Sachs and some other conditions are found more frequently among the Jewish population, individuals from other ethnic groups can still be carriers, although this is much less common. For this reason, even if only one member of a couple is Jewish, both should still be tested. Here is a list of genetic disorders for which screening is available to couples of Jewish descent:

- ✔ Tay-Sachs
- ✔ Cystic Fibrosis
- ✔ Canavan
- ✔ Gaucher
- ✔ Neimann-Pick

Another ethnically selective medical condition is *sickle-cell anemia,* a blood disorder that's especially prevalent among people with African or Hispanic ancestors. This condition, too, is recessive, and so both members of a couple need to be carriers for the baby to be at risk of inheriting the disease.

People whose ancestors come from Italy, Greece, and other Mediterranean countries are at elevated risk of having — and passing to their children — genes for the blood disorder *beta-thalassemia,* also known as *Mediterranean anemia* or *Cooley's anemia.* Among Asians, the analogous blood problem is *alpha-thalassemia.* Both of these disorders produce abnormalities in hemoglobin (the protein in red blood cells that holds onto oxygen) and therefore result in varying degrees of anemia. Like Tay-Sachs and sickle-cell anemia, both parents have to carry the gene in order for there to be a risk that their baby has the disease.

The risks of inheritable diseases overlap from one ethnic or geographic group to another. Genes get passed around among the various populations whenever the parents are from different ethnic groups. But you can roughly gauge whether your ancestry puts you at an elevated risk of carrying certain disease genes. Although not exhaustive, the map in Figure 5-3 shows approximately which populations are identified with which conditions. If your ancestors come from any of the shaded areas, bring up the subject with your practitioner.

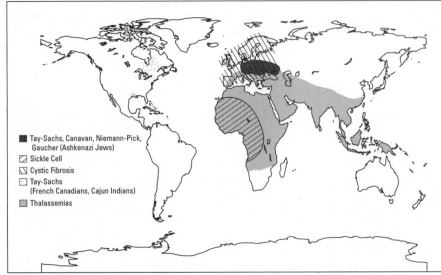

Figure 5-3:
Find the areas where your ancestors came from.

Legend:
- Tay-Sachs, Canavan, Niemann-Pick, Gaucher (Ashkenazi Jews)
- Sickle Cell
- Cystic Fibrosis
- Tay-Sachs (French Canadians, Cajun Indians)
- Thalassemias

Some people don't know very much about their ethnic background or family medical history, perhaps because they were adopted or have not had much contact with their biological families. If this situation is true in your case, don't worry. Keep in mind that the chances that both you and your partner carry a gene for a particular disorder are extremely low.

Physical exam

At your first prenatal visit, your practitioner examines your head, neck, breasts, heart, lungs, abdomen, and extremities. He or she also performs an internal exam (see Figure 5-4). During this exam, your practitioner evaluates your uterus, cervix, and ovaries, and performs a Pap test.

After the exam is a good time for you to discuss the overall plan for your pregnancy and talk about any possible problems. You can also discuss what medications you can take while you're pregnant, when you should call for help, and what tests you can expect to undergo throughout your pregnancy.

If possible, go with your partner for this initial visit. Your family medical history and ethnic roots are important, too. Also, you should have a chance to ask questions, address your concerns, and find out what to look forward to in the coming months. You should play an integral role in the pregnancy, so attend if you can, to show that she has your full support and involvement.

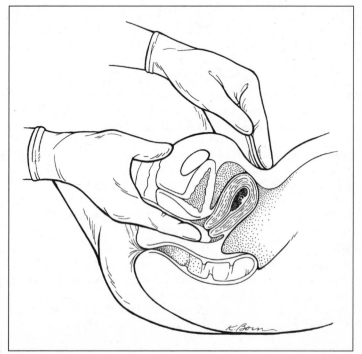

Figure 5-4:
A typical
pelvic exam.

Blood tests

During your first prenatal visit, your practitioner needs to draw your blood for certain tests. The following tests are routine:

- **A standard test for blood type, Rh factor, and antibody status.** The blood type refers to whether your blood is type A, B, or O and whether you are Rh-positive or Rh-negative. The antibody test is designed to tell whether special blood-group antibodies to certain antigens (like the Rh antigen) are present. (See Chapter 14 for more about the Rh factor and the implications of blood incompatibilities.)

- **Complete blood count (CBC).** This test checks for *anemia,* which refers to a low blood count. At the same time, this test also checks your *platelet count* (a component of blood important in clotting).

- **VDRL.** This test checks for *syphilis,* a sexually transmitted disease. VDRL is a very accurate test, but it sometimes produces a false positive result. A false positive test can result from the patient having other conditions, such as lupus or the antiphospholipid antibody syndrome (see Chapter 15). However, these kinds of false positive results are usually weakly positive. The VDRL test is nonspecific, and so in order to confirm the diagnosis of syphilis, another, more specific blood test should be performed. Because it is essential that syphilis be adequately treated, it is important that this test be performed. In fact, it's required in most states.

- **Hepatitis B.** This test checks for evidence of the hepatitis viruses. These viruses come in several different types, and the hepatitis B virus is one that can be present without producing actual symptoms. In fact, some women are diagnosed only during a blood test, such as the one performed during pregnancy.

- **Rubella.** Your practitioner also checks for immunity to *rubella* (also called *German measles*). Most women have been vaccinated against rubella, or because they have had the illness in the past, their blood carries antibodies, which is why the risk of contracting German measles during pregnancy is so rare. Most practitioners test to see that the mother is immune to rubella during the very first prenatal visit. Any woman who is found not to be immune is counseled to be very careful to avoid contact with anyone who has the illness. These women are also advised to get vaccinated against rubella soon after they deliver, so that they are not susceptible in subsequent pregnancies.

- **HIV.** Some states require that health care providers routinely ask whether you want to be checked for HIV, the virus that causes AIDS. Because medication is available to reduce the risk of transmission to the baby, as well as to slow disease progression in the mother, being aware of your HIV status is very important. This test can usually be performed at the same time as the other prenatal blood tests.

Doctors sometimes need to perform other tests during your first prenatal visit. These additional tests include the following:

- ✔ **Glucose screen.** This test is usually done around 24 to 28 weeks, but sometimes it is done in the first trimester if you are at a high risk of developing *gestational diabetes.* Check out Chapter 6 for the details of how the testing is done and Chapter 15 to find out why treating gestational diabetes is important.

- ✔ **Varicella.** Your doctor may conduct this test to check for immunity to *varicella* (chicken pox). If you are unsure whether or not you had chicken pox or you know that you did not have it, let your practitioner know so that you can be tested for immunity. For more detailed information on varicella, see Chapter 15.

- ✔ **Toxoplasmosis.** A test is sometimes done in order to check for immunity to *toxoplasmosis,* which is a type of parasitic infection. In the United States, testing for toxoplasmosis is not considered routine unless you are at a higher risk for toxoplasmosis. For example, if you have an outdoor cat and you are the one to change the litter box, your practitioner is likely to send off a test to check for past or recent exposure. If you are in France, where the incidence of toxoplasmosis is much higher, your practitioner will probably recommend that you be tested. See Chapter 15 for more information on toxoplasmosis.

- ✔ **Cytomegalovirus (CMV).** Testing for CMV infection, a common childhood infection, is not routine during pregnancy. However, if you have a lot of contact with school-age children who may have the infection, your practitioner may suggest you have this test performed. As with toxoplasmosis, the blood test looks for evidence of past or recent infection. See Chapter 15 for more details on CMV.

Urine tests

Each time you visit your practitioner during your pregnancy, including the first prenatal visit, you are asked to leave a sample of urine. The urine sample is needed in order to check for the presence of glucose (for a possible sign of diabetes), and protein (for evidence of preeclampsia).

Ultrasound

An *ultrasound* uses sound waves to create a picture of the uterus and the baby inside it. Ultrasound examinations do not involve radiation, and the procedure is safe for both you and your baby. Your practitioner may suggest that you undergo a first-trimester ultrasound exam. Often, this ultrasound is performed *transvaginally,* which means that a special ultrasound probe is inserted into the vagina. The advantage to this technique is that the probe, or *transducer,* is closer to the fetus, so a much clearer view is attained than with a standard *transabdominal* ultrasound examination.

Some women worry that a transvaginal probe inserted into the vagina could harm the baby. While understandable, there is no truth to this concern. The probe is completely safe.

The following are evaluated during a first trimester ultrasound exam:

✔ **The accuracy of your due date:** An ultrasound can show whether the fetus is any larger or smaller than the date of your last menstrual period would suggest. If the *crown-rump measurement* (which measures the fetus from the crown of the head to the rump; refer to Figure 5-2) is more than three or four days off your due date, your doctor may change your due date. An ultrasound in the first trimester is actually more accurate than a later ultrasound in confirming or establishing your due date.

✔ **Fetal viability:** By five to six weeks into your pregnancy, an ultrasound should be able to detect a fetal heartbeat. After a fetal heartbeat has been identified, the risk of miscarriage drops significantly (to about 3 percent). Prior to five weeks, the fetus itself may not be visible; instead, the ultrasound may show only the gestational sac.

✔ **Fetal abnormalities:** Although a complete ultrasound examination to detect structural abnormalities in the fetus is usually not performed until about 20 weeks, some problems may already be visible by 11 to 12 weeks. Much of the brain, spine, limbs, abdomen, and urinary tract structures may be seen with transvaginal ultrasound. In addition, the presence of a thickening behind the neck of the fetus (known as *increased nuchal translucency*) may help to indicate an added risk for certain genetic or chromosomal conditions (see the sidebar "Coming soon: New first trimester screening tests" later in this chapter).

✔ **Fetal number:** An ultrasound shows whether you are carrying more than one fetus. In addition, the appearance of the membrane separating the babies, as well as the placental locations, helps to indicate whether the babies share one placenta or have separate placentas. We go into greater detail about this topic in Chapter 13.

✔ **The condition of your ovaries:** An ultrasound can also reveal abnormalities or cysts in your ovaries. Sometimes a small cyst, called a *corpus luteal cyst,* is seen. This is a cyst that forms at the site where the egg was released. Over the course of three or four months, it gradually goes away. Two other types of cysts, called *dermoid cysts* and *simple cysts,* are unrelated to the pregnancy and may be found incidentally during an ultrasound exam. Whether removal of these types of cysts is necessary and when they should be removed depends on the size of the cyst and any symptoms you may be having.

✔ **The presence of fibroid tumors:** Also called *fibroids,* these are benign overgrowths of the muscle of the uterus. We go into more details about these in Chapter 15.

> ✔ **Location of the pregnancy:** Occasionally, the pregnancy may be located outside the uterus. This is called an *ectopic pregnancy* (see the "Ectopic pregnancy" section later in this chapter for more information).

Routine prenatal visits

Your first prenatal visit usually lasts 30 to 40 minutes or more because your doctor has so much information to provide and so many topics to discuss. Subsequent visits are usually much shorter, sometimes only 5 to 10 minutes long. The frequency of your visits depends on your particular needs and any special risk factors you may have, but in general they're about every four weeks during the first trimester. At these visits, your urine, blood pressure, and weight and the baby's heartbeat are checked.

Tests for Prenatal Diagnosis

Depending on your age, your medical and obstetrical history, your family history, and other factors, you may want to undergo one or more tests designed to detect certain genetic diseases or conditions. A number of such tests are available, including chorionic villus sampling (CVS), amniocentesis, and fetal blood sampling. CVS and early amniocentesis are the only ones that can be done during the first trimester. (We discuss CVS and early amniocentesis in the next section. Routine amniocentesis, which is performed after 15 weeks, and fetal blood sampling are covered in Chapter 6.)

These prenatal tests involve testing the chromosomes of the developing baby. Chromosomes carry the genetic information that determines what a person is like. People normally have 46 chromosomes — 23 inherited from their mother and 23 from their father (see Figure 5-5). The 23 from each side are paired inside the nucleus of each human cell. Twenty-two of these pairs are what's known as *autosomes,* which are the chromosomes that aren't gender-related. The 23rd pair of chromosomes are the sex chromosomes, which can be either XX (girl) or XY (boy).

A woman has two X chromosomes and so can only give an X chromosome to her offspring. A man has one X and one Y chromosome and can therefore give either to his offspring. As you can see, it is the man who determines the gender of the baby, so you know who is to blame if you don't get the little girl or little boy you were hoping for!

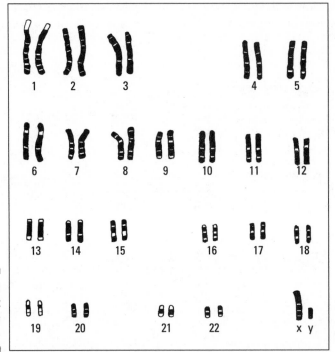

Figure 5-5:
A typical set
of human
chromosomes.

Certain abnormalities in chromosome number or structure can lead to problems in the baby. For example, Down syndrome, one of the more common chromosomal abnormalities that is associated with severe mental retardation, may occur if the fetus has an extra copy of chromosome 21. (The condition is also known as *Trisomy 21,* because the fetus has three copies of chromosome number 21.) The amniocentesis, CVS, and other tests detect such abnormalities in chromosome number and structure by yielding an enlarged picture of the individual chromosomes called a *karyotype* (refer to Figure 5-5). In addition, if a couple is known to be at risk for carrying a child with a genetic disease that runs in that couple's family or ethnic group (Tay-Sachs or cystic fibrosis, for example), the material obtained during these procedures can also be used to test for such diseases. However, unless a couple is specifically at risk for one of these rare genetic disorders, this testing is not routinely done; the chromosomes are checked only for number and structure.

Traditionally, women who are age 35 or older (or who will be at their due date) are offered the chance to undergo prenatal diagnosis to check the fetal chromosomes. Thirty-five is the target age because a woman's risk of having a baby with a chromosomal abnormality increases significantly after she reaches that age. It is also the age at which the risk of miscarriage from the procedure itself is equal to the chance that the fetus has a chromosomal abnormality. However, although the risk of a chromosome abnormality is much less for women under the age of 35, most babies with Down syndrome are born to women under the age of 35 because far more women under 35 have babies than women over 35.

Note: The cutoff age of 35 is somewhat arbitrary and not followed in all countries. In Great Britain, for example, women are offered prenatal chromosomal testing at age 37 or after.

Even among women at risk for a chromosomal problem, some choose not to be tested, either because they don't want to run any risk of miscarriage associated with the test (see the following sections for more specific information) or because of their personal beliefs about terminating a pregnancy

Even if pregnancy termination is not something you would consider, prior knowledge of a fetus's abnormalities can give you time to make preparations for a child that may have special needs.

If you are under the age of 35 and still want your fetus to be tested for chromosomal abnormalities, you have that right. However, be aware that your insurance carrier may not cover the cost (which can amount to several hundred dollars or more, depending on where you live). All women are offered screening tests for Down syndrome. The traditional screening test used is a blood test called the *triple screen,* which measures certain substances that help detect fetuses at risk for Down syndrome (see Chapter 6). The difference between a *screening test* and an invasive test for *prenatal diagnosis* is that no risks of pregnancy loss are associated with a screening test, because it is simply a blood test or ultrasound exam performed on the mother. But a screening test doesn't diagnose a chromosomal problem 100 percent of the time, whereas an invasive test of prenatal diagnosis usually does.

Chorionic villus sampling

Chorionic villi are tiny, budlike pieces of tissue that make up the placenta. Because they develop from cells arising out of the fertilized egg, they have the same chromosomes and genetic makeup as the developing fetus. By checking a sample of chorionic villi, your doctor can see whether or not the chromosomes are normal in number and structure, determine the fetal sex, and test for some specific diseases (if the fetus is thought to be at risk for these diseases).

Chorionic villus sampling (CVS) is performed by withdrawing placental tissue (containing chorionic villi) either through a hollow needle inserted through the abdomen *(transabdominal CVS)* or through a flexible catheter inserted through the cervix *(transcervical CVS,* shown in Figure 5-6). Ultrasound equipment is used to guide the doctor as he or she performs the procedure. The tissue is then examined under a microscope, and the cells are cultured in a laboratory.

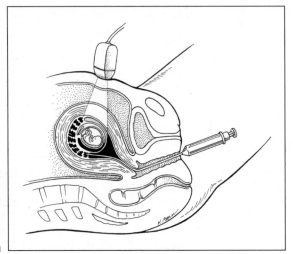

Figure 5-6:
In transcervical CVS, your doctor uses a flexible catheter inserted into the cervix to withdraw a tiny amount of placental tissue, using ultrasound as a guide.

The decision on whether to perform CVS through the abdomen or the cervix depends on where the placenta is located within the uterus and the general shape and position of the uterus itself. Regardless of whether CVS is performed through the cervix or the abdomen, like amniocentesis it raises the risk of miscarriage slightly. Neither method is more risky than the other. The risk for miscarriage with CVS is, on average, 1 percent greater than it would be if the test was not performed. The person performing the test should have plenty of experience doing the procedure; experience helps reduce the risk of miscarriage.

Many women assume that the risk of miscarriage after CVS is much higher than after amniocentesis. But in fact, the risks are quite similar; between ½ and 1 percent.

CVS results are typically available in seven to ten days. The main advantage that CVS has over amniocentesis is that it can provide information earlier in the pregnancy. This time factor may be important to some women who feel that termination is an option if severe abnormalities are present.

Several years ago, people were concerned that babies tested with CVS may be at a greater risk for certain limb defects. Since then, an international registry has collected data on more than 200,000 mothers who underwent the testing after their ninth week of pregnancy and has found no evidence of an increase in limb defects among their babies. That is why CVS is usually performed between weeks 10 and 12.

Unlike amniocentesis, CVS cannot measure AFP (*alpha-fetoprotein;* see Chapter 6). However, this measurement can be taken from maternal blood drawn at 15 to 18 weeks into the pregnancy.

If you undergo CVS and are Rh-negative, you should receive an injection of Rhogam following the procedure.

Early amniocentesis

For amniocentesis, a thin, hollow needle is inserted through your abdomen and into the amniotic sac so that some amniotic fluid can be withdrawn. Cells taken from the fluid are cultured, and information about genetic diseases and chromosome abnormalities is obtained. A traditional amniocentesis is performed at 15 to 20 weeks (see Chapter 6 for more information), but an early one can be done at 11 to 14 weeks. The advantage of doing the test early is simply that the results come sooner. The disadvantage is that the rate of miscarriage is greater than with either routine amniocentesis or CVS. Very recently, studies from Canada and Great Britain indicate a higher incidence of club feet in babies whose mothers had early amniocentesis. For these reasons, we believe that CVS is the better option during the first trimester.

Be sure that you understand the risks of early amniocentesis if your doctor recommends one for you. Under certain circumstances where CVS is not possible and an early diagnosis is absolutely essential, a woman may still decide to undergo this test, even with the aforementioned risks.

Causes for Concern

In each trimester, a few things may, in some cases, go less than smoothly. The following sections describe some of the things that can happen during the first trimester of your pregnancy and what they may mean to you.

Bleeding

Early in pregnancy, around the time of your missed period, it is not uncommon to experience a little bleeding from the vagina. The amount of bleeding is usually less than what you would expect with a period and lasts for only one or two days. This is called *implantation bleeding,* and it happens when the fertilized egg attaches to the lining of the uterus. Bleeding due to implantation is not a cause for concern, but many women may be confused by it and mistake it for their period.

Coming soon: New first trimester screening tests

CVS and early amniocentesis are the only tests that can give definitive information about fetal chromosomes during the first trimester. But researchers are trying to develop noninvasive, risk-free screening tests that could help determine whether a fetus is at increased risk for certain problems, primarily Down syndrome. Here are a few promising possibilities, though none of these tests is yet in everyday use:

✔ **Nuchal translucency:** This test involves using ultrasound to measure a special area behind the fetal neck. Experiments with this procedure in England have suggested that Down syndrome can be identified this way in about 80 percent of cases. A nuchal translucency test can only be done by physicians specially trained in the procedure. When measurements of nuchal translucency are combined with blood screening tests, the accuracy of these tests is probably increased.

✔ **Serum screening:** Tests that check the levels of PAPP-A, a substance produced by the placenta, and hCG, a hormone in the mother's blood, may be able to help screen for Down syndrome in the first trimester. But studies are still underway to determine the rate at which such a test can identify Down syndrome.

✔ **Fetal cells in maternal circulation:** Medical scientists are looking at ways to identify cells from the fetus that have escaped into the mother's bloodstream. Such cells could be cultured and screened for genetic abnormalities. This technique is still experimental.

Bleeding also may occur later in the first trimester, but it doesn't necessarily indicate a miscarriage. About one-third of women experience bleeding during the first trimester, and the majority of them go on to have perfectly healthy babies. Bleeding is especially common in those carrying more than one fetus — and again, most go on to have normal pregnancies. Bright red bleeding usually indicates active bleeding, while dark staining usually indicates old blood that is making its way out from the cervix and vagina. Most of the time, an ultrasound exam does not show any evidence of the source of the bleeding. However, sometimes a collection of blood, known as a *subchorionic* or *retroplacental collection,* is visible and indicates an area of bleeding from behind the placenta. It usually takes several weeks before this blood is reabsorbed. During this time, some dark blood continues to pass out through the cervix and vagina.

In some cases, bleeding can be the first sign of an impending miscarriage (see the next section for more information). In this case, the bleeding is often accompanied by abdominal cramping. However, keep in mind that the vast majority of women who experience bleeding go on to have a completely normal pregnancy.

If you notice some bleeding, you should let your practitioner know. If it is a small amount and not associated with a lot of abdominal cramping, it is not an emergency. If you are bleeding very heavily (much more than a period), you should call your practitioner as soon as you can. She or he may want to do an ultrasound and perform a pelvic exam to investigate the cause of the bleeding and see whether the pregnancy is still viable and located inside the uterus. Most of the time, your practitioner can do very little about the bleeding. Some doctors may suggest that you rest at home for a few days and avoid exercise and sex. No scientific data supports these instructions, but given that no really good alternatives exist, they certainly don't hurt.

Miscarriage

The great majority of pregnancies proceed normally. But about one in five end in early miscarriage. Some women miscarry before they ever know they're pregnant. If a miscarriage occurs this early in a pregnancy, you may mistake it for a regular menstrual period. About half the time, chromosomal abnormalities in the embryo cause the miscarriage. In another 20 percent of cases, the embryo may have structural defects that are too small to be detectable by ultrasound or pathological examination.

Miscarriage may lead to cramping and bleeding. You may feel abdominal pains that are stronger than menstrual cramps, and you may pass fetal and placental tissue. In cases where all the tissue is passed, your practitioner doesn't need to do anything else. Often, though, some tissue remains in your uterus, and you may need to have a D&C (dilation and curettage) procedure, designed to empty the uterus. This is done by dilating, or gently opening, the cervix with surgical instruments and then emptying the remaining contents of the uterus with a suction device and/or a scraping of the uterus. Sometimes a D&C is done in the doctor's office, and sometimes it is done in an operating suite, depending on the doctor, the gestational age, and any other important medical problems.

Sometimes, you may have no overt signs of miscarriage. Your practitioner may discover during a routine prenatal visit that the fetus is no longer alive. This is what is known as a *missed abortion*. If you have a missed abortion very early in your pregnancy, a D&C may not be necessary. But if it happens later in the first trimester, you may need to have a D&C to reduce the risk of heavy bleeding or incomplete passage of tissue. Depending on your obstetrical history and your desire to try to determine the cause of the miscarriage, you may decide to have the tissue sent for genetic analysis (to find out whether the chromosomes were normal or abnormal). Because half of all miscarriages are due to chromosomal abnormalities, it may be useful to find out if this is the cause.

Unfortunately, most miscarriages cannot be prevented. Many, if not most, of them may simply be nature's way of handling an abnormal pregnancy. However, having a miscarriage does not mean that you can't have a perfectly normal pregnancy in the future. In fact, even in women who have had two consecutive miscarriages, the chances are very good (about 70 percent) that the next pregnancy will be successful, even without any special treatment.

However, any woman who experiences two or three consecutive miscarriages *may* have some underlying condition that can be identified and possibly treated. She should have a complete physical examination and undergo special tests to look for causes. Some women who have even one miscarriage may want to be examined. If you miscarry, discuss with your practitioner the possibility of undergoing certain tests — or sending fetal or placental tissue to a laboratory for chromosomal analysis.

Ectopic pregnancy

An *ectopic pregnancy* occurs when the fertilized egg implants outside the uterus — in one of the fallopian tubes, the ovary, the abdomen, or the cervix. An ectopic pregnancy is a serious problem and a threat to the mother's health. Fortunately, ultrasound has advanced to the point that it can detect ectopic pregnancies very early. Signs of an ectopic pregnancy include vaginal bleeding, abdominal pain, dizziness, and feeling faint. Your doctor can treat the problem in one of several ways, depending on the location of the embryo or fetus, how far along the pregnancy is, and the particular symptoms you are experiencing. Unfortunately, the embryo or fetus cannot be moved to the uterus so that the pregnancy can continue as normal.

Ovarian torsion

If you have an ovarian cyst, it may cause the ovary to twist and turn, which is called *ovarian torsion*. Ovarian torsion can also happen in women who took fertility drugs and may have large ovaries and lots of follicles. The main symptom of ovarian torsion is excruciating pain, which may come and go, on one side of the abdomen. If you experience these symptoms, call your doctor.

Chapter 6

The Second Trimester

• •

In This Chapter

▶ Looking — and feeling — like you're going to have a baby

▶ Understanding ultrasound, amniocentesis, and other second-trimester examinations

▶ Knowing when to be concerned

• •

The second trimester, which encompasses the three months between week 13 and week 26, is often the most enjoyable part of pregnancy. The nausea and fatigue so common during the first trimester are usually gone, and you feel more energetic and comfortable. This is a very exciting time because you can feel the baby moving within you and you are finally starting to show. During the second trimester, blood tests, prenatal tests, and ultrasound (sonogram) can confirm that the baby is healthy and growing normally. And many women find that they are finally able to grasp the concept that they will soon be having a baby. This is often the time you start sharing the exciting news with family, friends, and coworkers.

In this chapter, we give you a clear idea of what your second trimester is going to feel like and the things you begin to notice — from your baby's movements to your skin and hair changes to your own clumsiness. We also tell you about ultrasounds, amniocentesis, and all the other medical tests and measurements you have. Finally, we go over some signs of possible trouble.

Discovering How Your Baby Is Developing

Your baby grows rapidly during the second trimester, as you can see in Figure 6-1. The fetus measures about 3 inches long (8 cm) at 13 weeks. By 26 weeks, it's about 14 inches (35 cm) and weighs about 2¼ pounds (1,022 grams). Somewhere between weeks 14 and 16, the limbs begin to elongate and start to look like arms and legs. Coordinated arm and leg movements are observable on ultrasound, too. Between 18 and 22 weeks, you may begin to feel fetal movements, although they don't necessarily occur regularly throughout the day (see "Fetal movements" later in this chapter).

The baby's head, which was large in relation to the body during the first trimester, becomes more in proportion as the body catches up. The bones solidify and are recognizable on ultrasound. Early in the second trimester, the fetus looks something like an alien (think ET), but by 26 weeks, it looks much more like a human baby. The fetus also performs many recognizable activities. It not only moves, but it also undergoes regular periods of sleeping and wakefulness and can hear and swallow. Lung development increases markedly between 20 and 25 weeks. By 24 weeks, lung cells begin to secrete *surfactant,* a chemical substance that enables the lungs to stay expanded. Between 26 and 28 weeks, the eyes — which had been fused shut — open, and hair (called *lanugo*) appears on the head and body. Fat deposits form under the skin, and the central nervous system matures dramatically.

At 23 to 24 weeks, the fetus is considered *viable,* which means that if it were born at this time, it would have a reasonable chance of surviving if born in a center with a neonatal unit experienced in caring for very premature babies. A premature baby born at 28 weeks (nearly three months early) and cared for in an intensive care unit has an excellent chance of survival.

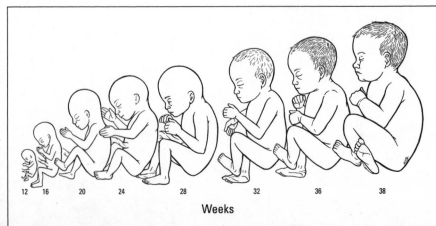

Figure 6-1: Notice that during the second trimester (13-26 weeks), your baby grows and develops at an astounding rate.

12 16   20   24   28   32   36   38

Weeks

Fetal movements

It's difficult to know for sure when you first feel your baby moving inside you. Many women sense fluttering movements (called *quickening*) at about 16 to 20 weeks. Not every woman can tell that sensation is actually the baby moving. Some think it's just gas — but most likely, it's the baby. Around 20 to 22 weeks, the fetal movements are much easier to identify but still are not consistent. Over the course of the next four weeks, they fall into a more regular pattern. Different babies have different movement patterns. You may notice that your baby tends to move more at night — perhaps to prepare you for all the sleepless nights you'll have after she or he is born! Or you may simply be more aware of the baby's movements at night because you are more sedentary at that time. If this is your second (or third or fourth . . .) child, you may start to feel movements a couple of weeks earlier.

If you haven't felt your baby move at all by 22 weeks, let your practitioner know. He or she may recommend an ultrasound, especially if you haven't had one already, to check the baby. A common explanation for not feeling the baby's movements is that the placenta is implanted on the anterior (front) wall of the uterus between the baby and your skin. The placenta acts as a cushion and delays the time when you first feel movements.

After 26 to 28 weeks, if you stop feeling the baby move as much as usual, call your practitioner. By 28 weeks, you should feel movement at least six times an hour after you eat dinner. If you are not sure whether the baby is moving normally, lie down on your left side and count the movements. If the baby moves — any movement counts — at least six times in an hour, be reassured that the baby is okay. On the other hand, if you feel that the baby's movements are still less than they should be, call your practitioner.

Understanding Your Changing Body

By 12 weeks, your uterus begins to rise out of your pelvis. Your practitioner can feel the top of the uterus through your abdominal wall. By 20 weeks, the top of your uterus reaches the level of your navel. Then each week, your uterus grows by about one centimeter (½ inch). Your doctor may run a tape measure from your pubic bone to the top of your uterus to measure the *fundal height* (refer back to Figure 3-1) to see that your uterus, and the baby, are growing appropriately. Many women begin to show at 16 weeks, although looking pregnant varies a great deal. Some women look pregnant at 12 weeks; others are not obvious until 28 weeks.

Many of the changes you experience have little to do with the size of your belly. Rather, they involve your baby's development and your body's continuing adaptation to pregnancy. You may experience some, none, or all of the symptoms described in this section.

Maternity clothing

Thank goodness the fashion industry has recognized that women continue to care about looking chic and professional when they're pregnant — which doesn't necessarily mean wearing those choir-boy blouses with big bows at the neck. Many women look forward to shopping for maternity clothes, while others aim to stay in their usual clothes for as long as possible. Keep in mind that you're only going to need maternity clothes for a few months, and they're not cheap. Here are a few suggestions:

- **Don't plan too far ahead; buy clothes only as you need them.** Anticipating how big you'll become and whether you'll carry the baby high up in your belly or down low is difficult. When you do shop, buy clothes that fit comfortably but have enough room to accommodate further growth.

- **Don't be shy about accepting hand-me-downs.** Women rarely wear out their maternity clothes. Your friends are probably happy to see their clothes get more use.

- **Look for consignment shops and second-hand stores in your area.** They're good places to find inexpensive maternity clothes.

- **If you have trouble finding maternity clothes in your style, remember that you can often go a long way through your pregnancy in regular leggings and big shirts or sweaters.** (Joanne never had to buy any maternity clothes at all.)

- **Perhaps the most important items to buy are comfortable shoes and roomier bras.** Both shoe size and bra size can increase during pregnancy.

- **You don't have to wear special maternity underwear — unless you find it especially comfortable.** Many kinds of regular underwear, especially the bikini kind, fit well under a bulging belly.

Forgetfulness and clumsiness

Until she was pregnant herself, Joanne never would have believed that misplacing keys, bumping into furniture, and dropping things could be real side effects of pregnancy. We don't know of any medical explanation for these effects, but some women do feel that they are more scatterbrained and clumsy. If it happens to you, don't worry. You're not losing your mind. Look at it this way: Now you have an excuse for having forgotten your best friend's birthday. And rest assured that you'll go back to being your brilliant, coordinated self after your baby is born.

Gas

You may find that you develop the annoying and embarrassing tendency to burp and pass gas at inopportune times during this trimester. If it's any consolation, you're not the first pregnant woman to run into this problem. Unfortunately, though, you can do very little about it — besides getting a dog to blame it on. Try to avoid becoming constipated (see Chapter 3), because that can make things worse. Also avoid eating large meals that may leave you feeling bloated and uncomfortable or foods that you know make the problem even worse.

Hair and nail growth

While you're pregnant, your fingernails and toenails may become stronger than they've ever been before and grow at an unprecedented rate. Manicures are safe when done in a reputable, clean salon and often relieve stress, so sit back and enjoy your beautiful nails!

Pregnancy also speeds up hair growth. Unfortunately, some women find that hair also begins growing in unusual places — on their face or stomach, for example. Waxing, plucking, or shaving the unwanted hair is safe, but hair removal creams (depilatories) contain chemicals that have not been extensively studied. Because safer alternatives are readily available, we suggest avoiding these creams. Take comfort in the likelihood that the unwanted hair disappears after your baby is born.

Heartburn

Heartburn — the burning sensation you feel when stomach acids rise into your esophagus — is common during pregnancy. Heartburn has two basic causes. First, the high level of progesterone that your body is producing can slow digestion and relax the sphincter muscle between the esophagus and the stomach, which normally prevents the upward movement of stomach acids. Second, as the uterus grows, it presses upward on the stomach, which can push stomach acids into the esophagus. (See Figure 6-2.)

Some well-meaning person may tell you that heartburn is a sign that your baby will have a lot of hair, but this old adage isn't true.

You may be able to get relief from heartburn by following these suggestions:

- ✔ Eat small, frequent meals rather than large ones.
- ✔ Carry an antacid when you're away from home.
- ✔ Carry a package of dry crackers to munch on when you feel heartburn. They may neutralize the gas.
- ✔ Avoid spicy, fatty, and greasy foods.

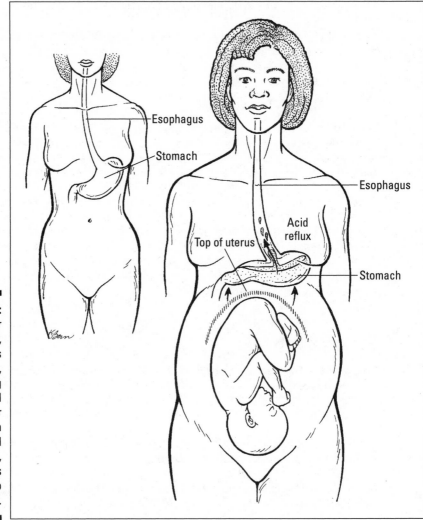

Figure 6-2:
As your baby grows, your uterus expands, pushing upward on your stomach and esophagus, sometimes leading to heartburn.

Labels in figure: Esophagus, Stomach, Esophagus, Acid reflux, Top of uterus, Stomach

✔ Avoid eating just before bedtime, because heartburn occurs most readily when you lie down. Also, try sleeping with your head elevated on several pillows.

✔ If your heartburn becomes intolerable, talk to your doctor about taking a prescription treatment that has been shown to be safe during pregnancy.

Lower abdominal/groin pain

Between 18 and 24 weeks, you may feel a sharp pain or a dull ache near your groin on either or both sides. It's often worse when you move quickly or stand, and it may fade if you lie down. This pain is called *round ligament pain.* The round ligaments are bands of fibrous tissue on each side of the uterus that attach the top of the uterus to the labia. The pain occurs because as the uterus grows, the ligaments stretch. The pain can be quite uncomfortable, but it's normal. The good news is that it usually goes away or at least lessens considerably after 24 weeks.

Sometime in the middle of the second trimester (the exact time varies), you may start to feel mild, short-lived contractions or cramps. These are referred to as *Braxton-Hicks contractions* and are nothing to worry about. They often are more noticeable when you are walking or physically active and then go away when you get off your feet. If they become uncomfortable and regular (more than six in an hour), call your practitioner.

Nasal congestion

The increased blood flow that occurs during pregnancy can also cause stuffiness and some swelling of the mucous membranes inside your nose. This, in turn, can lead to postnasal drip and, ultimately, a chronic cough. Nasal saline drops may provide some relief and are perfectly safe to use during pregnancy. Keeping the air in your home or office well humidified also helps. Nasal sprays and decongestants work, too, but avoid using these medications for more than a few days at a time. You (or your partner especially) may notice that all of a sudden, you are snoring like never before! This common symptom again has to do with the increase in nasal congestion. Our advice? Buy your partner a good set of earplugs!

Nosebleeds and bleeding gums

Because of the higher volume of blood coursing through your body to support your pregnancy, you may experience some bleeding from small blood vessels in your nose and gums. This bleeding usually stops by itself, but you can help by applying slight pressure to the point of bleeding. If bleeding becomes particularly heavy or frequent, call your doctor.

Using a softer toothbrush may help to minimize bleeding when you brush your teeth.

Skin changes

You may notice a dark line, called the *linea nigra,* on your lower abdomen running from your pubic bone up to your navel. This line may be more noticeable in women with relatively dark skin. Fair-skinned women often don't develop this line at all.

The skin on your face may also darken in a masklike distribution around your cheeks, nose, and eyes. This darkening is called *chloasma* or the *mask of pregnancy.* Sun exposure makes it even darker.

Both of these skin changes, shown in Figure 6-3, are due to hormonal influences on the skin pigment cells in these areas. These changes don't occur in all women, and if they do happen to you, rest assured that this new coloring usually fades away after the baby is born.

Red spots, called *spider angiomas,* may suddenly appear anywhere on your body. Press on them, and they probably turn white. These spots are concentrations of blood vessels caused by the high level of estrogen in your body. They'll probably disappear after delivery.

Some women notice a reddish coloring on the palms of their hands. Known as *palmar erythema,* this coloring is another estrogen effect, and it, too, will go away.

Skin tags are also a common occurrence, although it isn't totally clear why they develop. Fortunately, they, too, fade away or disappear after pregnancy. Because they are likely to resolve in time, it's probably not a good idea to rush to the dermatologist to have them removed, unless they are really bothersome.

Prenatal Visits

In the second trimester, you're likely to see your practitioner about once every four weeks. At each visit, he or she checks your weight, your blood pressure, your urine, and the fetal heart rate. You may want to bring up any questions you have about fetal movement, childbirth classes, your weight gain, and any unusual symptoms or discomforts you may have.

Your practitioner routinely performs a number of tests during your second trimester to find out whether you are at risk for such complications as diabetes, anemia, or birth defects. You may also have an ultrasound exam, so that your practitioner can see things such as whether you're having twins, whether your baby is growing normally, and whether you have plenty of amniotic fluid.

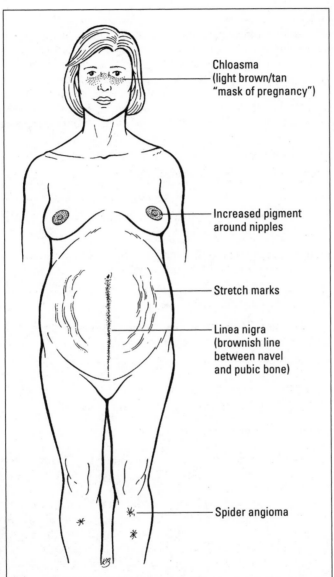

Chloasma
(light brown/tan
"mask of pregnancy")

Increased pigment
around nipples

Stretch marks

Linea nigra
(brownish line
between navel
and pubic bone)

Spider angioma

Figure 6-3:
Some common
skin changes
associated
with
pregnancy.

Second trimester blood tests

The following blood tests are usually performed during the second trimester.
Ideally, your results are normal right away. If they are at all unusual, you may
need further testing — an ultrasound examination, perhaps. But keep in mind
that further testing does not necessarily mean that anything is wrong — only
that your practitioner is being careful to ensure that everything is okay.

Alpha-fetoprotein screen

MSAFP stands for *maternal serum alpha-fetoprotein,* a protein made by the fetus that also circulates in the mother's bloodstream. Doctors use a simple blood test to check the level of MSAFP, usually sometime between 15 and 18 weeks. The test result is affected by weight, race, and preexisting diabetes, so it has to be adjusted for those factors. MSAFP can usually indicate whether a pregnancy is at risk for certain complications. An elevated MSAFP (expressed as more than 2.0 or 2.5 *multiples of the median,* or MOMs) *may* indicate:

✔ Underestimation of the age of the fetus (how far along you are).

✔ The presence of twins or more.

✔ Bleeding that may have occurred earlier in the pregnancy.

✔ Neural tube defects (spina bifida, anencephaly, and others). See the "Neural tube defects" sidebar.

✔ Abdominal wall defects (protrusion of the fetus's abdominal contents through a defect in the abdominal wall).

✔ Rh disease (see Chapter 14) or other conditions associated with *fetal edema* (abnormal fluid collection in the fetus).

✔ Increased risk for low birthweight, preeclampsia, or other complications (see Chapter 14).

✔ A rare fetal kidney condition known as *congenital nephrosis.*

✔ Fetal death.

✔ Death of one or more fetuses in a multiple pregnancy.

✔ Other fetal abnormalities.

Remember that the MSAFP test is only a screening test. Most women with an elevated MSAFP have a normal fetus and continue to have a completely normal pregnancy. Only about 5 percent of women with a positive maternal serum screen actually have a fetus with a neural tube defect. On the other hand, the test is not perfect, and therefore it can't identify all abnormal fetuses. To reduce the risk of getting a false positive result (that is, an abnormal test result but a normal fetus), a positive test should be repeated (especially if it is only mildly elevated or under 3.0 MOMs), and an ultrasound should be performed to confirm the age of the fetus. If a test comes back elevated a second time or if it is greater than 3.0 MOMs on the first screen, a detailed ultrasound exam should be done to look for any detectable abnormalities.

If you have two elevated MSAFP tests or a very high single test, you may want to have an amniocentesis to check the level of AFP in the amniotic fluid (see the section "Amniocentesis," later in this chapter). The amniotic fluid can also be checked for a substance called *acetylcholinesterase,* which is present if the fetus has an open neural tube defect (see the "Neural tube defects" sidebar). In most cases, the amniotic fluid AFP is negative and the pregnancy continues normally. Some studies suggest, however, that women who have an abnormal MSAFP and then a normal amniotic fluid AFP *may* be at risk for preterm delivery, low birthweight babies, or hypertension. So if you fit the pattern, your doctor may suggest that you and your fetus be closely observed, either with ultrasound or with other tests of fetal well-being, such as non-stress tests (see Chapter 7). This area is fairly controversial in the field of obstetrics, and not all practitioners follow the same routine.

Note: In mothers of twins, MSAFP greater than 4.0 or 4.5 MOMs is considered elevated. In triplets and quadruplets, the measurement has not been well studied.

The double, triple, and now quadruple screen for Down syndrome

Another test that can be performed with the same sample of blood that's used for the MSAFP is a screening test for Down syndrome — the most common chromosome abnormality in babies. This test can also help to identify women at risk of having babies with other chromosomal abnormalities, like Trisomy 18 or Trisomy 13 (an extra copy of either the number 18 or 13 chromosome).

This test is performed by measuring two or three substances in the blood: MSAFP, hCG (human chorionic gonadotropin), and sometimes *estriol* (a form of estrogen). The results of two or three of these tests are used to calculate a risk for Down syndrome. In women under the age of 35, the test detects Down syndrome about 60 percent of the time when it is present. (In other words, if 100 women carrying fetuses with Down syndrome had the test, the condition would be diagnosed in about 60 of them.) In mothers over the age of 35, the accuracy goes up to 60 to 80 percent. This test is only a screening, so even if the result is abnormal, the fetus is normal in the majority of cases. If your test is abnormal, your practitioner will discuss with you the possibility of having an amniocentesis to check the baby's chromosomes.

Recently, doctors have been looking at the utility of adding a fourth test, called *Inhibin-A,* to this screen. Although it is too early to tell definitively, it is hoped that by adding this test, the Down syndrome detection rate will be even higher than it is with the double or triple screen. Preliminary studies show that it may be as high as 70 percent in women under 35.

Unlike the screen for neural tube defects, which yields a high MSAFP and is often repeated when abnormal, the triple (or double) screen for Down syndrome should *not* be repeated, because it will only provide a less accurate result.

Glucose screen

The glucose screen is a test to identify women who may have gestational diabetes. We discuss why treating gestational diabetes is important in Chapter 15.

The test is done by first having you drink a nasty-tasting glucose mixture (it tastes like flat soda) and then, exactly one hour later, drawing a sample of

Neural tube defects

The baby's central nervous system begins as a flat sheet of cells that rolls up into a tube as it matures. The front of the tube, which closes at about day 23 of life, is destined to become the brain. The other end of the tube, which closes at about day 28 of life, becomes the lower end of the spinal cord. If either end fails to close for some reason (it isn't known why it sometimes doesn't), a *neural tube defect* occurs. The most common neural tube defects are *spina bifida* (an opening in the spine), *anencephaly* (an absence of the skull), and *encephalocele* (an opening in the skull). These defects are serious because they cause abnormalities in the nervous system such as paralysis, extra fluid in the brain, or mental retardation. In fact, fetuses with anencephaly usually do not survive more than a few days after birth.

This all sounds pretty scary, but fortunately, these defects are rare. We go into detail about them here because screening programs are in place in most countries to help identify those fetuses that might have one of these defects and because there are ways to reduce the likelihood of having a baby with a neural tube defect —

by taking folic acid, starting before conception (see Chapter 1), for example, and by getting your blood sugar under control if you have diabetes.

In the United States, a neural tube defect occurs about once in every 1,000 babies born. The incidence in the United Kingdom is higher: four to eight cases in every 1,000 babies. In Japan, the incidence is quite low, at about one case per 2,000 babies. No one knows exactly why the incidence varies among countries, but it has something to do with the interaction between the environment and one's genetic makeup. If you or your baby's father have a family history of neural tube defects, let your practitioner know, because that slightly raises your risk of having a baby with a neural tube defect, and you can discuss your options for prenatal diagnosis (ultrasound or amniocentesis). Also, if you had a previous pregnancy in which a neural tube defect was diagnosed or if you have a family history of this condition, the amount of folic acid you should take at the beginning of pregnancy is much higher (4 mg per day).

blood. This sample is checked for the level of glucose (sugar). High levels indicate that you are at risk for gestational diabetes.

The one-hour screening test is usually performed between 24 and 28 weeks, though some doctors do it twice — once early in the pregnancy and again at 24 to 28 weeks. About 75 percent of obstetricians screen all their patients for gestational diabetes, though such universal testing is not yet recommended by the American College of Obstetricians and Gynecologists. About 25 percent of obstetricians test only those women who are at risk for gestational diabetes (see the "Risk factors for gestational diabetes" sidebar). As you can see, these risk factors are broad, and about 50 percent of all pregnant women have one of the risk factors.

If your initial glucose screening test is abnormal, it doesn't necessarily mean that you have gestational diabetes. (Remember, it's only a screening test.) Your practitioner will recommend another test, a three-hour one, that tells whether gestational diabetes is really present. The three-hour test involves drawing blood after you fast overnight, having you drink a different glucose mixture, and then drawing blood three more times, at one, two, and three hours later. Some practitioners recommend eating an extra helping of pasta or rice for the three days before the test (this is called *carbohydrate loading*) in order to get your body ready for the test. A test is considered positive — or abnormal — if two of the four blood levels are in the abnormal range. If you test positive for gestational diabetes, your doctor will put you on a special diet and check your glucose levels throughout the remainder of your pregnancy. If your glucose levels are still elevated despite adhering to this special diet, you may need to be on insulin to keep your sugars well controlled. (See Chapter 15 for more on this topic.)

Complete blood count (CBC)

Many obstetricians check a complete blood count at the same time that they do your glucose test in order to see whether you've developed significant anemia (iron deficiency) or a variety of other less common problems. Anemia is common during pregnancy, and some women need to take extra iron.

Ultrasound

An ultrasound (or *sonogram*) exam is an incredibly useful tool that allows you and your doctor to see the baby inside your uterus. Sound waves are emitted by a device called a *transducer*. The sound waves are reflected off the fetus and converted into an image that appears on a monitor. (See sonogram photos in Chapter 21.) You can see almost all the structures in the fetus's body, and you can see the fetus moving around and performing all its normal activities — kicking, waving, and so on. The best time to view the baby's anatomy is around 18 to 22 weeks.

An ultrasound exam doesn't hurt. Gel or lotion is spread over the abdomen, and the transducer is moved around through the gel (see Figure 6-4). A full bladder is not necessary because the amniotic fluid surrounding the fetus

---

Risk factors for gestational diabetes

Predicting whether any woman is going to develop gestational diabetes is impossible. However, your risk of developing the condition is greater if you match any of the following descriptions. If you do, be sure to mention it to your practitioner.

✔ Maternal age greater than 25 years

✔ Previous birth of a large infant

✔ Previous unexplained fetal death

✔ Previous pregnancy with gestational diabetes

✔ Strong family history of diabetes

✔ Obesity

provides the liquid needed to transmit the sound waves to create a clear or detailed picture. Picture quality varies, depending on maternal fat, scar tissue, and the position of the fetus.

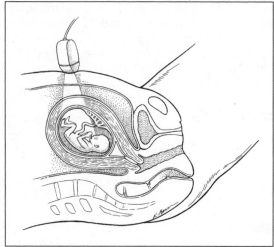

Figure 6-4: An ultrasound test being performed during the second trimester.

Ultrasound is like a checkup for the fetus. It can provide information about the following:

- ✔ Number of babies.
- ✔ Gestational age.
- ✔ Rate of fetal growth.
- ✔ Fetal position, movement, and breathing exercises (the fetus moves its chest and abdomen as if it were breathing air).
- ✔ Fetal heart rate.
- ✔ Amount of amniotic fluid.
- ✔ Location of placenta.
- ✔ Fetal anatomy, including the identification of some birth defects.
- ✔ The baby's gender (after 15 to 16 weeks), although this is not always possible to see.

Although ultrasound has truly revolutionized obstetrics, providing invaluable help in identifying, managing, and sometimes even treating certain problems, it isn't perfect. It can detect only about half of all birth defects (although many of the ones it misses are minor), and it can't always identify fetuses with chromosomal abnormalities. (For example, even when done by someone with a great deal of experience, ultrasound can detect only about half of all cases of Down syndrome in women at risk for this problem.)

A doctor (an obstetrician, a perinatologist, or a radiologist) or an ultrasound technologist may perform the ultrasound. Sometimes a technologist does a preliminary exam, and the doctor comes in later to check on images or review the printed pictures. Typically, the examiner measures the fetus first and then studies its anatomy. The extent and degree of detail of the exam varies from woman to woman and doctor to doctor. A detailed ultrasound can examine these structures:

- ✔ Brain and skull
- ✔ Heart, chest cavity, and diaphragm
- ✔ Stomach, abdominal cavity, and abdominal wall
- ✔ Face
- ✔ Kidneys
- ✔ Bladder
- ✔ Arms and legs
- ✔ Genitalia
- ✔ Spine

Whether and how often you need an ultrasound depends on your particular risk factors, your doctor's preferences, and your insurance coverage. Some doctors recommend that all women have an ultrasound exam at about 20 weeks; others feel that it's unnecessary if your risks for having problems are low. Multiple ultrasound examinations may be needed if any of the following conditions arise:

- ✔ If you are carrying twins or more
- ✔ If your doctor suspects that the baby is too small or too large for its age
- ✔ If your doctor suspects that you have too little or too much amniotic fluid
- ✔ If you are at risk for preterm labor or incompetent cervix (see Chapter 14)
- ✔ If you have diabetes, hypertension, or other underlying medical conditions (see Chapter 15)
- ✔ If you are bleeding
- ✔ If your doctor wants to do a *biophysical profile,* which is an assessment of fetal well-being that looks at movement, breathing exercises, amniotic fluid volume, and fetal tone (ability to flex its muscles). See Chapter 7.

Recently, doctors have also used ultrasound to get an accurate measurement of the cervix (the opening of the uterus) in women at risk for preterm delivery and incompetent cervix. This procedure is usually done by placing a transducer in the vagina and measuring the length of the cervix and by checking the appearance of the lower part of the uterus.

Amniocentesis

Amniocentesis is a test that is performed by inserting a thin, hollow needle into the amniotic fluid and then withdrawing some of the fluid through the needle into a syringe (see Figure 6-5). The amniotic fluid can then be tested in a variety of ways. If a *genetic amniocentesis* — a check of fetal chromosomes — is performed, it is usually done at 15 to 20 weeks. Amniocentesis for other reasons, like checking for lung maturity in the baby, may be performed at any time later on in the pregnancy.

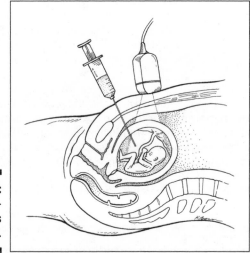

Figure 6-5:
An amnio-
centesis
procedure.

During the amniocentesis procedure, you lie flat on your back on top of a table. Your abdomen is cleaned with an iodine solution. When an ultrasound image of the fetus and the amniotic sac is showing on the ultrasound screen,

Our patients want to know . . .

Q: "Is ultrasound safe?"

A: The technology has been in widespread use for more than 30 years, and most studies have shown no harmful consequences for the baby or mom. In addition, the information provided by an ultrasound examination has been shown to have many health benefits.

a thin needle is inserted through your abdomen and uterus into the amniotic sac. When enough amniotic fluid is withdrawn (usually about 15 to 20 cc, or 1 to 2 tablespoons), the needle is removed.

A common misconception is that the needle is inserted through the navel. It isn't. The exact point of insertion depends on where the fetus, the placenta, and the amniotic sac are located within the uterus. Many women have heard that an amniocentesis needle is exceptionally long, and they fear that such a long needle causes pain. But the needle's length, which enables it to reach the amniotic sac, does not make it painful. It is the thickness of a needle that determines how uncomfortable it is, and an amniocentesis needle is very thin.

The procedure typically lasts no longer than one to two minutes, but it may seem like an eternity to an anxious woman. It is mildly uncomfortable but not terribly painful. Many women feel a slight, brief cramping sensation as the needle goes into the uterus and then a weird pulling sensation as the fluid is withdrawn through the needle. Having an amniocentesis performed is not altogether pain-free, but most women report that it isn't as bad as they expected it to be. Afterward, your doctor may advise that you rest and avoid strenuous activity and sex for one to two days.

Some women experience cramping for several hours after the procedure. The best treatment for this cramping is rest. Some practitioners recommend a single glass of wine to help ease the discomfort.

For a genetic amniocentesis, the amniotic fluid cells must be incubated, which takes some time. Results are usually available in one to two weeks.

If prenatal blood studies show that you are Rh-negative, your doctor will give you an injection of Rhogam (Rh-D immune globulin), which helps prevent Rh sensitization (see Chapter 14).

A genetic amniocentesis primarily tests to see that 23 chromosome pairs are present and that their structure is normal. It does not routinely test for all possible genetic diseases or birth defects.

Risks and side effects of amniocentesis

Not all patients have these symptoms or problems after an amniocentesis, but it is important to be aware that they can occur.

- ✔ **Cramping:** Usually goes away within a day.

- ✔ **Spotting:** May last one to two days.

- ✔ **Amniotic fluid leak:** A leakage of 1 to 2 teaspoons of fluid through the vagina occurs in 1 to 2 percent of patients. In the great majority of these cases, the membrane seals over within 48 hours. Leakage stops and the pregnancy continues normally. If you experience a large amount of leakage or persistent leakage, call your doctor.

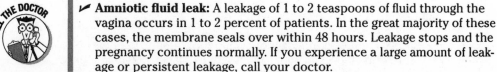

✔ **Fetal injury:** Injury to the fetus is extremely rare, given the use of ultrasound guidance.

✔ **Miscarriage:** Although amniocentesis is considered very safe, it's still invasive, and it is associated with an increased risk of pregnancy loss of about one-half percent. (That is, your basic risk of miscarriage goes up by one-half of one percent when you have amniocentesis.) Your decision to undergo the procedure must weigh both risks and benefits, which vary according to the individual. For example, a 40-year-old woman with a history of infertility may not want to undergo any test that carries an increased risk of miscarriage, even though she stands an even higher risk of carrying a fetus with a chromosomal abnormality. On the other hand, a 32-year-old maternal-fetal medicine specialist who sees patients with a multitude of problems every day — we're thinking of Joanne, at the time of her first pregnancy — may opt to undergo an amniocentesis even though her risk of having a fetus with a chromosomal abnormality is relatively low — lower, in fact, than her risk of miscarriage because of the test. The peace of mind was worth the small risk of miscarriage.

Reasons for having an amniocentesis

Genetic amniocentesis may be recommended for the following conditions or situations:

✔ Your age is 35 or more at your due date. This may vary from country to country and also depends on the number of babies you are carrying. For example, if you are carrying twins, you may be offered amniocentesis at age 33.

✔ You had an elevated MSAFP (see the section "Alpha-fetoprotein screen," earlier in this chapter).

✔ You had abnormal results from the Down syndrome screening.

✔ Your ultrasound exam was abnormal, indicating, for example, poor fetal growth or suspected structural abnormalities.

✔ You had a previous child or previous pregnancy with a chromosomal abnormality.

✔ You are at risk of having a baby with a certain genetic disease (if both parents are carriers for cystic fibrosis, Tay-Sachs, or sickle-cell anemia, for example, or if one parent is a carrier for a genetic disease that can be passed along by just one parent, such as Huntington's disease).

✔ You and your partner have concerns and want to confirm that the chromosomes are normal.

Amniocentesis is also performed for other reasons:

✔ **Preterm labor:** An infection within the amniotic fluid may be a cause of preterm labor. The fluid can be sent to a lab for tests to look for any such infection. If an infection is present, your doctor may want to deliver your baby right away to minimize harm to you and the baby.

✔ **Other infections:** Some patients may find that they are at risk of developing such infections as toxoplasmosis, CMV (cytomegalovirus), or parvovirus (see Chapter 15). The amniotic fluid can be tested for evidence of such problems in patients at risk.

✔ **Rh sensitization:** Patients with Rh sensitization are sometimes followed with a test known as *delta OD-450,* in which the amniotic fluid is examined for evidence of broken-down fetal red blood cells. See Chapter 14.

✔ **Lung maturity studies:** Sometimes your doctor needs to find out whether the fetus's lungs are mature enough for the baby to be delivered. Certain tests on the amniotic fluid can determine the maturity of the lungs. See Chapter 7.

An amniocentesis that is done later on in the pregnancy — later than 20 weeks — doesn't carry the same risk of miscarriage. It carries only a very, very small risk of infection, rupture of membranes (breaking the water), or onset of labor.

Other prenatal tests and procedures

The tests or procedures described in this section are not done in all pregnancies — only when a specific problem is present. In fact, most of these tests are rarely done and are usually done in centers that specialize in fetal medicine. They may sound scary, but they're included here just to let you know what might be available if you do develop a problem.

Fetal blood sampling

For fetal blood sampling, which is also known as *PUBS (percutaneous umbilical blood sampling)* or *cordocentesis,* fetal blood is withdrawn from the umbilical cord. This test lets your doctor obtain blood for rapid chromosomal diagnosis when time is critical. It is also sometimes done in order to diagnose some fetal infections, to detect evidence of fetal anemia, or to diagnose and treat a condition called *non-immune hydrops,* in which fluid accumulates abnormally in the fetus. The procedure, performed by an experienced maternal-fetal medicine specialist, is done under ultrasound guidance. It's similar to an amniocentesis except that the needle is directed into the umbilical cord rather than into the amniotic fluid. Risks are low but include infection, rupture of the membranes, or fetal loss. (The risk of fetal loss is about 1 percent.)

Some fetuses develop anemia, which can be treated *in utero* (within the womb) with a blood transfusion. The procedure is done during a fetal blood sampling, and blood is actually transfused into the umbilical cord. Conditions that may lead to anemia include certain infections (like parvovirus), genetic diseases, or certain blood group incompatibilities (see Chapter 14).

Fetal tissue biopsy

In the very few instances in which a fetus is known to be at risk for some rare genetic disease, a biopsy of fetal tissue (skin, muscle, or liver) may be needed for diagnosis. A maternal-fetal medicine specialist trained in the procedure performs this test. It is done using ultrasound to guide a biopsy device through the abdomen and uterine wall.

Fetal shunt placement (and other fetal surgery)

Occasionally, a fetus may develop a condition that can actually be treated in utero. For example, a fetus may develop an obstruction in its bladder outlet so that urine can't pass from its bladder to the amniotic fluid. In such a case, a *shunt* can be placed from the bladder to the amniotic fluid under ultrasound guidance, preventing damage to the fetus's kidneys. The shunt is a tiny plastic conduit that allows urine trapped behind an obstruction to escape into the amniotic fluid, thereby relieving the obstruction. It should be placed by a maternal-fetal medicine specialist who has expertise in this area. Recently, you may have heard of or seen articles on *fetal surgery.* Fetal shunt placement is one type of fetal surgery.

Fetal echocardiogram

A *fetal echocardiogram* is basically a sonogram focused on the fetal heart. It's usually performed by a maternal-fetal medicine specialist, a pediatric cardiologist, or a radiologist. You may be sent for a *fetal echo* if you have a history of diabetes or a family history of congenital heart disease, or if an ultrasound shows any signs of a heart abnormality. Sometimes a fetal echo is recommended if *any* structural problem is seen on ultrasound, because heart abnormalities are often associated with other birth defects.

Doppler studies

Ultrasound can be used to perform Doppler studies of fetal and umbilical blood flow. These studies are a way of assessing blood flow to various organ systems and also within the placenta. A Doppler study is sometimes used as a test of well-being in fetuses with IUGR (intrauterine growth restriction). (See Chapter 14 for more on IUGR.)

Causes for Concern

In this section, we talk about certain problems that can develop during the second trimester and symptoms that you should discuss with your practitioner.

Bleeding

Some women experience bleeding in the second trimester. Possible causes include a low-lying placenta *(placenta previa),* premature labor, cervical incompetence, or placental abruption (all covered in Chapter 14). Sometimes no cause can be found. If you do experience bleeding, it doesn't necessarily mean that you will have a miscarriage, but you should call your doctor. Most often he or she recommends that you have an ultrasound exam and be monitored to make sure that you're not contracting. Bleeding may increase the risk for premature delivery, so your doctor may recommend that your pregnancy come under extra-close surveillance.

Fetal abnormality

Although the vast majority of pregnancies proceed normally, about 2 to 3 percent of infants are born with some abnormality. Most of these abnormalities are minor, although some do lead to significant problems for the newborn. Some are due to chromosomal problems, and others stem from abnormal development of organs and structures. For example, some newborns may have heart defects or abnormalities of the kidneys, bladder, or gastrointestinal tract. Many of these problems, though not all of them, can be diagnosed on a prenatal ultrasound exam. When confronted with any such problem, the most important first step is to gather all the available information about it, so that you know what to expect and what the treatment options are.

Incompetent cervix

During the second trimester, usually between 16 and 24 weeks, some women develop a problem known as an *incompetent cervix*. The cervix opens up and dilates, even though the woman feels no contractions. This condition may lead to miscarriage. Indeed, an incompetent cervix is most often diagnosed *after* the miscarriage occurs. A woman who develops this condition ordinarily doesn't notice any symptoms, although sometimes she may report feeling pelvic heaviness or pressure that's out of the ordinary, or she may notice some spotting. Most women who experience an incompetent cervix do so for no identifiable reason. Others may have one of the following risk factors:

- ✔ **DES exposure:** DES *(diethylstilbestrol)* is a medication that was prescribed to some pregnant women decades ago, mainly in the 1950s, '60s, and '70s. Some female children born to women who took DES may have developed certain problems, including abnormalities in the shape of their uterus, cervix, or fallopian tubes. When they become pregnant, they are at an increased risk of experiencing cervical incompetence.

- ✔ **Cervical trauma:** Some evidence suggests that multiple *D&Cs* (dilation and curettage) or procedures called *cervical cone biopsy* or LEEP (in which a cone-shaped portion of the cervix is removed in the diagnosis or treatment of cervical abnormalities) can lead to cervical incompetence. A significant tear of the cervix during a prior delivery may also increase the risk for cervical incompetence.

✔ **Multiple gestations:** Some obstetricians believe that carrying multiple babies, especially triplets or more, may increase the risk for an incompetent cervix. This issue is very controversial; some obstetricians recommend placing a *cerclage* (a stitch in the uterus — see the explanation that follows) in all patients with triplets or more, but others perform the procedure only in patients that they think are at high risk for incompetent cervix. Some patients who have undergone a procedure called *multifetal pregnancy reduction* (see Chapter 13) may also be at an increased risk for an incompetent cervix, although routine cerclage placement is not recommended for them at this time.

✔ **Prior history of incompetent cervix:** Once you have had an incompetent cervix, your risk of having it again in a subsequent pregnancy is increased.

In cases in which an incompetent cervix is diagnosed before the pregnancy is lost, the woman's cervix can be held shut with a stitch, called a *cerclage,* around the cervix. The cerclage is usually placed at 12 to 14 weeks, although it's occasionally performed as an emergency procedure later in the pregnancy. It's most commonly performed in the hospital under spinal or epidural anesthesia, but the woman is usually discharged later the same day. Some women with a cerclage notice that they have a heavy discharge throughout pregnancy. If you need to have a cerclage, talk to your doctor about how active you can be — whether you can have sex and how much exercise is advisable. Complications associated with *elective* cerclage (not emergency cerclage) are unusual but can include infection, contractions, rupture of membranes, bleeding, and miscarriage.

Symptoms to call your doctor about during the second trimester

The following is a list of second-trimester symptoms that require some attention. If you experience any of them, call your practitioner.

✔ Bleeding

✔ An unusual sense of pressure or heaviness

✔ Regular contractions or strong cramping

✔ A lack of normal fetal movement

✔ High fever

✔ Severe abdominal pain

Chapter 7

The Third Trimester

● ●

In This Chapter

▶ Your baby grows and prepares to enter the real world

▶ Dealing with your changing body

▶ Gauging the effects of working while pregnant

▶ Assessing the baby's well-being

▶ Preparing for the main event at childbirth classes

▶ Knowing when to be concerned

● ●

You're finally ready for the third act — the final trimester of your pregnancy. By now, you're probably accustomed to having a protruding belly, your morning sickness is long gone, and you've come to expect and enjoy the feeling of your baby moving around and kicking inside you. In this trimester, your baby continues to grow, and your practitioner continues to monitor your and your baby's health. You also begin making preparations for the new arrival, which may mean anything from getting ready to take a leave of absence from your job to taking childbirth classes (and other ways of finding out what to expect during labor and delivery).

Your Baby Gets Ready for Birth

At 28 weeks, your baby measures about 14 inches (about 35 cm) and weighs about 2½ pounds (about 1,135 grams). But by the end of the third trimester — at 40 weeks, your due date — it measures about 20 inches (50 cm) and weighs 6 to 8 pounds (about 2,700 to 3,600 grams) — sometimes a bit more, sometimes a bit less. The fetus spends most of the third trimester growing, adding fat, and continuing to develop various organs, especially the central nervous system. The arms and legs get chubbier, and the skin turns bluish-pink and smooth. Your baby is less susceptible to infections and to the adverse effects of medications, but some of these agents may still affect its growth. The last two months are usually spent getting ready for the transition to life in the world outside the uterus. The changes are less dramatic than they were early on, but the maturation and growth that happen now are very important.

By 28 to 34 weeks, the fetus generally assumes a head-down position (called a *vertex* presentation), as shown in Figure 7-1. This way, the buttocks and legs (the bulkiest parts of its body) occupy the roomiest part of the uterus — the top part. In about 4 to 6 percent of singleton pregnancies, the baby may be positioned buttocks-down *(breech)* or lie across the uterus *(transverse)*. (See later in this chapter for more information about breech presentation.)

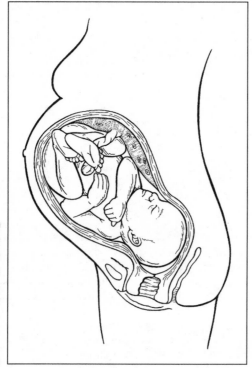

Figure 7-1: How your baby may look inside your uterus during the third trimester.

By 36 weeks, growth slows, and amniotic fluid volume is at its maximum level. After this point, the amount of amniotic fluid may start to decline. In fact, most practitioners routinely check the amniotic fluid volume on ultrasound or by feeling your abdomen during the last few weeks to make sure that a normal amount remains.

Patterns of fetal growth

The rate at which your baby grows varies throughout your pregnancy. At 14 to 15 weeks, for example, the baby puts on weight at about 0.18 ounce (5 grams) per day, and at 32 to 34 weeks, 1.06 to 1.23 ounces (30 to 35 grams) per day (that's about half a pound — 0.23 kilograms — each week). After 36 weeks, the fetal growth rate slows, and by 41 to 42 weeks (you're *over*due at this point), minimal or no further fetal growth may occur.

The following factors affect fetal growth:

- ✔ **Cigarette smoking.** Smoking can reduce the birthweight by about half a pound (about 200 grams).
- ✔ **Diabetes.** The mother's being diabetic can make the baby too big or too small.
- ✔ **Genetic or family history.** In other words, basketball players usually don't have children who grow up to be professional jockeys!
- ✔ **Fetal infection.** Some infections affect growth, while others don't.
- ✔ **Illicit drug use.** Drug abuse can slow fetal growth.
- ✔ **Maternal weight gain.** If you gain too much or too little, it can affect the baby's growth.
- ✔ **Mother's medical history.** Some medical problems, like hypertension or lupus, can affect fetal growth.
- ✔ **Multiple pregnancy.** Twins and triplets are often smaller than single babies.
- ✔ **Placental function.** Placental blood flow that's below par can slow down the baby's growth.

Your practitioner keeps an eye on your baby's growth rate, most often by measuring fundal height and paying attention to your weight gain. If you put on too little or too much weight, if your fundal height measurements are abnormal, or if something in your history puts you at risk for growth problems, your doctor is likely to send you for an ultrasound exam to more accurately assess the situation.

Fetal movements

Sometimes in the third trimester, you may feel as if a volcano is erupting inside your uterus. Look down at your belly during times of fetal activity, and it may appear that an alien from outer space is doing an aerobic dance inside you. Toward the end of pregnancy, fetal movements may feel less like jabs and more like tumbles or rolls. The timing of movement also changes; there are longer periods of quiet. The fetus is adapting to a more newborn-like pattern, taking longer naps and having longer active cycles.

Many pregnant women have heard that it's normal for fetal movements to diminish close to the due date. This is not true, although the quality of movement may change from sharp, forceful punches to heavier, slower rolls.

If you don't sense a normal amount of activity, let your practitioner know. A good general rule is that you should feel about six movements in one hour after dinner, while resting. Any movement, no matter how subtle, counts. Some women find that they go for periods of feeling less fetal movement, but then the movements pick up again and are normal. This is very common and is not a reason to be concerned. However, if you notice a pattern of diminishing fetal movements or you feel absolutely no fetal movements over several hours (despite resting or eating), you should give your practitioner a call right away.

Breathing movements

Fetuses undergo what are called *rhythmic breathing movements* from 10 weeks onward, although these movements are much more frequent in the third trimester. The fetus doesn't actually breathe, but its chest, abdominal wall, and diaphragm move in a pattern that is characteristic of breathing. These movements are not noticeable to you, but they can be observed with ultrasound and are thought to be a sign that the baby is faring well. During the third trimester, the amount of time a fetus spends performing the breathing movements increases, especially after meals.

Fetal hiccups

At times, you may feel a quick, rhythmic pattern of fetal movements, occurring every few seconds. These movements are most likely hiccups. Some women feel fetal hiccups several times throughout the day; others sense them only rarely. These hiccups often continue after the baby is born and are completely normal.

Keeping Up with Your Changing Body

As the baby grows, so does your belly! And while big is beautiful, it can become uncomfortable. You may notice that your uterus pushes up on your ribs, which can be quite uncomfortable. Sometimes you notice kicking in one spot in particular — that is probably where the baby's extremities are, either feet or arms. If you are pregnant with twins or more, the discomforts are, of course, even more pronounced. It is not uncommon for women with twins to feel one baby move more than the other. This is usually related to the position of the babies — one position is more noticeable than the other.

Whether you have one, two, or more babies inside, as you get bigger, it becomes more and more difficult to move around like you used to.

If you find it difficult to rise from lying on your back and no one is around to help, try turning on your side first and then pushing yourself up to a sitting position, as shown in Figure 7-2.

Accidents and falls

Being pregnant may make you more cautious about taking obvious risks, but it doesn't prevent you from stumbling or otherwise having an occasional mishap. If you do fall, don't worry. Chances are good that the baby remains well protected within your uterus and within its sac of amniotic fluid, which is an excellent natural cushion. But just to be careful, let your practitioner know. He or she may want you to come in to check that the baby is fine.

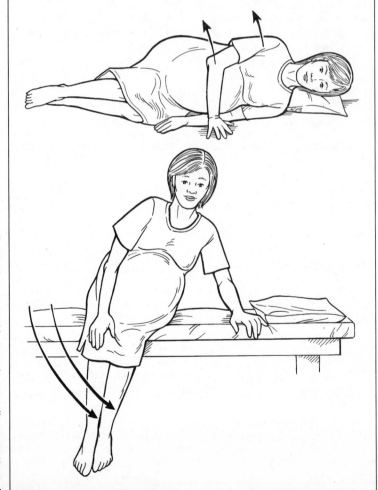

Figure 7-2: Make it easy on your back: Before trying to get up from lying down, first roll over to your side and then push yourself up while swinging your legs down.

A pregnant woman knows no strangers

You may find that your belly has suddenly become public property. Perfect strangers feel compelled to put their hands on your abdomen and tell you how pleased they are that you're about to have a baby! Although some women find this kind of thing caring and supportive, others find it annoying, embarrassing, and uncomfortable.

Many people consider it perfectly polite also to comment on your appearance. They may tell you that you look too fat or too thin; that you are carrying too wide or all in your buttocks. They may say that this or that is a sign that the baby is a boy or a girl. "Whoa, you must be about ready to pop!" they may exclaim, or "My goodness, you're enormous!" Try, if you can, *not* to pay attention to what they say. Indeed, the very best piece of advice we can offer is that you don't let other people drive you crazy. They may have the best of intentions, but they rarely realize how their words sound to you.

We tell our patients all the time to talk to us if they have concerns. So don't hesitate to ask your doctor or other health care provider if what you hear does worry you. But also remember what you know: If someone tells you that you look too small, remember that if you had an ultrasound exam recently and the size of your fetus was perfectly appropriate, you have nothing to worry about. If you have not had an ultrasound recently and you are concerned about the size of your baby, talk with your practitioner about it. He or she may reassure you that your belly is measuring perfectly normal.

Many women feel compelled to tell you all the horror stories of their own pregnancies — or all the pregnancy horror stories they've ever heard. If you pay too much attention, you'll only suffer anxiety and needless worry. Just tell the person politely that you really prefer not to hear their story; it's upsetting to you. (Unless, of course, you don't mind these stories.)

If, after your fall, you suffer severe abdominal pain, contractions, bleeding, or leakage of amniotic fluid, or if you notice a decrease in fetal movements, call your practitioner immediately. If the fall or injury involves a direct blow to your uterus (for example, the steering wheel hits your belly in a car accident), your practitioner will probably want to monitor your baby for a while to make sure that everything is okay.

Braxton-Hicks contractions

In the late second trimester or beginning of the third trimester, your uterus may, from time to time, become momentarily hard or feel as though it is balling up. Most likely, you're experiencing Braxton-Hicks contractions. They're not the kind of contractions you have in labor; they're more like practice ones.

Braxton-Hicks contractions are usually painless, but at times they may be uncomfortable, and they may occur with more frequency when you are active and subside when you rest. Women who have already had children tend to

notice more Braxton-Hicks contractions. You may have a hard time distinguishing Braxton-Hicks contractions from fetal movements, especially if this
is your first pregnancy. Other times, Braxton-Hicks contractions can become
uncomfortable and lead to false labor.

If you are less than 36 weeks along and you experience contractions that are
persistent, regular, and increasingly painful, call your doctor to make sure that
you're not in premature labor.

Carpal tunnel syndrome

If you feel numbness, tingling, or pain in your fingers and wrist, you're probably experiencing *carpal tunnel syndrome*. It occurs when swelling in the wrist
puts pressure on the *median nerve,* which runs through the *carpal tunnel*
from the wrist to the hand. It can happen in one or both hands, and the pain
may be worse at night or upon awakening.

If carpal tunnel syndrome becomes persistent or bothersome, discuss it with
your practitioner. Wrist splints, available at some drug stores or surgical
supply stores, can relieve the problem. Try not to be discouraged if it doesn't
seem to get better, though, because it usually improves (often dramatically
fast) after delivery.

Fatigue

The fatigue that you felt early in your pregnancy may return in the third
trimester. You may feel as if you're just slowing down. You're tired all the time,
you're carrying around more weight, you're not very comfortable much of the
time, and you may feel that you can't accomplish everything you need to.
Women may find their second or third pregnancies more tiring than the first
because they have to care for one or more older children.

Try to be realistic about what you can do and don't feel guilty about what
you can't get done. No one wants you to be Superwoman. Take time for yourself and get as much rest as you can. Delegate tasks. Whenever possible, let
other people help with household chores and other responsibilities. Do whatever you can to take advantage of the quiet times. Rest as much as you can
now, because after delivery, the work really picks up!

Dad, this is one of the key times when you can help your partner during pregnancy. It is fairly obvious that she is tired — if not fully exhausted. So hey,
pitch in even more than usual. Do her chores and errands as much as you can.
Try to help her get the rest she needs and assure her that she's not a wimp for
being tired.

Hemorrhoids

No one wants to talk about them, it seems, but *hemorrhoids* — dilated, swollen veins around the rectum — are a common problem for pregnant women. They are essentially varicose veins of the rectum (see the section on varicose veins later in this chapter). As with varicose veins in the legs, they are caused by the uterus pressing on major blood vessels, which leads to pooling of blood, and ultimately makes the veins enlarge and swell. Progesterone relaxes the veins, allowing the swelling to increase. Constipation makes hemorrhoids worse. Straining and pushing hard during bowel movements puts added pressure on the blood vessels, causing them to enlarge and possibly protrude from the rectum.

Hemorrhoids sometimes bleed. This bleeding doesn't harm the pregnancy, but if it becomes frequent, talk to your doctor and possibly see a colorectal specialist. If hemorrhoids become very painful, you may want to discuss whether treatment is necessary. Meanwhile, you can try the following:

- **Avoid constipation (see Chapter 5).**
- **Exercise.**
- **Get off your feet when you can**. Doing so alleviates extra pressure on your veins.
- **Try over-the-counter topical medications such as Preparation H or Anusol.**
- **Take warm baths two to three times a day.** Soaking in warm water can help relieve the muscle spasms that most often cause the pain.
- **Use over-the-counter hemorrhoidal pads (such as Tucks) or witch hazel pads to clean and medicate the area.**

Pushing during the second stage of labor (see Chapter 8) can make hemorrhoids worse or make them appear where they were not before. But most of the time, hemorrhoids go away after delivery.

Insomnia

During the last few months of pregnancy, many women find it very difficult to sleep. Let's face it — it's hard to find a comfortable position when you're eight months along. You feel a little like a beached whale. Getting up five times a night to go to the bathroom doesn't make things any easier. However, you may find relief in the following:

- **Drink warm milk with honey.** Warming the milk releases *tryptophan,* a naturally occurring amino acid that makes you sleepy; the honey causes you to produce insulin, which also makes you drowsy.

✔ **Get in some exercise during the day.**

✔ **Go to bed a little later than usual.**

✔ **Limit your liquid intake after 6 p.m.** Don't limit it to the point that you become dehydrated, however.

✔ **Invest in a body pillow.** You can tuck it around your body in various places, making it easier to find a comfortable position. You can get a body pillow in almost any department store.

✔ **Take a warm, relaxing bath before going to bed.**

I think I've dropped

During the month before delivery, a woman may notice that her belly feels much lower and that suddenly it is much easier to breathe. This is due to the fact that the baby has *dropped,* or descended lower into the pelvis. This movement is also called *lightening.* It typically happens two to three weeks before delivery in women who are having their first child. Those who have had children before may not drop until they are in labor. When dropping happens, you may find that you're suddenly much more comfortable. Your uterus doesn't press up on your diaphragm or stomach as much as it used to, so breathing is easier, and heartburn may improve. At the same time, however, you may feel more pressure in your vaginal area — many women say they feel heaviness there. Some women report feeling strange, sharp twinges as the baby's head moves and exerts pressure on the bladder and pelvic floor.

You may not notice that you have dropped. During your prenatal visit, your doctor may be able to tell by external or internal exam how low down the baby's head is and whether it's *engaged,* meaning that the fetal head has reached the level of the *ischial spines,* which are bony landmarks in your pelvis that can be felt during an internal exam (see Figure 7-3).

When the fetal head is at this level, it's said to be at *zero station.* Most practitioners divide the pelvis into descending stations from –5 to +5 (although some use –3 to +3). Often at the beginning of labor, the head may be at –4 or –5 station (fairly high — sometimes called *floating,* because the fetal head is still floating in the amniotic cavity). Labor proceeds until the head descends all the way to +5, when delivery is about to begin.

If the baby's head is engaged prior to labor, you're more likely to deliver vaginally, although obviously there are no guarantees. Similarly, while a floating (unengaged) head isn't every obstetrician's dream, it doesn't mean that you won't have a completely normal delivery.

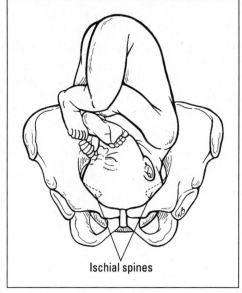

Figure 7-3:
When the baby's head reaches the bony ischial spines in your pelvis, it is said to be engaged.

Ischial spines

If you are having your second child or more, the baby's head may not engage until well into labor.

Pregnancy rashes and itches

Pregnant women are subject to the same rashes that nonpregnant women get. One rash is unique to pregnancy, however. It is called *Pruritic Urticarial Papules of Pregnancy,* or PUPP. It sounds scary, but it's really more of a nuisance than anything else, because it can cause some intense itching. It occurs more often during a first pregnancy and in women having twins or more (the more fetuses, the greater the likelihood). PUPP tends to occur late in pregnancy and is characterized by hives or red patches that first appear in the stretch marks on your abdomen. These patches can spread to other areas on the abdomen and to the legs, arms, chest, and back. They almost never spread to the face. (Thank heaven for small favors.) The good news is that the condition poses no risk to the baby. But if you develop this rash, your doctor may recommend that you have some blood tests to make sure that you don't have other conditions that can be associated with itching.

The only surefire way to make PUPP go away is to deliver. Some women tell us that the itching goes away within hours of giving birth. If delivery is still weeks away, it sometimes helps to bathe in a solution of colloidal oatmeal (Aveeno makes a good one). Skin lotions containing Benadryl (the ones you used to treat poison ivy when you were a kid) can also help, but these products can sometimes dry the skin, which only makes the itching worse. Some women get relief from taking Benadryl orally, but check with your doctor before doing so. Finally, in very severe cases (which are rare), the doctor may prescribe a short-term course of steroids.

Even if you don't have a rash, you may notice that you itch a lot, especially over your belly. This itching is very common and usually is caused by the stretching of your skin as the baby gets bigger. It often itches most where stretch marks develop.

Up to 2 percent of pregnant women develop *cholestasis of pregnancy*. This is a condition in which the itching is associated with an increase of bile acids in the blood. If the itching is mild, it can be treated with skin moisturizers, topical anti-itching medications, or oral antihistamines such as Benadryl. If the itching is severe, your doctor may recommend oral medications that help to clear the bile acids from the bloodstream. Some studies have suggested that the baby should be monitored with non-stress tests (see the section later in this chapter) when the mother has this condition, because it is associated with an increased risk of complications. The good news is that the itching goes away shortly after delivery. The bad news is that the condition may recur in future pregnancies.

Preparing for breastfeeding

If you plan on breast-feeding, you may want to take steps to toughen the skin around your nipples. This may be helpful in preventing the nipples from cracking and becoming sore when you are breast-feeding. Because cracked nipples can be painful, preparing them helps reduce any discomfort you may have. You can try very gently rubbing or massaging your nipples between your fingers, exposing them to air, rubbing them gently with a wash cloth, or wearing a nursing bra with the flaps down so that your nipples rub against your clothes. Creams or oil work against toughening, so avoid using them on your nipples.

Some women worry that they don't have the right type of breasts for breast-feeding, but no breast type is right or wrong. Breasts both large and small can produce adequate milk. Some women with retracted or inverted nipples can make breast-feeding easier by massaging their nipples so that they protrude more. (See Chapter 12 for more information.) Some maternity or baby stores sell special breast shells that use suction to help the nipples come out.

Many women notice from early on in pregnancy that their breasts occasionally secrete a yellowish discharge. This discharge is *colostrum,* and it's what the newborn baby sucks out and swallows in the first few days of life before actual milk comes in. Colostrum has a higher protein and lower fat content than milk; most importantly, it contains antibodies from your immune system that help protect your baby against certain infections until his or her own immune system matures and can take over.

Don't worry if you don't produce colostrum during pregnancy; not producing colostrum in no way means that you won't produce adequate milk. Each woman is different; some leak from the breasts during pregnancy, and some don't.

Sciatica

Some women experience pain extending from their lower back to their buttocks and down one leg or the other. This pain or, less commonly, numbness is known as *sciatica,* because it's due to pressure on the sciatic nerve, a major nerve that branches from your back, through your pelvis, to your hips, and down your legs. Mild cases of sciatica can be relieved by bed rest (shift from side to side to find the position that is most comfortable), warm baths, or heating pads applied to the painful areas. If you develop a severe case, you may need prolonged bed rest or special exercises. Ask your doctor.

Shortness of breath

You may find that as pregnancy proceeds, you become increasingly short of breath. The hormone progesterone affects your central breathing center and may cause these feelings of breathlessness. What's more, as your enlarging uterus presses upward on your diaphragm, your lungs have less room to expand normally.

(When Joanne was pregnant with her second child, she used to be so short of breath that the only books she could read to her daughter were ones with very short sentences. Dr. Seuss had to sit on the shelf until after she delivered.)

In most cases, shortness of breath is perfectly normal. But if it comes on very suddenly or if it comes with chest pain, call your doctor.

Stretch marks

Stretch marks are an almost inevitable part of pregnancy, though some women do avoid them. They are caused by the skin stretching to accommodate the enlarging uterus and the weight gain. Some women probably also have some genetic predisposition for stretch marks. The marks typically appear as pinkish-red streaks along the abdomen and breasts, but they fade to silvery gray or white several months after delivery. Their exact color depends on your skin tone — they appear more brown on dark-skinned women, for example.

No cream or ointment is completely effective in preventing stretch marks. Many people think that rubbing vitamin E oil on the belly helps prevent stretch marks or helps them fade faster, but the effectiveness of vitamin E has never been proven scientifically. Women have used numerous other concoctions to avoid stretch marks, but again, none of these products works for all women. Your best bet is to avoid excessive weight gain and to exercise regularly to maintain muscle tone, which eases the pressure of the uterus on the overlying skin.

Recently, some dermatologists have started offering a special laser procedure that may be helpful in reducing stretch marks *after* delivery. If yours are particularly noticeable, you can consult with a dermatologist a few months after your pregnancy is over.

Swelling

Swelling (also called *edema*) of the hands and legs is very common in the third trimester. It most often occurs after you've been on your feet for a while, but it can happen throughout the day. Swelling tends to be even more common when the weather is warm.

No evidence indicates that lowering your salt intake prevents swelling or makes it go away.

Although swelling is a normal symptom of pregnancy, it can occasionally be a sign of preeclampsia (see Chapter 14). If you notice a sudden increase in the amount of swelling, or a sudden, large weight gain — 5 pounds or more in a week — or if the swelling is associated with significant headache or right-sided abdominal pain, call your practitioner immediately.

For ordinary swelling, try the following:

- ✔ **Keep your legs elevated whenever possible.**
- ✔ **Stay in a cool environment.** In summer, avoid spending prolonged periods of time in the hot weather.
- ✔ **Wear supportive pantyhose or stockings — but nothing that is too tight around your knees.**
- ✔ **When in bed, don't lie flat on your back; try to lie on your side.**

Urinary stress incontinence

Leaking a little urine when you cough, laugh, or sneeze isn't unusual when you're pregnant. This kind of *urinary stress incontinence* occurs because your growing uterus is putting pressure on your bladder. Relaxation of the pelvic floor muscles increases the problem during the late second and third trimesters. And sometimes the baby may give the bladder a swift kick and cause it to leak urine. Kegel exercises — in which you repeatedly contract the pelvic floor muscles as if you're trying very hard not to urinate — can prevent or markedly reduce the problem. Some women continue to experience a little stress incontinence even after delivery, but it usually goes away after about 6 to 12 months. If you had a particularly difficult labor, where you pushed for a long time, or had a very large baby, the stress incontinence may not completely go away. It's a good idea to give it a least six months to see whether it goes away. After that, talk to your doctor about how to proceed.

Varicose veins

You may notice that a small road map has suddenly appeared on your lower legs (and sometimes the vulvar area). These marks are dilated veins, referred to as *varicose veins*. They are caused by the pressure of the uterus on major blood vessels — the *inferior vena cava* (the vein that returns blood to the heart) and the pelvic veins, in particular. Pregnancy also causes the muscle tissue inside your veins to relax and your blood volume to increase, and these conditions add to the problem. Women with light skin or with a family history of varicose veins are particularly susceptible. Very often, the bluish-purple highways fade after delivery, but sometimes they do not disappear completely. They are most often painless, but occasionally they may be associated with discomfort, achiness, or pain. In rare instances, a blood clot develops in the superficial veins of the legs, which can lead to *superficial thrombophlebitis*. This is not a serious problem; it's often successfully treated with rest, leg elevation, warm compresses, and sometimes special stockings. A clot that forms in the deep veins of the leg is more serious (see Chapter 15 for a discussion of *deep vein thrombosis*).

There's no way to prevent getting varicose veins — you can't fight heredity — but you may be able to reduce their number and severity by following these tips:

- ✔ **Avoid standing for prolonged periods of time.** Get off your feet several times a day.

- ✔ **Avoid wearing clothes that are very tight around one part of your leg** (tight garters or socks with tight elastic tops, for example).

- ✔ **If you must be relatively stationary, move your legs around from time to time to stimulate circulation.** Flexing your feet up and down also helps keep the blood from pooling.

- ✔ **Keep your legs elevated whenever you can.**

- ✔ **Wear support stockings or talk to your doctor about a prescription for special elastic stockings.**

Thinking about Labor

Toward the end of your third trimester, you're likely to think more about delivery and anticipate what that's going to be like. Many of our patients want to know, more specifically, when their labor may start and whether they can do anything to influence the timing or to bring it on sooner. In this section, we give some answers to these rather complicated questions.

Timing labor

"When am I going to have this baby?" It's a question we hear very frequently as the end approaches. We wish we had a foolproof way of knowing, but not even a crystal ball works. Sometimes a woman whose cervix is long and closed goes into labor within 12 hours of an internal exam, while other women can walk around with a cervix dilated to 3 centimeters for weeks! Some signs that suggest that something *may* happen include loss of the *mucous plug* (not really a plug but thick mucous produced in the cervix), *bloody show* (a blood-tinged mucous discharge), increasing frequency of Braxton-Hicks contractions, and diarrhea. But nothing is a sure sign. Loss of the mucous plug or bloody show may occur hours, days, or weeks before labor, or in some cases, not at all. This unpredictability may add to your anxiety, but it also makes the whole process more exciting.

Bringing on labor?

Women have tried all kinds of tricks to induce labor on their own. But nothing — short of medical induction — really has been proven to work. Here are some strategies you may hear about:

✔ **Chinese food:** It may provide a great meal, but it won't jump-start your labor.

✔ **Enema:** This procedure cleanses the bowel and may trigger some contractions, but it doesn't usually induce labor.

✔ **Nipple stimulation:** Vigorously rubbing or massaging the nipples can cause contractions, but it should not be performed at home because it can lead to *hyperstimulation* of the uterus (that is, too-frequent contractions), which is not healthy for you

or your baby. It's not a sure thing, in any case, because as soon as you stop the nipple stimulation, the contractions usually also stop.

✔ **Raspberry leaf tea:** This tea can cause the uterus to contract, but it has not been shown to trigger labor.

✔ **Sex:** Lovemaking may cause your uterus to contract, but it doesn't usually put anyone into labor. It may make for a lovely evening, however, assuming you have any libido left!

✔ **Walking:** Go out for a walk or other light exercise, and you may contract more. You definitely get the benefit of fresh air and exercise, but that's about it.

Using perineal massage

In the past few years, a great deal of interest has been generated about *perineal massage*. This process involves using an oil or cream on the *perineum* (the area between the vagina and the rectum) and massaging the area in preparation for childbirth. Although studies show that this practice decreases the need for *episiotomies* (cutting the perineum to allow room for the baby to pass during childbirth) or lacerations, the number of cases in which it has made a clear difference is not very large. (See Chapter 9 for more information on episiotomies.) There's no harm in trying it, though. If you think perineal massage may help and it's comfortable for you, go right ahead.

Working during Pregnancy

Almost half of all working Americans are women, and more than one million of them become pregnant each year. For most women, work has no adverse effects on pregnancy. On the contrary, by keeping you busy and stimulated, work may help you avoid dwelling on the discomforts of pregnancy or eating too much. If you're not at high risk for complications and your pregnancy is going smoothly, you can work until you deliver. Some women prefer to take a few weeks off before their due date to finish last-minute shopping and take care of certain obligations before the baby arrives.

Many women find it easy to balance their job responsibilities with the needs of pregnancy. But many also have concerns about how their job may affect their pregnancy. Specific issues that you should discuss with your practitioner include:

- ✔ Effects of long periods of standing or walking
- ✔ Job-related stress
- ✔ Occupational hazards

Stress in pregnancy, whether related to work or to home situations, is not well studied. Some doctors believe that very high levels of stress may increase the risk of developing preeclampsia or preterm labor (both of which are discussed in Chapter 14). Too much stress is obviously not good for anyone. Do whatever you can to decrease the stress in your life (see Chapter 3).

Some jobs may expose pregnant women to certain health risks (see Chapter 3). If you have a job that exposes you to toxic substances, high levels of radiation, and so on, you need to talk with your practitioner.

Banking cord blood

Cord blood banking involves extracting blood from the umbilical cord and saving it for possible use in the future (see Chapter 9). If you're considering cord blood banking, now is the time to find out about your options and make arrangements with an agency. Also, because some hospitals now have their own cord blood programs, find out whether the hospital where you will deliver offers this service.

 Remember that your health and the baby's health are the highest priority. Don't feel that you're a wimp because you have to attend to your pregnancy. Some women believe that if they complain about certain symptoms or take time out from a busy schedule to eat or go to the bathroom, they will garner the disapproval of their superiors at work. Don't let yourself feel guilty about your special needs during this time, and don't let work cause you to ignore any unusual symptoms. If you need time off to deal with complications, take it, and don't feel bad about it. People who haven't been pregnant never completely understand the physical strains you're dealing with.

The Home Stretch: Prenatal Visits in the Third Trimester

Between 28 and 36 weeks, your doctor probably wants to see you every two to three weeks and then weekly as you close in on delivery. The usual measurements are taken: blood pressure, weight, fetal heart rate, fundal height, and urine tests. These visits are also a good time to discuss with your practitioner issues related to labor and delivery.

If you don't deliver by your due date, your doctor may want to start performing non-stress tests (see the section on this topic later in this chapter). These tests assess fetal well-being. After 40 to 41 weeks, placental function and amniotic fluid may decline, and ensuring that both remain adequate to support the pregnancy is important. By 42 weeks, many practitioners recommend inducing labor (see Chapter 8) because the risk of problems for the baby rises significantly after that time.

Group B strep cultures

The only routine test that may be performed during one of your final prenatal visits is a culture for *Group B strep,* a bacteria commonly found in the vagina and rectum. Within the scientific community, controversy exists over whether or not women should be routinely screened for Group B strep. Some obstetricians perform this test at 36 weeks, but others don't. About 15 to 20 percent of women harbor this organism. If the culture is positive at 36 weeks, your doctor may recommend that you receive antibiotics during labor to reduce the risk of transmitting the bacteria to the baby. Treating this bacteria any earlier doesn't help, because it can come back by the time you're in labor. Currently, no tests that yield immediate results are available, so you can't test for Group B strep at the time of labor; it must be done in advance.

Amniocentesis for lung maturity

If you're planning a repeat cesarean delivery (meaning that you had one in an earlier pregnancy) or elective induction at less than 39 weeks, practitioners currently recommend that you have an amniocentesis to establish that the fetus's lungs are mature and ready to function.

The most commonly performed test for lung maturity is called *L/S ratio,* meaning the ratio of *lecithin* to *sphingomyelin* (both are substances found in the amniotic fluid). If the L/S ratio is 2.0 or greater and/or PG (*phosphatidyl glycerol,* a substance produced by mature lung cells) is present in the amniotic fluid, the baby's lungs are considered mature.

Assessing the Fetus

At certain times, your practitioner may suggest that you undergo tests for the baby. These tests, also referred to as *antepartum fetal surveillance,* are designed to check the baby's well-being. The tests can be performed at any time after about 24 to 26 weeks if cause for concern exists, or after 41 weeks if delivery has not yet occurred. Several different tests can be used; we describe these tests in the following sections.

Non-stress test (NST)

Non-stress testing consists of measuring the fetal heart rate, fetal movement, and uterine activity by a special monitoring machine (see Figure 7-4). You are hooked up to this device, which is designed to pick up uterine contractions and the baby's heart rate and to generate a tracing of both. It's similar to the device used during labor to monitor the fetal heart rate and contractions. You are also given a button to press each time you perceive fetal movement. The monitoring goes on for about 20 to 40 minutes. The doctor then looks at the tracing for signs of *accelerations,* or increases, in the fetal heart rate. If accelerations are present and occur often enough, the test is considered *reactive,* and the fetus is thought to be healthy and should continue to be so for three to seven days. (The fetus is healthy in more than 99 percent of cases.)

If the accelerations are not adequate (that is, the test is *nonreactive*), you still have no cause for alarm. In 80 percent of cases, the fetus is fine, but further evaluation is needed. Most practitioners repeat the NST once or twice a week.

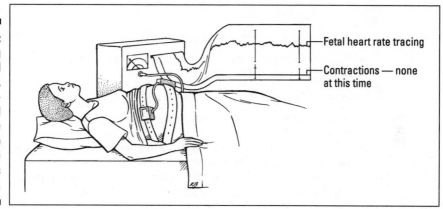

Figure 7-4: Monitoring the fetal heart rate, fetal movements, and uterine activity to see that the baby is healthy.

Fetal heart rate tracing

Contractions — none at this time

Contraction stress test (CST)

The contraction stress test is similar to a non-stress test except that the fetal heart is timed in relation to uterine contractions. The contractions sometimes occur on their own but more often are brought on with low doses of oxytocin (Pitocin) or by nipple stimulation. Three good contractions in a ten-minute period need to be present in order for the test to be interpreted. If the fetal heart rate doesn't drop after the contractions, the test is considered negative, and the baby is thought to be fine for at least one more week. If the test is positive (that is, the fetal heart rate does drop after the contractions) or suspicious, your practitioner investigates the situation further. Proper management depends on your particular situation.

Under certain circumstances, a CST should *not* be performed, such as if the mother has placenta previa (see Chapter 14) or if she is at risk of preterm delivery.

Nipple stimulation to bring on contractions should not be performed at home. It should be performed only under your doctor's supervision, because it is important that you be monitored to make sure that the uterus does not contract too much.

Biophysical profile (BPP)

The biophysical profile evaluates the following:

- ✔ **Fetal movements, observed by ultrasound.** Ideally, three distinct movements of body, arms, or legs are observed within a period of 30 minutes.
- ✔ **Fetal body tone, observed by ultrasound.**
- ✔ **Fetal breathing movements (chest motions that mimic breathing), observed by ultrasound.**
- ✔ **Quantity of amniotic fluid, observed by ultrasound.**
- ✔ **Non-stress test (see section earlier in this chapter).**

The baby receives 2 points for each parameter that's normal. A perfect score is 10 out of 10. Babies who score 8 out of 10 or better are considered okay. A score of 6 out of 10 is probably fine but usually calls for follow-up testing. A score of less than 6 out of 10 needs further evaluation.

Vibracoustic stimulation

A vibracoustic stimulation test may be performed during a non-stress test, but the fetus's response to stimulation by sound or vibrations is observed. The practitioner "buzzes" the mother's belly with a vibrating device, which causes a transmission of sound or vibrations to the fetus. Normally, the fetal heart rate accelerates when the fetus is stimulated in this way. A vibracoustic stimulation can often cut down the time necessary to perform a non-stress test, because you see accelerations in the heart rate more quickly.

Doppler velocimetry

A Doppler velocimetry test is done only in certain situations — if certain fetal problems (like intrauterine growth restriction — see Chapter 14) exist, for example, or if you have high blood pressure. Basically, for this test a special type of ultrasound exam is performed, and the blood flow through the umbilical cord is assessed.

Fetal kick counts

Fetal kick counts is a way that you can test for fetal well-being at home. If you have certain risk factors or if you need specific guidelines to track the adequacy of fetal movements, your practitioner may suggest that you keep a diary to chart fetal movement, starting at 28 weeks. You can track fetal movements in several different ways. One way is to lie down on your left side after dinner and count fetal movements. You should feel at least six movements within one hour. (You don't have to count for the full hour if you feel six movements in less than an hour.) Another way of doing the test is to count fetal movements while lying down for an hour each day and to plot the movements on a chart given to you by your practitioner. With this method, you can see the pattern of the baby's movements.

Going Back to School: Taking a Childbirth Class

Childbirth education has dramatically changed the average woman's experience of labor and delivery. Today's birthing experience is a far cry from earlier in this century, when women were knocked out with anesthesia for the delivery and the expectant father's only job was to pace around the waiting room like Ricky Ricardo anticipating the arrival of Little Ricky. Today, a great majority of first-time expectant parents attend childbirth classes. The parents-to-be find out what experiences to anticipate, as well as meet other expectant parents. They also find out about techniques — such as breathing, relaxation, and massage — to alleviate the fear, anxiety, and even the pain associated with labor.

The greatest benefit of childbirth classes is probably the opportunity they provide to find out what to anticipate during labor, because a little information goes a long way in reducing anxiety and fear about the big event. Following are some other benefits to the classes:

- **The chance to bring your partner into the process of pregnancy.** If attending your prenatal visits isn't always possible for your partner, a class may be the best time for him (or her) to find out about what's ahead and ask his own questions.

- **The chance to meet other parents-to-be.** You may make friends and, ultimately, find playmates for your child.

- **The chance to practice techniques for breathing, relaxation, and muscle control — all of which may help you deal with some of the pain during labor.**

- **The chance to ask questions that come up between prenatal visits.**

Most couples find childbirth education classes helpful. However, you may occasionally run into a teacher who's extremely dogmatic or judgmental or who may preach a philosophy that you or your practitioner do not subscribe to. Keep in mind that you don't have to believe everything you hear at a childbirth class. If you anticipate using medication or anesthesia to reduce the pain of labor and the teacher warns you that all such medications are evil, don't be bullied into accepting any particular point of view. You gain no advantage for being a martyr during labor. Just find out in class whatever you can that may be helpful and take the rest in stride. Ultimately, it's your labor, and you need to do what you feel comfortable with.

If you decide to take a class, make sure that the one you choose provides reliable and accurate information. Ask your health care provider for recommendations or ask friends who have already attended classes.

A tour of the hospital or childbirth center where you plan to deliver often occurs as part of your childbirth education class. (If it does not, ask your practitioner about arranging a tour.) Seeing where it's all going to happen is often very helpful.

Childbirth education isn't for everyone. Some women feel that to be fully informed about what's ahead only adds to their nervousness — and that's a perfectly fine way to look at it. Every woman should make her own decision about whether to attend childbirth classes.

Several methods of childbirth preparation are available. They're all designed to help you discover how to deal with pain and to lower your anxiety and discomfort about what lies ahead, but they vary somewhat in technique. Some offer a range of instruction, without adhering to any one philosophy, and a few take a particular approach. The following sections describe some of the most common childbirth preparation philosophies.

Lamaze

Lamaze, perhaps the most well known of all the techniques, focuses on shallow, rapid breathing to make the pain endurable. This technique teaches you ways to concentrate and to relax by practicing planned responses to contractions. Your coach — the baby's father or other person close to you — helps you practice, and ultimately apply, the techniques.

Bradley method

The Bradley method is a collection of techniques for deep abdominal breathing and relaxation to decrease the pain of labor. The emphasis is on developing the ability to concentrate on what's going on inside your body. Your partner participates to help you focus on your body and deal with the pain. Although the goal of this method is to enable you to deliver without anesthesia, don't feel like a failure if labor turns out to be more difficult than you expected and you end up asking for medication.

Using a doula to help you through the process

A *doula* is a professional who has had special training in providing emotional and educational support to women (and couples) throughout pregnancy. They are also called *childbirth assistants* or *birth assistants*. Doulas should not make medical decisions about your pregnancy or labor, but they do provide you with information about the course of pregnancy and the process of labor and delivery. They usually accompany you to the hospital and help tend to your emotional needs during labor. A doula can supplement the support you get from your partner or even replace it if he or she is unable to tolerate the whole process.

If you do decide to hire a doula (most people don't), have a discussion early in the interview process to make sure that everyone involved knows his or her role. That way, your partner doesn't feel left out. Also, make it clear that you want your practitioner making the medical decisions, not the doula.

Grantly Dick-Read

The basic premise of the Grantly Dick-Read technique is that the pain of labor results largely from the mother's fear of the unknown. Educating the patient about the childbirth process decreases that fear and its associated tension, and thereby decreases the pain of labor.

Causes for Concern

During the final weeks and months of pregnancy, you see your practitioner more often than before. Still, certain questions and problems may arise between visits. This is when things start heating up, with both the baby and your body preparing for delivery. Here are some of the key things that may lead you to call your doctor.

Bleeding

If you experience any significant bleeding, let your practitioner know immediately. Some third-trimester bleeding is harmless to you and your baby, but sometimes it can have serious implications. Getting evaluated to be sure that everything is fine makes sense. Possible causes of third-trimester bleeding include

- Preterm labor.
- Inflammation or irritation of the cervix or the harmless rupture of a superficial blood vessel on the cervix, either of which can occur after intercourse or after a pelvic exam.

- ✔ Placenta previa (see Chapter 14) or a low-lying placenta.

- ✔ Placental separation or abruption (see Chapter 14).

- ✔ Bloody show (see Chapter 8). This show is usually less than the amount of blood you would see during a normal menstrual period, and it's often mixed with mucous.

Breech presentation

A baby is in a so-called *breech* position when its buttocks or legs are down, closest to the cervix. Breech presentation happens in 3 to 4 percent of all singleton deliveries. A woman's risk of having a breech baby decreases the further along she goes in her pregnancy. (The incidence is 24 percent at 18 to 22 weeks but only 8 percent at 28 to 30 weeks. By 34 weeks, it's down to 7 percent, and by 38 to 40 weeks, 3 percent.) The fetus is more likely to assume a breech position for one of the following reasons:

- ✔ If the fetus is preterm or especially small

- ✔ If an increased amount of amniotic fluid exists (all the more room to turn around in)

- ✔ If a congenital malformation of the uterus is present (for example, a bicornuate, or T-shaped, uterus)

- ✔ If fibroids that impinge on the uterine cavity are present

- ✔ If placenta previa (see Chapter 14) is present

- ✔ If you're having twins or more

- ✔ If the mother's uterus is relaxed from having had several babies already

If your baby is in a breech position, your doctor talks with you about the potential risks and benefits of a vaginal breech delivery. Special concerns about a breech delivery include the following:

- ✔ Trapping the baby's head (which comes out last in a breech delivery) in a cervix that has been incompletely dilated by the passage of the baby's body, which is smaller than the head. (This situation is especially troublesome if the baby is very small or premature.)

- ✔ Trauma resulting from an *extended fetal head* (meaning the head is tilted back).

- ✔ Difficulty delivering the arms, which can lead to potential arm injuries.

Because of these potential problems, many practitioners recommend that all breech babies be delivered by cesarean section. However, many fetuses in breech position are actually good candidates for vaginal delivery. Conditions that should be present for you and your doctor to consider a vaginal breech delivery include the following:

✔ Estimated fetal weight between 4 and 8 pounds.

✔ The baby is in a *frank* breech position, which means that the buttocks, not the feet, are in position to come out first.

✔ The buttocks are engaged in the pelvis.

✔ Your doctor doesn't detect (by physical exam or by x-ray) any problem with the baby's head fitting through the birth canal.

✔ Ultrasound shows that the fetal head is either flexed or in the *military* position (looking straight ahead, not tilted back).

✔ Immediate anesthesia is available so that cesarean delivery can be done in an emergency.

✔ The doctor is experienced in vaginal breech deliveries.

If you and your practitioner decide that a vaginal breech delivery is not right for you, another option is *external cephalic version,* a procedure in which the doctor tries to turn the baby into normal delivery position by externally manipulating the mother's abdomen. This is a common and usually safe procedure. Sometimes it's fairly uncomfortable, but it works in about 50 to 70 percent of cases. This procedure shouldn't be done if you have any of the following conditions:

✔ If you have uterine abnormalities

✔ If you've been bleeding during the third trimester

✔ If you're having twins or more

✔ If the volume of amniotic fluid is decreased

✔ If the placenta is working poorly or there is any evidence of fetal compromise

✔ If an ultrasound shows that the umbilical cord is wrapped around the baby's neck

✔ In some cases, if the woman has had a previous cesarean delivery or other uterine surgery

Decreased amniotic fluid volume

The medical term for decreased amniotic fluid volume is *oligohydramnios.* (It also used to be called *dry birth*.) This condition may not be associated with an identifiable cause or it can occur in association with intrauterine growth restriction (described in a later section of this chapter), preterm rupture of the membranes, or other conditions. Usually, a mild decrease in amniotic fluid is not a major cause for concern; your practitioner begins to monitor you more closely — with non-stress tests and ultrasound exams — to make sure that no problem arises. If you're very close to your due date, your practitioner may feel that it's best to deliver the baby. On the other hand, if you are only 30 weeks along, the best option may be increased rest and close observation. Of course, the management of the problem also depends on its cause. See Chapter 14 for more details about problems with amniotic fluid.

Decreased fetal movement

If you're not feeling the amount of fetal movement that you've been accustomed to, let your doctor know. Fetal movement is one of the most important things to pay attention to as you near your due date (see the section "Fetal kick counts," earlier in this chapter).

Fetal growth problems

You may find out at a routine prenatal visit that your practitioner thinks that your uterus is measuring either too big or too small. This finding is *not* a cause for immediate alarm. Often in this situation, your practitioner suggests that you have an ultrasound exam to get a better idea of how big the baby is. Ultrasound is used to measure parts of the baby — the size of the head, the circumference of the abdomen, and the length of the thigh bone *(femur).* These measurements are plugged into a mathematical equation that estimates the fetal weight (EFW). That estimate is then entered on a curve plotting the baby's age in weeks against weight, as shown in Figure 7-5, which represents the average growth of thousands of fetuses at each gestational age. Your practitioner can check to see where your baby's weight falls on the curve and thus tell which percentile the baby is in. If the baby's weight is anywhere between the 10th and the 90th percentiles, the weight is considered normal. If the weight is above the 90th percentile, the baby is exceptionally large, and if it's below the 10th percentile, it's exceptionally small. Remember, not every baby is at the 50th percentile, so the 20th percentile is still normal and no reason to worry.

Keep in mind that although ultrasound is an excellent tool for assessing fetal growth, it isn't perfect. Judging the baby's weight by an ultrasound exam is not the same as putting the baby on a scale. Weight estimates can vary by as much as 10 to 20 percent in the third trimester due to variations in body composition. So if your baby is outside the normal range, it's not always a cause for alarm.

If your baby measures very large, your practitioner may suggest that you have another glucose screen to check for gestational diabetes (see Chapter 14).

If your baby measures especially small, your doctor may suggest that you be followed more closely — that you undergo non-stress tests and repeat ultrasound exams to keep an eye on fetal growth. Too little growth is a condition known as *intrauterine growth restriction,* or IUGR (see Chapter 15). Most of the time, fetuses that measure less than the 10th percentile on ultrasound are completely normal, just a bit on the small side. Just like people, fetuses come in all shapes and sizes. In any case, after delivery, most babies catch up and grow normally.

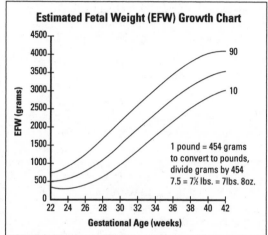

Figure 7-5: This graph shows how much the average fetus weighs at different points during pregnancy.

But in some cases, a fetus may be small due to an infection, certain maternal conditions, or abnormal placental function, and these reasons are causes for concern. That's why IUGR calls for further evaluation and close monitoring. The severity of the problem depends on how far along the pregnancy is, how small the fetus is, and the underlying cause. A low-weight fetus at 23 weeks is a greater cause for concern than one at 38 weeks. We go into problems with fetal growth and how to manage them in greater detail in Chapter 14.

Leaking amniotic fluid

If you notice that your underwear is wet, several explanations are possible. It may be a little urine, vaginal discharge, the release of the mucous plug in the cervix, or actual leakage of amniotic fluid (also known as *rupture of the membranes*). Often, you can tell what it is by examining the fluid. Mucous discharge tends to be thick and globby, while vaginal discharge is whitish and smooth. Urine has its characteristic odor and isn't continuous. Amniotic fluid, on the other hand, is normally clear and watery and often is lost in spurts. Sometimes you have a big gush of water when membranes rupture, but if the membrane has only a small hole, the leakage may be scant.

If you leak what you think may be amniotic fluid, call your practitioner right away. If you are not preterm and the amniotic fluid is clear, leaking fluid is not an emergency. However, most practitioners want you to call them to let them know so that they can tell you what to do. If the fluid is bloody or greenish-brown, be sure that you let your practitioner know. Greenish fluid means that the baby has had a bowel movement, known as *meconium,* inside the uterus. Most of the time, such an event doesn't indicate a problem, but sometimes it means that the baby is being stressed. Your practitioner makes sure that the baby is okay by monitoring the baby's heart beat (probably by performing a non-stress test).

Macrosomia

Although a big, healthy, chubby baby is beautiful and wonderful, you *can* get too much of a good thing. A fetus is considered *macrosomic* (exceptionally large) if it weighs in above the 90th percentile (meaning that it's heavier than 90 percent of babies) or weighs at least 8 pounds, 13 ounces (4,000 grams). Macrosomia can mean extra long labor, may put a woman at risk of needing a cesarean delivery, and increases the chance of having a difficult delivery. The way in which your doctor responds to the problem depends on exactly how large the baby is, whether you have diabetes, your medical history, and an examination. Ultrasound is not that great at predicting macrosomia; half the time when a baby appears to be too large on ultrasound, it really isn't. Also, if you are overweight yourself, performing an ultrasound exam is technically even more difficult, making the prediction of macrosomia even harder. See Chapter 14 for more details on macrosomia.

Preeclampsia

Preeclampsia, in which high blood pressure is associated with the spilling of protein into the urine and sometimes swelling *(edema)* in the hands, face, and legs, is a condition unique to pregnancy. Preeclampsia (also called *tox-emia* or *pregnancy-induced hypertension*) isn't uncommon; it occurs in 6 to 8 percent of all pregnancies. It can range from being very mild to being a serious medical condition. Chapter 14 provides you with the signs and symptoms of preeclampsia.

Preeclampsia usually comes on gradually. Your practitioner may at first notice only a slight elevation in your blood pressure. He or she may then tell you to rest more, to lie on your side as much as possible, and to come in for more frequent visits. But occasionally, preeclampsia happens suddenly.

Preterm labor

The strict technical definition of preterm labor is when a woman begins to have contractions and changes in her cervix before she's 37 weeks along. Many women have contractions but no cervical change — in which case it isn't real preterm labor. However, in order to find out whether your cervix is changing, you need to be examined. In addition, your practitioner determines how often you are contracting by placing you on a uterine contraction monitor (like the one used to perform a non-stress test — see the section on this topic earlier in this chapter).

The contractions associated with preterm labor are regular, persistent, and can be uncomfortable. They often start out feeling like bad menstrual cramps. (Braxton-Hicks contractions, in contrast, are not regular or persistent, and they are usually not uncomfortable.) Preterm labor may also be associated with increased mucous discharge, bleeding, or leakage of amniotic fluid. It is important to diagnose preterm labor as early as possible. Medications aimed at arresting premature labor work best if the cervix is dilated less than 3 cm.

If labor occurs after 35 weeks, your practitioner probably won't try to stop your contractions except in rare circumstances (such as poorly controlled diabetes).

If you find that you're having regular, uncomfortable, persistent contractions (more than five or six in an hour) and you're not yet 35 to 36 weeks pregnant, call your practitioner. The only way to tell whether you are experiencing real preterm labor is to be examined. Also, if you think your membranes have ruptured (your water has broken) or if you're having any bleeding, call your practitioner right away. See Chapter 14 for more detailed coverage on preterm labor.

When the baby is late

You think, for nearly nine months, that your baby is going to come on a certain date. But in fact, only about 5 percent of women actually deliver on their due date. Eighty percent deliver between 37 and 42 weeks, which is considered full term. Ten percent don't deliver even by 42 weeks. These pregnancies are known as *post-date* or *post-term* pregnancies. At one time, these pregnancies were often simply a reflection of incorrectly estimated due dates. But today, with the widespread use of ultrasound, the due dates are usually pretty accurate. An ultrasound performed during the first trimester is especially accurate, usually within three to four days. A third trimester ultrasound, in contrast, may be off by two to three weeks.

Many practitioners advise that labor be induced if the pregnancy reaches 42 weeks. If it goes on any longer, the baby is likely to still be fine, but greater health risks are possible, including:

- **Decreased amniotic fluid volume:** Because the amniotic fluid tends to decrease after about 36 weeks, it may be very low by 42 weeks. This condition can increase the chance that the umbilical cord becomes compressed during contractions or fetal movements, thereby limiting blood flow to the baby.

- **Increase in perinatal morbidity:** The rate of fetal death increases significantly after a mother passes her 42nd week. That's why, in many cases, after a woman passes her due date, her doctor may start to monitor the pregnancy by performing non-stress tests (see earlier in this chapter). She or he also checks to see whether the woman's cervix is favorable for labor induction (see Chapter 8). If the cervix is unfavorable (thus lowering the chances for a successful induction) and the results of the non-stress tests and amniotic fluid volume checks are good, it may be safe to continue the pregnancy. If the fluid is low, the cervix is favorable, or the non-stress test results are not reassuring, induction is probably the best course of action.

- **Macrosomia:** The baby weighs more than 8 pounds, 13 ounces (4,000 grams) — which is more than what 90 percent of babies weigh at birth. See the coverage earlier in this chapter for more information.

- **Meconium aspiration:** The medical term for what happens when the baby breathes in *(aspirates)* the *meconium* (an early fetal bowel movement). Meconium aspiration is more common in post-date pregnancies because passage of meconium is more common in these pregnancies.

Part III
The Big Event: Labor, Delivery, and Recovery

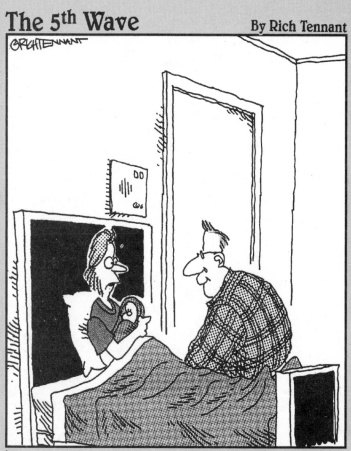

The 5th Wave   By Rich Tennant

"Even the doctors were surprised at how involved you were in there. Especially right near the end when you turned on that tape of the 'William Tell Overture.'"

In this part . . .

And now for the moment you've all been waiting for. . . . Like pregnancy itself, childbirth can go more smoothly if you know what's going to happen. You can benefit by being aware, for example, of the various ways in which you may deliver or the choices you may make about anesthesia. Also, it helps to know ahead of time what caring for a newborn is like. We filled the chapters in this section with details about childbirth and child care. We don't intend for this part to be overwhelming, just comprehensive enough to prepare you for the big event.

Chapter 8

Honey, I Think I'm in Labor!

● ●

In This Chapter

▶ Packing for the trip to the hospital or birthing center

▶ Determining whether you're in labor

▶ Being admitted to the hospital or birthing center

▶ Monitoring the baby during labor

▶ Helping things along: Inducing labor

▶ Knowing what happens in each of the three stages of labor

▶ Understanding the complications that may occur during labor and delivery — and knowing how they can be handled

▶ Managing the pain of childbirth with several techniques

● ●

Despite the incredible advances that have been made in science and medicine, no one really knows what causes labor to begin. Labor may be triggered by a combination of stimuli generated by the mother, the baby, and the placenta. Or labor may begin because of rising levels of steroid-like substances in the mother or other biochemical substances produced by the baby. Because we don't know exactly how labor starts, we also can't pinpoint exactly when it will occur.

It's pretty common for women to be unsure whether or not they are really in labor. Even a woman expecting her third or fourth child doesn't always know when she's genuinely in labor. This chapter helps you better identify your own labor (but you still may find yourself calling your practitioner several times or even making many trips to the hospital or birthing center, only to find out that what you think is labor really is not).

In this chapter, we cover the three stages of labor so that you can be better prepared every step of the way. We also let you know what complications may arise and how your practitioner may handle them. This chapter gives you a great deal of information on managing your pain during labor — something every expectant mother thinks about! And we even start off with suggestions for things to pack in your suitcase.

Packing Your Suitcase

Many women find it comforting to know that their bag is packed for the trip to the hospital or birthing center. Having your bag ready allows you to concentrate on watching for signs of labor and helps keep you from worrying about being prepared.

You may want to have a few things on hand while you're in labor, including the following:

- ✔ **A camera — plus film and batteries.**

- ✔ **Telephone numbers of the people you may want to call and a calling card.**

- ✔ **Insurance information.**

- ✔ **Socks.**

- ✔ **Glasses.** (They may be less trouble than contact lenses during labor.)

- ✔ **A snack for your partner or coach.**

- ✔ **Hard candies or lollipops.** You may have to go for some time without eating or drinking.

- ✔ **Something your partner can use to massage your back during labor.** Some people find that a tennis ball, a narrow paint roller, or a lightweight rolling pin works well.

- ✔ **Radio or cassette or CD player, if you find music relaxing.** Don't forget to bring your favorite cassettes or CDs!

- ✔ **Change for parking meters, telephones, or vending machines.**

After delivery, some additional items can help make your life easier, more comfortable, or fun:

- ✔ **A post-delivery snack for yourself.**

- ✔ **Champagne for a post-delivery toast, if you like.**

- ✔ **Sanitary napkins** (the modern, stick-on kind with wings). Most hospitals provide only the old-fashioned pads that you fasten to a belt, and they aren't very comfortable.

- ✔ **Sturdy cotton underwear.** Bring several pair that you don't mind ruining with blood stains. (No thongs or lacy, flimsy panties!)

- ✔ **A bathrobe and nightgown.** Hospitals provide gowns, but they're usually about as flattering and comfortable as a suit of armor.

- ✔ **Toiletries.** Throw in a hairbrush, toothbrush and toothpaste, shampoo, makeup, deodorant, and any other things that you use regularly. Remember that you may have many guests during your stay at the hospital.

- **Extra-large shoes.** Most women become very swollen after delivery, particularly in their feet, because of all the fluid shifts that occur. You may find that your regular shoes don't fit, so take along extra-big ones to go home in. The swelling usually goes away within four to five days.

- **Clothes to go home in.** But don't bring you favorite prepregnancy jeans. They still won't fit, and you'll want to wear something softer if you have an episiotomy during delivery. Leggings and loose tunics or any clothes that are soft and ample work great.

- **Clothes for your baby — or babies! — to go home in.** Easy-on, easy-off clothes are obviously most convenient. Keep in mind that your baby will still have his or her umbilical cord stump, so two-piece outfits will be easier to deal with than one-piece. If it's cold outside, be sure to dress the baby in layers — as a general rule, one more layer than you would wear yourself.

- **An infant car seat.** Your partner or a family member can bring the car seat just before you take the baby home. It makes sense to have the seat all strapped in and ready to go *before* bringing the baby out to the car.

Knowing When Labor Is Real — and When It Isn't

You may experience some of the early symptoms of labor before labor actually begins. Rather than indicating that you're in labor, these symptoms suggest that labor may occur in the next few days or weeks. Some women experience these labor-like symptoms for days or weeks, and others experience them only for several hours. Most of the time, going into labor isn't as dramatic as it is portrayed on sitcoms (picture Lucy saying, "Ricky, this is it!"). Women very rarely lack the time they need to get to the hospital before they deliver.

If you think you're in active labor, don't run to the hospital right away. Instead, telephone your practitioner first.

Noticing changes before labor begins

As you near the end of your pregnancy, you may recognize certain changes as your body prepares for the big event. You may notice all of these symptoms, or you may not notice any of them. Sometimes the changes begin weeks before labor begins, and sometimes they begin only days before.

- ✓ **Bloody show:** As changes in your cervix take place, you may expel from your vagina some mucous discharge mixed with blood. The blood doesn't come from your uterus, where the baby is; the blood comes from small, broken capillaries in your cervix.

- ✓ **Diarrhea:** Usually a few days before labor, your body releases *prostaglandins,* which are substances that help the uterus contract and may cause diarrhea.

- ✓ **Dropping and engagement:** Especially in women who are giving birth for the first time, the fetus often drops into the pelvis several weeks before labor (see Chapter 7 for more information). You may feel increased pressure on your vagina and sharp pains radiating to your vagina. You also may notice that your whole uterus is lower in your belly and that you are suddenly more comfortable and can breathe more easily.

- ✓ **Increase in Braxton-Hicks contractions:** You may notice an increase in the frequency and strength of *Braxton-Hicks contractions,* which are described in Chapter 7. These contractions may become somewhat uncomfortable, even if they don't grow any stronger or more frequent. Some women experience strong Braxton-Hicks contractions for weeks before labor begins.

- ✓ **Mucous discharge:** You may secrete a thick mucous discharge, which is known as the *mucous plug.* During your pregnancy, this substance plugs your cervix, protecting your uterus from infection. As your cervix starts to thin out *(efface)* and dilate in preparation for delivery, the plug may wash out.

Our patients want to know . . .

Q: "I've never had a contraction, so how do I know what one feels like?"

A: A *contraction* occurs when the muscle of the uterus tightens and pushes the baby toward the cervix. Usually, contractions are uncomfortable and, therefore, unmistakable. But many women worry that they won't know that they're having contractions. You can tell whether you're experiencing contractions by using a quick and easy trick.

With your fingertips, touch your cheek and then your forehead. Finally, touch the top part of your abdomen, through which you can feel the top part of your uterus (the *fundus*). A relaxed uterus feels soft, like your cheek, and a contracting uterus feels hard, like your forehead. This exercise is also good to try if you think you may be in preterm labor (see Chapter 14 for more information).

Recognizing the differences between false labor and true labor

Distinguishing true labor from false labor isn't always easy. But a few general characteristics can help you determine whether the symptoms you're experiencing mean you're in labor.

In general, you're in false labor if your contractions

 ✔ Are irregular and don't increase in frequency

 ✔ Disappear when you change position, walk, or rest

 ✔ Occur only in your lower abdomen

 ✔ Do not become increasingly uncomfortable

On the other hand, you're more likely to be in actual labor if your contractions

 ✔ Grow steadily more intense and more uncomfortable

 ✔ Don't go away when you change position, walk, or rest

 ✔ Occur along with leakage of fluid (due to rupture of the membranes)

 ✔ Make normal talking difficult or impossible

 ✔ Stretch across your upper abdomen or are located in your back, radiating to your front

Table 8-1 provides the characteristics of both true labor and false labor.

Table 8-1	True versus False Labor	
Characteristic	*False Labor*	*True Labor*
Contraction frequency	Irregular; no increase in frequency	Regular; contractions become closer and closer together
Contraction length	Irregular	40 to 60 seconds
Contraction intensity	No increase; not particularly uncomfortable	Grow increasingly more painful
When you change position	Contractions go away	No change, or an increase in contractions
Location of contraction	Lower abdomen	Upper abdomen or lower back, radiating to the lower abdomen

Sometimes the only way you can know for sure whether you are in labor is by seeing your practitioner or going to the hospital. When you arrive at the hospital, your doctor, a nurse, a midwife, or a resident physician performs a pelvic exam to determine whether you're in labor. The practitioner also may hook you up to a monitor to see how often you are contracting and to check how the fetal heart responds. Sometimes you find out right away whether you are truly in labor. But the practitioner may need to keep you under observation for several hours to see whether the situation is changing. You are considered to be in labor if you are having regular contractions and your cervix is changing fairly rapidly — effacing, dilating, or both. Sometimes women walk around for weeks with a partially dilated or effaced cervix but are not considered to be in labor because these changes are occurring over weeks instead of hours.

Checking the situation with an internal exam

When a practitioner is trying to determine whether you're in labor, he or she performs an internal exam to look for several things:

- **Dilation:** Your cervix is closed for most of your pregnancy but may gradually start to dilate during the last couple of weeks, especially if you've had a baby before. After active labor begins, the rate of cervical dilation speeds up, and the cervix dilates to 10 centimeters by the end of the first stage of labor. Often, you are considered to be in active labor when your cervix is about 4 centimeters dilated or 100 percent effaced.

- **Effacement:** Effacement is a thinning out or shortening of the cervix, which happens during labor. Your cervix goes from being thick (uneffaced) to 100 percent effaced. This progression is illustrated in Figure 8-1.

- **Station:** When you are in labor, the practitioner uses the term *station* to describe how far your baby's head (or other presenting part) has descended in the birth canal in relation to the *ischial spines*, a bony landmark in your pelvis. These stations are numbered from –5 (or sometimes –3) to +5 (or +3). A station of –5 (or –3) indicates that the baby's head is at the highest point on the scale, and a station of +5 (or +3) indicates that the baby's head is at the lowest point on the scale and closest to delivery (see Chapter 7 for more information on station).

- **Position:** When labor begins, the baby typically starts out facing to the side (left or right; see a baby facing left, in the position known as *left occiput anterior,* in Figure 8-2a). As labor progresses, he or she rotates until the head assumes a face-down position called *occiput anterior* (see Figure 8-2b) so that the baby comes out looking at the floor. Occasionally, the baby rotates to the oposite position and comes out sunny-side up, looking at the ceiling (also known as *occiput posterior,* shown in Figure 8-2c).

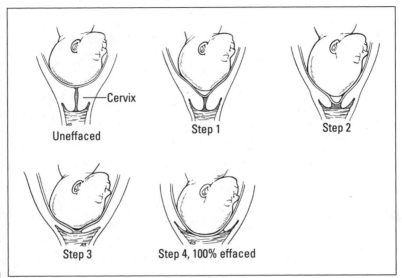

Figure 8-1:
During cervical effacement, the cervix progresses from an uneffaced state to 100 percent effaced and partially dilated.

Cervix

Uneffaced

Step 1

Step 2

Step 3

Step 4, 100% effaced

Figure 8-2:
As labor begins, the baby's head faces to the side (a); during labor the face usually rotates to the back (b) but may rotate to the front (c).

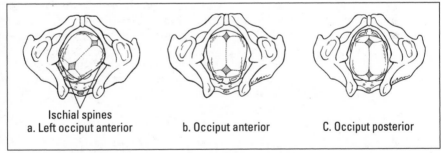

Ischial spines
a. Left occiput anterior

b. Occiput anterior

C. Occiput posterior

When to call your practitioner

If you think you are in labor, call your practitioner. Don't be embarrassed if he or she tells you that you're probably *not* in labor (it happens to many women). Timing your contractions for several hours before you call, to see whether they are getting closer together, is a good idea because your practitioner can use this information to help determine whether you're in true labor. If your contractions are occurring every 5 to 10 minutes and they are uncomfortable, definitely call. If you are less than 37 weeks and feeling persistent contractions, don't sit for hours counting their frequency — call your practitioner immediately.

Call your practitioner if any of the following apply to you:

✔ Your contractions are coming closer together, and they're becoming increasingly uncomfortable.

✔ You have ruptured membranes. Having your water break may come as a small amount of watery fluid leaking out, or it may be a big gush. If the fluid is green, brown, or red, let your practitioner know right away.

✔ You have heavy bleeding (more than a heavy menstrual period) or are passing clots.

✔ You are not feeling an adequate amount of fetal movement (see Chapter 7 for more information).

✔ You have constant, severe abdominal pain with no relief between contractions.

✔ You feel a fetal part or umbilical cord in your vagina. In this case, go to the hospital right away!

Getting Admitted to the Hospital

When you are in labor or if you are being induced or are having an elective cesarean delivery, you need to be admitted to the hospital's labor floor. If you are preregistered (ask your practitioner about the process for doing this in your hospital or birthing center), your records are already on the labor floor when you arrive, and a hospital unit number is assigned to you. When you arrive at the hospital or birthing center, you go through an admission process and get assigned to a room.

Settling into your hospital room

Although each hospital or birthing center has its own system, getting you settled in usually follows this routine after you get to your room:

✔ A nurse asks you to change into a gown.

✔ A nurse asks you questions about your pregnancy, your general health, your obstetrical history, and when you last ate. If you think your bag of water has broken or you are leaking fluid, let your nurse know.

✔ A nurse, midwife, resident, or other practitioner performs an internal exam to see how far along in labor you are.

✔ Your contractions and the fetal heart rate are monitored.

✔ Blood may be drawn, and an IV *(intravenous)* line may be started in your arm (for delivering fluids and, possibly, medications). See "Other Concerns, Worries, and Labor-Related Questions You May Have" later this chapter for more information on routine IVs.

✔ You are asked to sign a consent form for routine hospital care, delivery, and possibly cesarean section. (You sign the consent form when you are admitted in case you need an emergency cesarean during labor and there's no time to sign consent forms.)

You may want to hand over any valuables you have with you to your partner or other family member (or simply leave them at home).

Checking out the accommodations

Some women go through labor in the same room in which they deliver the baby, and others are moved to a different room for delivery. Most hospital rooms include some standard features, which you can see in Figure 8-3. The room you are placed in probably includes all of the following:

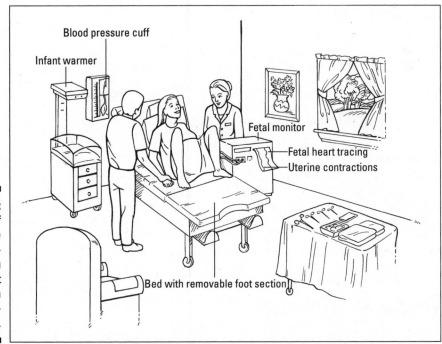

Figure 8-3:
The kinds of furniture and equipment you can expect to see in your hospital room.

✔ **Bed:** In a room used for both labor and delivery (also known as a *birthing room*), the bed is specially designed to come apart and be turned into a delivery table. Some hospitals have rooms where you labor, deliver, and even remain for your postpartum recovery. These rooms are called *LDR* (an acronym for *labor, delivery, and recovery*) *rooms* or *LDRP rooms* (the "P" stands for *postpartum*).

✔ **Doppler/stethoscope:** Portable tools used for listening periodically to the fetal heartbeat, instead of using the continuous fetal monitor.

✔ **Fetal monitor:** This machine has two attachments, one to monitor the baby's heart rate and one to monitor your contractions. The fetal monitor generates a *fetal heart tracing,* which is a paper record of how the baby's heart rate rises and falls in relation to your contractions, as shown in Figure 8-4.

✔ **Infant warmer:** This has a heat lamp to keep the newborn's body temperature from dropping.

✔ **IV line:** This tube is connected to a bag of *saline* (salt water) containing a glucose mixture to keep you properly hydrated.

✔ **Rocking chair or recliner:** The extra chair is for the father, your coach, or other family member.

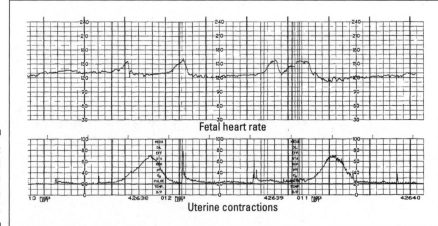

Figure 8-4:
The fetal heart rate and uterine contractions.

Testing, Testing

While you are in labor, your practitioner may monitor your baby in a number of different ways, to make sure that he or she is tolerating the whole process well. In this section, we describe the kinds of tests that are commonly used to determine whether everything is going along smoothly for you and the baby during labor.

Fetal heart monitoring

Labor puts stress on both you and the baby. Fetal heart monitoring provides a way to make sure that the baby is handling the stress. In some hospitals, all patients in labor are routinely monitored. In others, patients who are at low risk for complications may be monitored only intermittently.

Monitoring can be done through several techniques, including external and internal monitoring.

External monitoring

Electronic fetal heart monitoring uses either two belts or a wide, elastic band placed around the abdomen. A device attached to the belt or under the band uses an ultrasound-Doppler technique to pick up the fetal heartbeat. A second device uses a gauge to pick up the contractions. An external contraction monitor can show the frequency and duration of contractions, but it can't provide information about how strong they are. An external fetal heart monitor gives information about the fetus's response to contractions. An external fetal heart monitor records *long-term variability* — that is, periodic changes in heart rate (which is a good sign).

You may hear your practitioner use the following terms to describe the fetal heartbeat:

- **Normal:** About 120 to 160 beats per minute.

- **Bradycardia:** A decrease in the fetal heart rate, to below 120 beats per minute, that lasts for more than two minutes.

- **Tachycardia:** An increase in the fetal heart rate to above 160 beats per minute for more than two minutes.

- **Accelerations:** Brief increases above baseline in the fetal heart rate, often after a fetal movement. Accelerations are a reassuring sign.

- **Decelerations:** These are intermittent decreases below the baseline fetal heart rate. The significance of decelerations depends on their frequency, how far the heart rate drops, and when they occur in relation to contractions. Decelerations are classified as early, variable, or late, according to when they occur in relation to contractions.

    - *Early* decelerations occur along with contractions (they begin early in the contraction, hence their name). These decelerations represent the fetus's reflexive response to having its head compressed during contractions. They tend to occur later in the labor process, when the baby is low in the birth canal, but they can occur any time during labor. Early decelerations are benign and not a cause for concern.

    - *Variable* decelerations occur with or without contraction. They are due to a temporary compression of the umbilical cord. Variable decelerations are usually of no concern unless they become very frequent or the heart rate drops very low. They often go away if you change your position in bed.

- *Late* decelerations start well after you're into a contraction, and the heart rate stays down temporarily after the contraction ends. They occur when the uterus and placenta aren't getting enough blood and oxygen to the baby. If they occur only occasionally, they may be of little concern. However, if they occur after *every* contraction, they may indicate that the baby is not receiving enough oxygen and that he or she may not be tolerating the process of labor. Your nurse and practitioner may take steps to improve the flow of oxygen to the baby. They may, for example, increase your intravenous fluids (to improve your blood flow), give you extra oxygen to breathe through a mask, or shift your position in bed. If these measures make the decelerations go away, your practitioner may allow your labor to continue. If not, he or she may recommend further tests or even a cesarean delivery.

The level of concern your practitioner has about any of these decelerations depends on how far along you are in your labor, how the baseline fetal heart rate pattern looks between contractions, and any special problems you or your baby may have. Some decelerations occur during the pushing stage (see Chapter 9) and aren't always a cause for concern — it depends on how long they last and what the heart rate pattern looks like between pushes.

Babies are amazingly resilient and usually tolerate the labor process well. One or two decelerations aren't going to harm him or her. It's only the persistent and severe ones that are troublesome.

- **Long-term variability:** Periodic accelerations in the fetal heart rate, signifying that your baby is tolerating labor.

- **Short-term (beat-to-beat) variability:** Moment-to-moment changes in heart rate — a good sign. Short-term variability can be evaluated accurately only with an internal fetal heart monitor (see the next section for more information).

Internal monitoring

An internal fetal heart monitor is used when closer observation than is possible with external monitoring is needed. Your practitioner may be concerned about how the fetus is tolerating labor, or he or she may simply be having difficulty picking up the heart rate externally — if, for example, you're having more than one baby. In order for an internal fetal monitor (also called an *internal scalp electrode*) to be placed, the membranes (bag of water) must be ruptured and the cervix dilated to at least 1 or 2 centimeters. During an internal exam, the monitor is passed through the cervix via a flexible plastic tube. This procedure is no more uncomfortable than a pelvic exam. The tiny electrode is then attached to the baby's scalp. The process is quite safe and is only rarely associated with a local infection or a slight rash on the baby's head.

An internal monitor for contractions (called an *internal pressure transducer,* or IPT) is used to better assess how strong the contractions are. This monitor is used when the progress of labor is slow, in order to determine whether you require oxytocin to strengthen your contractions (see "Inducing labor" later in this chapter for more information). The monitor consists of thin, flexible, fluid-filled tubing, which is inserted between the fetal head and the uterine wall during an internal exam. Sometimes, this same device is used to infuse saline into the uterus — if very little amniotic fluid is present, if the fetal heart tracing indicates that the umbilical cord is getting compressed, or if very thick meconium is present.

Deciding whether to monitor your baby

Most hospitals, and most practitioners, have their own ways of deciding when it's time to place fetal monitors and which ones to place. Although some low-risk patients may require only intermittent monitoring, other patients are better off with continuous monitoring. Sometimes knowing whether it makes sense to use continuous monitoring isn't possible until you are in labor and your practitioner can see how the baby is responding.

Other tests of fetal health

If the information from the fetal monitor raises concerns or is ambiguous, your practitioner can perform other tests to help determine how to proceed with your labor.

Scalp pH

If your practitioner is concerned about how well the baby is tolerating labor, he or she may want to perform a *scalp pH test.* The pH is a measure of the degree of acidity in the baby's blood. Stressed babies have more acidic blood. This test is possible only if the membranes are ruptured and the cervix is dilated at least 1 to 2 centimeters — and if the hospital where you are laboring has a pH testing machine.

When conducting a scalp pH test, a plastic cone is inserted into the vagina so that a tiny portion of the fetal scalp becomes visible. The scalp is gently wiped with a swab and then pricked with a small blade (similar to the way you may have a blood sample taken in a doctor's office with the use of a finger stick), and a tiny sample of fetal blood is collected into a glass tube. The blood sample is put into a pH machine to find out how well the baby is tolerating labor.

Scalp stimulation

Scalp stimulation is an easy test to see how the fetus is doing. The practitioner simply tickles the baby's scalp during an internal exam. If this touch causes the fetal heart rate to increase, the baby is usually doing fine.

Our patients want to know . . .

Q: "Is there any correlation between monitoring and cesarean deliveries?"

A: Women sometimes ask whether monitoring increases the chance that they will need a cesarean or some other kind of intervention with their delivery, such as the use of forceps or a vacuum extractor. Studies conducted many years ago suggested a correlation between monitoring and the chance of having a cesarean delivery. But the procedure of monitoring itself does not increase any mother's need to have a cesarean; it can only alert her practitioner to potential problems, which may, in turn, alert the practitioner to the need for a cesarean.

The correlation between monitoring and cesarean deliveries may also have been stronger in the past when practitioners were more likely to resort to intervention at the first sign of trouble. Today, physicians have many more ways of responding to signs of possible trouble that monitors may pick up. So the correlation between monitoring and cesarean delivery is not as clear as it once was.

Some practitioners, and some mothers, prefer not to monitor. But most doctors believe that monitoring is very useful and that the benefits monitors provide outweigh any risk that monitoring may lead to an unnecessary cesarean delivery.

Inducing Labor

To *induce* labor means to cause it to begin before it starts on its own. Induction may be elective (performed for the convenience of the patient or her practitioner) or it may be a necessity (due to some obstetrical, medical, or fetal complications).

Elective induction

Although some women like the idea of a planned delivery, others prefer that labor occur spontaneously. Some practitioners gladly perform elective inductions, and others are opposed to the whole concept of it. A patient may choose to undergo an elective induction for several reasons, including the following:

- ✔ She may find it easier to make arrangements for her other children, for her work or her partner's work, or for the convenience of other family members if she knows exactly which day she's going into labor.

- ✔ She may want to ensure that a particular physician in a group practice, with whom she has developed a special relationship, delivers her baby.

- ✔ She may be at risk for certain neonatal or labor complications and need to deliver when the maximum number of labor floor personnel or other specialists are present.

✔ She may have a history of poor pregnancy outcome (such as a previous full-term fetal death), and anxiety over this past experience may make her want to deliver earlier than she naturally would.

✔ She may live far away from the hospital and have a history of rapid deliveries.

Some studies in the medical literature suggest that elective induction of labor may lead to an increase in cesarean deliveries. If the cervix is neither dilated nor *effaced* (thinned out) or if the fetal head is not engaged in the pelvis, the risk of a cesarean delivery is probably higher. But if all conditions are favorable for induction, the risk of cesarean may not be increased at all. However, the length of time that the patient spends in the hospital probably does increase slightly when labor is induced.

If an elected induction of labor is planned for a woman who is less than 39 weeks along in her pregnancy, an amniocentesis to check fetal lung maturity is usually required. If you are considering elective induction of labor, you and your partner should fully understand that you may stand a slightly increased risk of needing a cesarean delivery. If both the expectant parents and the practitioner involved understand these risks, elective induction of labor can be appropriate for personal, medical, geographical, or psychological reasons.

Indicated induction

An induction is *indicated* (becomes a medical necessity) when the risks of continuing the pregnancy — for the mother or the baby — are greater than the risks of early delivery.

Problems with the mother's health that may warrant induction include

✔ Preeclampsia (see Chapter 14 for more information).

✔ The presence of certain diseases, such as diabetes or cholestasis (see Chapter 14), which may improve after delivery.

✔ An infection in the amniotic fluid, such as chorioamnionitis.

✔ Fetal death.

Potential risks to the baby's health that may warrant induction include

✔ The continuation of the pregnancy well past the due date.

✔ The membranes have ruptured but labor hasn't yet started, a situation that may place the baby at risk for developing an infection.

✔ Intrauterine growth restriction (see Chapter 14).

✔ Suspected *macrosomia* (large fetus).

✔ Rh incompatibility with complications (see Chapter 14).

✔ Decreased amniotic fluid (*oligohydramnios*).

✔ Tests of fetal well-being indicate that the fetus may not be thriving in the uterus.

Inducing labor

The way in which labor is induced depends upon the condition of the cervix. If your cervix is not favorable, or *ripe* (thinned out, soft, and dilated), various medications and techniques may be used to ripen it. Occasionally, this technique alone may put you right into labor.

The most common agent used for cervical ripening is a type of *prostaglandin* (a substance that helps soften cervical tissue and cause contractions), administered either as a gel or a tablet. The prostaglandin is placed into the vagina, and it may also cause mild contractions. Some practitioners prefer to use what's called a *Foley balloon,* a tiny balloon that is placed in the cervix through the vagina and inflated with saline or air to help the cervix open up.

If your cervix is not yet ripe and you require induction, you are likely to be admitted to the hospital in the evening and given medications to ripen the cervix at bedtime. Then *oxytocin* (a synthetic hormone similar to one that your body naturally releases during labor) can be administered to induce labor in the morning.

If you require induction and your cervix is already ripe, you are likely to be admitted in the morning, and labor is induced either by administering oxytocin intravenously or by rupturing your membranes (often called *breaking your water*). An *amniotomy,* or rupturing of the membranes, is done with a small plastic hook during an internal examination. This procedure is usually not especially painful.

Your practitioner instructs your nurse to administer oxytocin (usually known by its brand name, Pitocin) through an IV, and a special pump carefully adjusts and controls the dosage. You begin with very little medication, and then the level of medication increases at regular intervals until you have adequate contractions. Sometimes labor starts within a few hours after the induction is started, or it may take much longer. Occasionally, it may take as long as two days to really get things going.

A common misconception is that oxytocin makes labor more painful. It does not. Oxytocin is similar to the hormone that your body naturally releases during labor, and it is administered in about the same doses that your body would produce to cause normal labor.

Augmenting labor

Oxytocin also may be used to augment labor that is already happening. If your contractions are thought to be inadequate or if labor is taking an unusually long time, your practitioner may use oxytocin to help move things along. Again, the contractions produced as a result of this augmentation are no stronger and no more painful than contractions that occur during a spontaneous labor.

The Stages of Labor

Each woman's labor is, in some ways, unique. One individual woman's experience may even vary from pregnancy to pregnancy. Anyone who delivers babies knows all too well that labor can always surprise you. As doctors, we may expect a woman to deliver quickly and find that her labor takes a long time, and those who we think will take forever sometimes deliver very rapidly. Still, in the vast majority of pregnant women, labor progresses in a predictable pattern. It passes through easily discernible stages at a fairly standard rate.

Your practitioner can track your progress through labor by performing internal exams every few hours. How easily you progress through labor is measured by how quickly your cervix dilates and how smoothly the fetus descends downward through the pelvis and birth canal. By plotting cervical dilation and fetal *station* (see the section on false and true labor earlier in this chapter for more information) along a graph, practitioners can measure the progress of labor objectively. Your practitioner may track your progress through labor using a special graph, called a labor curve (shown in Figure 8-5), to illustrate how the labor is progressing by comparing your progress to a standard curve representing the average labor.

Doctors become concerned over the progress of labor if it is too slow or if the cervix stops dilating and the fetus doesn't descend. They have a shorthand system for describing the variables that determine how easily a woman makes her way through labor: the three Ps (passenger, pelvis, and power). In other words, the size and position of the baby (the passenger), the size of the pelvis, and the strength of contractions (the power) are all important factors. Your practitioner must pay attention to all of these factors, because if labor does *not* progress normally, it may be a sign that the baby would be better off delivered with assistance — with forceps or vacuum, or by cesarean delivery.

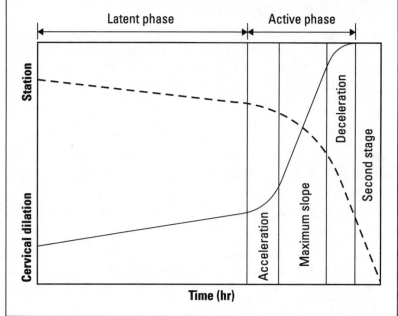

Figure 8-5:
Your practitioner may use a labor curve to track your progress.

If you are going through your first delivery (that is, you are what's known as a *nullipara*), the entire labor process is likely to last between 12 and 14 hours. For deliveries after the first one (for *multiparas*), labor is usually shorter (about 8 hours). Labor is divided into three stages:

- ✔ **The first stage** occurs from the onset of true labor to full dilation of the cervix. This stage takes an average of 11 hours for a first child and 7 hours for subsequent births.

- ✔ **The second stage** occurs from the point of full dilation of the cervix to delivery of the infant. This stage takes about 1 hour for a first child and 30 to 40 minutes for subsequent births. The second stage may be longer if you have an epidural.

- ✔ **The third stage** occurs from the time of delivery of the baby to delivery of the placenta — usually less than 20 minutes for all deliveries.

The first stage

The first stage of labor is by far the longest, and it is divided into three phases: the early (latent) phase, the active phase, and the transition phase. Each phase has its own unique characteristics.

Early or latent phase

During the early phase of the first stage of labor, contractions occur every 5 to 20 minutes in the beginning, and they increase in frequency until they are less than 5 minutes apart. The contractions last between 30 and 45 seconds at first, but as the first phase continues, they work up to 60 to 90 seconds in length. During the early phase, your cervix gradually dilates to 3 to 4 centimeters and becomes 100 percent effaced (thinned out).

The entire early phase of the first stage of labor lasts an average of 6 to 7 hours in a first birth and 4 to 5 hours for subsequent births. But the length of labor is unpredictable, because knowing when labor actually begins is difficult.

In the beginning of the early phase, your contractions may feel like menstrual cramps, with or without back pain. Your membranes may rupture, and you may have a bloody show (see the section on early symptoms of labor earlier in this chapter). If you have been admitted to the hospital, your doctor may use a small plastic hook to rupture your membranes for you, in order to help things along.

Early on in this phase, you may be most comfortable at home. You can try resting or sleeping, or you may want to stay active. Some women find that they have an overwhelming desire to clean or to perform some other house-hold chores. If you're hungry, eat a light meal (soup, juice, or toast, for example), but not a very heavy one — in case you later need anesthesia to deal with labor complications. You may want to time your contractions, but you don't need to be obsessive about it.

If you start to become more uncomfortable, the contractions occur with more frequency or intensity, or your membranes rupture (your water breaks), call your practitioner.

Many women find that walking around makes them more comfortable and distracts them from the pain during the early part of labor. Others prefer to rest in bed. Ask your practitioner whether your hospital has any restrictions on walking during labor.

Active phase

The active phase of labor is usually shorter and more predictable than the early phase. For a first child, it usually lasts 5 hours, on average. For subsequent babies, it lasts about 4 hours. Contractions occur in this phase every 3 to 5 minutes, and they last about 45 to 60 seconds. Your cervix dilates from 4 to 8 or 9 centimeters.

You may feel increasing discomfort or pain during this phase, and maybe a backache as well. By this time, you are likely already in the hospital or birthing center. Some patients prefer to rest in bed; others would rather walk around. Do whatever makes *you* comfortable, unless your practitioner asks that you stay in bed to be monitored closely. This is the time to use the breathing and relaxation techniques you may have practiced in childbirth classes.

If you need pain relief, let your practitioner know (for more information on pain relief, see later in this chapter). Your partner may help ease your pain by massaging your back, perhaps by using a tennis ball or rolling pin if you have one.

Above all, dad, you can be patient and understanding. The mother-to-be may, out of anxiety, fear, or pain, become somewhat angry or short-tempered — this reaction is completely normal during labor. You can help her use her breathing exercises and relaxation techniques. You can also help by

- ✔ Reassuring her that everything is going well
- ✔ Understanding when she gets frustrated or short-tempered
- ✔ Empathizing with her
- ✔ Distracting her (with games, humor, and so on)
- ✔ Helping to communicate her needs to the professional staff at the hospital or birthing center

Transition phase

Many practitioners consider the transition period as part of the active phase, but we prefer to label it separately. During the transition phase, contractions occur every 2 to 3 minutes and last about 60 seconds. The contractions during this phase are very intense. Your cervix dilates from 8 or 9 to 10 centimeters.

In addition to very intense contractions, you may notice an increase in bloody show and increased pressure, especially on your rectum, as the baby's head descends. During this last phase of the first stage of labor, you may feel as if you have to have a bowel movement. Don't worry; this sensation is a *good* sign and indicates that the fetus is heading in the right direction.

You may start to get frustrated or want to give up at this point, but remember, it's almost over!

If you feel the urge to push, let your practitioner know. You may be fully dilated, but try not to push until you are told to do so. Pushing before you're fully dilated can slow the labor process or tear your cervix.

Try to practice breathing exercises and relaxation techniques, if they work for you. When you want pain medication or an epidural anesthetic (both described later in this chapter), let your practitioner know. He or she decides which pain relief options are best for you based on how far along in labor you are and on other factors related to your and your baby's health.

During this phase of your labor, you can do a few things to help the mother-to-be:

✔ Be understanding.

✔ Promise her some expensive jewelry.

✔ Tell her she can name the baby whatever she wants.

✔ Promise to do all the cooking and cleaning for the next year.

✔ Do whatever she says, even if she tells you to shut up.

✔ Hold her hand.

✔ Feed her ice chips if her practitioner says it's okay.

Potential problems during the first stage of labor

Most women experience the first stage of labor without any problems. But if a problem arises, the following information prepares you with the information you need to handle it with a clear, focused mind.

Prolonged latent phase

The latent or early phase of labor is considered prolonged if it lasts more than 20 hours in a woman having her first child or more than 14 hours in someone who has delivered a previous child. Your practitioner may not be able to determine when labor actually starts, so knowing for sure when labor becomes prolonged also isn't always easy to determine.

When a practitioner determines that the labor is taking too long, he or she responds in one of two ways. One approach is to use medication, such as a sedative, to help you relax. In some cases, labor may then subside (which means that it was false labor all along), or active labor may begin. The other approach is to try to move labor along by performing an *amniotomy* (rupturing the membranes or breaking your water) or by administering oxytocin (Pitocin). Both procedures are covered in more detail earlier in this chapter.

Protraction disorders

Protraction disorders can occur if the cervix dilates too slowly or if the baby's head does not descend at a normal rate. For women who are having their first baby, the cervix should dilate at a *minimum* rate of 1.2 centimeters an hour, and the baby's head should descend about 1 centimeter an hour. For those who have delivered previously, the cervix should dilate at least 1.5 centimeters an hour, and the baby's head should descend about 2 centimeters an hour.

Protraction disorders may be caused by *cephalopelvic disproportion* (CPD), which is the name for a poor fit between the baby's head and the mother's birth canal. Protraction disorders may also occur because the baby's head is in an unfavorable position or because the number or intensity of contractions is inadequate. In both cases, many practitioners try administering oxytocin to improve labor progress.

Arrest disorders

Arrest disorders occur if the cervix stops dilating or if the baby's head stops descending for more than two hours during active labor. Arrest disorders are often associated with CPD (see the preceding section, "Protraction disorders"), but an infusion of oxytocin may solve the problem. If oxytocin does not alleviate the arrest disorder, you may need a cesarean section.

The second stage

The second stage of labor begins when you are fully dilated (at 10 centimeters) and ends with delivery of your baby. This is the "pushing" stage and, although technically it is part of labor, it is described in detail in Chapter 9.

The third stage

The third stage begins when the baby is out and ends with the delivery of the placenta. We go into more detail about this stage in Chapter 9.

Other Concerns, Worries, and Labor-Related Questions You May Have

As you probably already know from listening to your friends and relatives, each woman's labor is unpredictable and rarely does it progress just exactly as her best friend's or her sister's did. In this section, we describe some conditions that may or may not happen to you.

- **Back labor:** Some women experience most of their labor pain in the back, rather than in the abdomen. This pain is called *back labor,* and it occurs most commonly if the baby is in a position called *occiput posterior* (refer to Figure 8-2c), in which the back of the baby's head (the *occiput*) presses against the mother's lower spine. If you experience back labor, you may find some relief from the pain by changing your position (getting on all fours, squatting, or walking around, for example). Also try having your partner massage your lower back or apply heat or cold to it. If back labor becomes very uncomfortable, you may want to ask your practitioner for pain medication or an epidural. Often, as labor progresses, the baby's head rotates and the pain decreases.

- **Meconium:** *Meconium* is your baby's first bowel movement. This bowel movement usually happens after the baby is born, but 2 to 20 percent of babies pass meconium during labor, most commonly if they are born past their due date. If your water breaks spontaneously (without the help of your practitioner), you may notice that the fluid is greenish-brown in color rather than clear. Let your practitioner know if this happens. If your practitioner ruptures your membranes for you, he or she checks to see whether meconium is present. This color doesn't necessarily indicate that anything is wrong, but it can occasionally be associated with fetal stress. To be on the safe side in this situation, you and the baby should be closely monitored at the hospital.

✔ **Enemas:** Years ago, enemas were routinely administered to women in early labor. These days, an enema usually is not part of any practitioner's standard labor protocol. Still, some women prefer to have an enema because they don't want the embarrassment of having a bowel movement during labor. If you feel this way, you can ask for an enema at the hospital, or you can give yourself a warm-water enema in the comfort and privacy of your own home before going to the hospital.

✔ **Shaving:** Shaving the pubic area used to be a routine procedure during labor, but it is rarely done today. There is no medical reason for shaving the pubic area. Sometimes before a cesarean delivery, the doctor may shave a small portion of the pubic hair that grows along the area where the incision is made in order to keep the hair away from the incision when your doctor is sewing it up.

✔ **Routine IVs:** An IV is a small catheter, attached to plastic tubing, that is inserted into a vein and through which fluids and medications can be administered. In some hospitals, IVs are routinely started upon admission to the hospital. In other hospitals, IVs are not used until later on in labor. Some hospitals may not require an IV at all. Your practitioner knows the protocol at your hospital, so if you want more information on this matter, be sure to ask him or her. A major advantage to having an IV is that if complications arise suddenly, they can be treated immediately without waiting the time it takes to put the IV in place.

If you do need an IV (as many women do), don't worry — it isn't particularly uncomfortable.

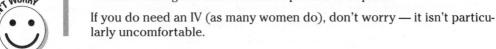

Managing the Pain of Labor

During the first stage of labor, pain is caused by contractions of the uterus and dilation of the cervix. The pain may feel like severe menstrual cramps at first. But in the second stage of labor, the stretching of the birth canal as the baby passes through it adds a different kind of pain — often a great feeling of pressure on the lower pelvis or rectum. But none of this pain needs to be excruciating, thanks to well-practiced breathing and relaxation exercises and, in many cases, modern techniques of anesthesia.

Most practitioners acknowledge that even for women who have diligently attended childbirth classes, labor is inherently painful. The degree of pain varies from woman to woman, as does the willingness and ability to tolerate pain. Some women choose to deal with the pain on their own or with the help of breathing and distraction techniques learned in childbirth classes — and that's a perfectly acceptable choice. Many other women want medication to help them deal with the pain, no matter how well prepared they are.

Do not feel that you are in any way falling short of being a perfect mother or that your pregnancy is not "natural" if you need medication to help with labor pain. We all respond to pain differently, both emotionally *and* physiologically, so even if your best friend, your sister, or your mother got through labor with little or no pain medication, you aren't weak if you choose to use it. Look at it this way: Women who are in excruciating pain usually don't breathe regularly. They also tense their muscles, and by doing so, they may only prolong labor. They also often thrash around, making monitoring the baby difficult.

In the past, many women were put under general anesthesia during the late stages of labor, but doctors rarely use that technique anymore. Today doctors generally can administer medication in two different ways to help you deal with labor pain: *systemically* — that is, by injection either into a blood vessel (intravenously) or into a muscle (intramuscularly) — or *regionally*, with the use of an epidural or other local anesthesia.

Systemic medications

The most common medications used systemically are relatives of the narcotic morphine — drugs such as meperidine (brand name Demerol), fentanyl (Sublimaze), butorphanal (Stadol), and nalbuphine (Nubain). These medications can be given every 2 to 4 hours as needed, either intravenously or intramuscularly. Giving them intravenously brings pain relief more quickly (often in five to ten minutes). But when the medicine is given intravenously, the pain relief doesn't last as long as it would if the medication were injected into a muscle. Also, providing medication intravenously is sometimes associated with a greater drop in blood pressure. Intramuscular injections give longer-lasting pain relief, because the medication is released into the circulating blood more slowly. But you may need to wait as long as 20 or 30 minutes before you feel any relief from pain. Many doctors use a combination of the two methods in order to provide both fast-acting and long-lasting pain relief.

Doctors often give pain medication along with promethazine (brand name Phenergan) or hydroxyzine (Vistaril) to limit the nausea and vomiting that these medications can cause. These extra medications also help prolong and enhance the painkiller's effect.

Any medication you take (even when you're not pregnant) has side effects, and pain relievers used during labor are no exception. Nausea, vomiting, drowsiness, and a drop in your blood pressure are the main side effects for the mother. The degree to which the fetus or newborn is also affected depends on how close to the time of delivery the medication is given. If a large dose is given within two hours prior to delivery, the newborn may be sleepy or groggy. In rare cases, his or her breathing may be weak. If this problem is significant, your doctor or the baby's doctor can give a medication that immediately reverses or counteracts the pain medication. There is no evidence to suggest that these medications, when given in appropriate doses and with proper monitoring, have any effect on the progress of labor or on the rate of cesarean deliveries.

Regional anesthetics

Systemic medications are distributed via the bloodstream to all parts of the body. Yet most of the pain of labor and delivery is concentrated in the uterus, vagina, and rectum. So regional anesthesia is sometimes used to deliver pain medication to those specific areas, rather than using systemic medication that affects the entire body. Regional anesthetics are a bit like getting a shot of painkiller in your gums when you go to the dentist. Medications used in regional anesthesia can be a local anesthetic (like lidocaine), a narcotic (such as those mentioned in the preceding section), or a combination of the two. Commonly used techniques for administering regional pain relief include epidural and spinal anesthesia and caudal, saddle, and pudendal blocks.

Epidural anesthesia

Epidural anesthesia is perhaps the most popular form of pain relief for labor. And almost universally, women who have had it say, "Why didn't I get this earlier?" or "Why was I hesitant about this?" An epidural must be administered by an anesthesiologist with special training in epidural catheter placement, so epidurals may not be available in every hospital.

In an epidural, a tiny, flexible, plastic catheter is inserted through a needle into your lower back and threaded into the space above the membrane covering the spinal cord. Before inserting the needle, the anesthesiologist numbs your skin with a local anesthetic. While the needle is going in, you may feel a brief tingling sensation in your legs. Most women find that having an epidural placed isn't really a painful process at all. After the catheter is in place, medication can be sent through it to numb the nerves coming from the lower part of the spine — nerves that go to the uterus, vagina, and perineum. The catheter (not the needle) stays in place throughout labor in case you need what's called a *top up* dose of the anesthetic to get you through the rest of labor and delivery.

A major advantage of epidural anesthesia is that smaller doses of pain medication are needed. However, because your sensory nerves run very close to your motor nerves, large doses of anesthetic can temporarily affect your ability to move your legs during labor.

The amount and type of medication you need can be adjusted according to the particular stage of labor you're in. During the first stage, pain relief focuses on uterine contractions, but during the second (pushing) stage, pain relief focuses on the vagina and perineum, which are distended by the baby passing through.

Years ago, anesthesiologists would not give epidurals during early labor because it confined patients to their beds for the remainder of their labor. Recently, however, *walking epidurals* — the kind that allow you to walk around, because they use medications that have little or no effect on motor function — have become more popular for this often painful stage of labor. Some anesthesiologists, however, question the effectiveness of this type of epidural in relieving pain.

Epidurals can also relieve pain in cesarean deliveries, although different medications in different doses are used. In fact, epidurals are very popular for cesareans because they enable the mother to be awake during her delivery, to experience the birth of her child. Not everyone who needs a cesarean can get an epidural, however. In cases in which cesarean delivery is an emergency or when the mother has blood clotting problems, an epidural may not be possible.

Epidurals, especially if they were placed too early, were once thought to prolong labor and increase the need for forceps, vacuum-assisted, or cesarean delivery. For this reason, many practitioners were reluctant to recommend epidurals to their patients. Most doctors today, however, accept that these problems are negligible when the epidural is placed by an experienced anesthesiologist after labor is well-established, and that the benefit outweighs the risk.

Sometimes the epidural takes away the sensation you feel when your bladder is full, so you may need a catheter to empty your bladder. In some cases, the epidural may block motor nerves to the point where you have difficulty pushing. You also may experience a rapid drop in blood pressure that can lead to a temporary drop in the baby's heart rate. A rare complication (occurring in less than 2 percent of epidurals) is a postpartum spinal headache, caused by inadvertent puncturing of the spinal cord membranes during epidural placement. Again, if the epidural is placed by an experienced anesthesiologist, these problems are less likely.

Overall, pain control simply makes the whole experience of labor and delivery much more enjoyable for the mother and her partner (and the person doing the delivery, too!). We definitely favor epidurals for pain management. In fact, when she was pregnant, Joanne joked that she wanted hers placed at 35 weeks as a preventive measure, so she wouldn't feel *any* pain.

Spinal anesthesia

Spinal anesthesia is similar to an epidural but different in that the medication is injected into the space *under* the membrane covering the spinal cord, rather than above it. This technique is often used for cesarean delivery, especially when a cesarean is needed suddenly and no epidural was placed during labor. The information provided in the preceding section about epidurals (regarding the amount of medication needed and the risks involved) applies to spinal anesthesia, too.

Caudal and saddle blocks

Caudal blocks (so called because they are placed in the *caudal* or lower part of the spinal canal) and saddle blocks (so called because the area that is anesthetized is the same area of your legs and groin that comes in contact with a saddle when you sit in it) involve placing the medications very low in the spinal canal, so that they affect only those pain nerves going to the vagina and perineum (the area between the vagina and anus). These methods have a more rapid onset of pain relief, but the relief wears off sooner. Placing these blocks also requires significant expertise on the part of the anesthesiologist, and they are not available everywhere.

Pudendal blocks

Your doctor can place a pudendal block by injecting an anesthetic inside the vagina, in the area next to the pudendal nerves. This technique numbs part of the vagina and the perineum, but it does nothing to relieve the pain from contractions.

General anesthesia

When you have general anesthesia, you are made fully unconscious by an anesthesiologist using a variety of medications. Doctors almost never use this technique for labor anymore, and it is only rarely used for cesarean deliveries because it is associated with a higher risk of complications. General anesthesia obviously also causes you to sleep through the delivery of your baby. But if, in a cesarean delivery, you have a clotting problem that rules out placing a needle into your spinal column or if the cesarean is an emergency and there isn't enough time to place an epidural, general anesthesia should be used.

Alternative forms of labor-pain management

Many women use various forms of nonmedical pain management to make their way through labor. Some women, for example, try hypnosis, which uses the power of suggestion to induce a state of altered awareness in which it's easier for the body to deal with pain. This state can be induced by a person trained in hypnosis, and some patients can be taught self-hypnosis.

However, a great deal of preparation and training is needed in the weeks prior to labor in order to achieve true pain relief through hypnosis, and it doesn't work for everyone. Unfortunately, only about one in every four or five individuals has the high level of suggestibility needed to achieve hypnosis. And if hypnosis is used inappropriately, it can be counterproductive.

Other methods of alternative pain management include acupuncture, various kinds of herbs, and massage, including *reflexology,* a specific kind of foot massage. Many books on all these practices are available in libraries or bookstores. Or you may want to talk to someone who practices the specific technique you're interested in.

Chapter 9

Special Delivery!

*W*hen you reach the end of the second stage of labor, you are very, very close to the point of delivery. Now is the time you've been waiting and preparing yourself for. Keep in mind that there's little need to worry too much ahead of time. You *can* prepare yourself — by taking childbirth classes and by reading this book, for example. And remember that your practitioner and his or her assistants in the delivery room guide you through the process. It's time to accept and rely on their help. It's also time to trust in yourself and let this natural process move along one step at a time. In this chapter, we describe the basic process of childbirth, both the traditional kind and cesarean delivery, to try to give you a clear and fairly detailed idea of what's going to happen.

Basically, babies are delivered in one of three ways: through the birth canal by your pushing, through the birth canal with a little assistance (that is, using forceps or a vacuum extractor), or by cesarean delivery. The method that's right for you depends on many different factors, including your medical history, the baby's condition, and the size of your pelvis relative to the size of your baby.

Having a Vaginal Delivery

Most expectant mothers spend a great deal of time during the 40 weeks of pregnancy thinking ahead to the actual delivery. If you are having a baby for the first time, it may seem pretty scary. Even if you have had a child before, it's normal to worry a bit until you see your beautiful baby. A little knowledge goes a long way, though, and being informed and prepared for all possibilities is always helpful.

The most common method of delivery is, of course, a vaginal delivery (Figure 9-1 gives you an overview of the process). Most likely, you'll experience what doctors call a *spontaneous vaginal delivery,* which means that it occurs as a result of your pushing efforts and proceeds without needing a great deal of intervention. If you do need a little help, it may come in the form of forceps or a vacuum extractor. A delivery requiring the use of one of these tools to help pull the baby out is called an *operative vaginal delivery.* We cover both courses of events in this chapter.

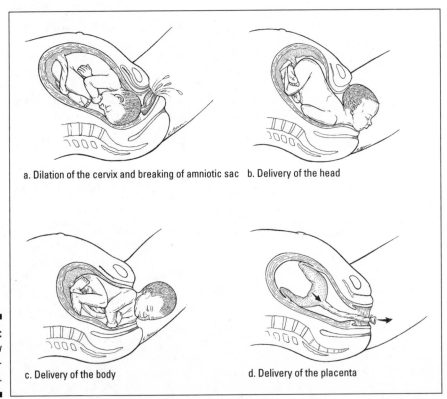

a. Dilation of the cervix and breaking of amniotic sac   b. Delivery of the head

Figure 9-1:
An overview
of the deliv-
ery process.

c. Delivery of the body   d. Delivery of the placenta

During the first stage of labor, your cervix dilates and your membranes rupture. When your cervix is fully *dilated* (open to 10 centimeters), you reach the end of the first stage of labor and are ready to enter the second stage, in which you push your baby through the birth canal (vagina) and actually deliver it. At the end of the first stage, you may feel an overwhelming sensation of pressure on your rectum. You may feel as if you need to have a bowel movement. This sensation is likely to be greatest during contractions. It's caused by the baby's head descending in the birth canal and putting pressure on neighboring internal organs. If you have an epidural (see Chapter 8), you may not feel this pressure, or the feeling may be less intense. If you do feel it, let your nurse or practitioner know, because it's probably a sign that your cervix is getting close to being fully dilated and that it may be time for you to push. Your nurse or doctor performs an internal exam to confirm that your cervix is fully dilated. If it is, he or she tells you to start pushing.

Note: Whether your nurse or doctor or midwife is actually coaching you during pushing varies from hospital to hospital and from practitioner to practitioner. The important thing is that someone is with you to help you through this stage of labor.

Occasionally, you may be fully dilated when the fetal head is still relatively high up in the pelvis. In this case, your practitioner may want you to wait until the contractions make the head descend more before you start to push.

Pushing the baby out

Pushing generally takes 30 to 90 minutes (though sometimes it takes as long as three hours), depending on the baby's position and size, whether you have an epidural, and whether you've had children before. Your nurse or practitioner gives you specific instructions on how to push. While you are pushing, your baby moves farther along its downward course. Women often begin pushing when the baby's head is at a station (see Chapter 7 for an explanation of *station*) of –1 or zero (mid-range), and pushing continues until the baby is at the lowest station — +3 or +5 (depending on which scale your practitioner uses). After you're at this stage, you can usually deliver the baby's head with one or two additional pushes. Then, after the baby's mouth is suctioned, the body usually comes out easily with one more push.

You have several possible positions in which to push (see Figure 9-2). The most common is the *lithotomy position.* In this position, you lean back and pull your flexed knees to your chest. At the same time, you bend your neck and try to touch your chin to your chest. The idea is to get your body to form a C. It's not the most flattering position in the world, but it does help to align the uterus and pelvis in a position that makes delivery relatively easy.

Other positions that may work are the squatting or knee-chest variations. The advantage of squatting is that you have gravity working with you. A disadvantage is that you may be too tired to hold the position for very long, and any monitoring equipment or an intravenous line you may have can be cumbersome. The knee-chest position is one in which you push while on all fours. This position is sometimes helpful if the baby's head is rotated in the birth canal in such a way that makes pushing the baby out in the lithotomy or squatting positions difficult. The knee-chest position may be awkward for some, however, and difficult to stay in for very long. Finding the one that feels best and works best for you may take a bit of experimentation.

If you find that you're not making progress, try changing positions.

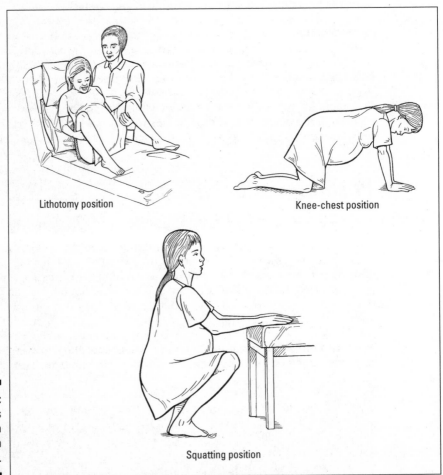

Figure 9-2:
Positions
you can
assume in
childbirth.

Lithotomy position

Knee-chest position

Squatting position

When you start to feel a contraction, your nurse or doctor probably tells you to take a deep, cleansing breath. After that, you inhale deeply again, hold in the air, and push like crazy. Focus the push toward your rectum and *perineum* (the area between the vagina and the rectum), trying not to tense up the muscles of your vagina or rectum. Push like you're having a bowel movement. Don't worry or be embarrassed if you pass stool while you're pushing. (If it happens, a nurse quickly cleans the perineum.) It's the rule rather than the exception, and all the people helping to take care of you have seen it many times before. In fact, passing stool is a sign that you're pushing correctly, so congratulate yourself. Trying to hold it in only impedes your efforts to push the baby out.

Try not to talk or groan during your push; when you do, some of the energy that would otherwise be available for pushing escapes. Also, try to focus your energy into the pelvic or rectal area, rather than wasting it on making faces or grimacing.

Try to hold each push for about ten seconds. Many nurses count to ten or ask your coach to count to ten to help you judge the time. After the count of ten, quickly release the breath you have been holding, take in another deep breath, and push again for another ten seconds, exactly as before. You probably push about three times with each contraction, depending on the length of the contraction.

Between contractions, try your best to relax and rest so that you can get ready for the next one. If it's okay with your practitioner, your coach may give you some ice chips or pat your forehead with a damp, cool cloth.

For the fathers-to-be, you can do a lot to help your partner through this stage:

✔ Help her count to ten during pushes.

✔ If necessary, let her know when a contraction is starting. (You can tell by watching the monitor.)

✔ Lift up her legs or hold her head forward, chin to chest. This position makes the pushes more efficient.

✔ Do whatever she asks to make her more comfortable. Offer to dab her forehead with a moist cloth if that makes her feel better.

✔ Be supportive and encouraging.

Some partners want to see everything that's happening; others feel uncomfortable even being in the delivery room. Likewise, some women want their partners to witness everything, and others prefer that their partners not see them in this situation. However you or your partner feel about it, communicate your feelings to each other so that you can make each other feel as comfortable as possible. The last thing you need is for you or your partner to be embarrassed during a time that should be one of joy and happiness.

After your baby gets far enough down the birth canal, the top of the head becomes visible during your pushing efforts. This first glimpse is called *crowning* because your practitioner can see the crown of the baby's head. Some labor rooms have mirrors so that you, too, can see the head crowning, but many women have no desire to look. (Don't feel bad or somehow inadequate if you don't want to — you're busy enough.) After the contraction, the baby's head may again disappear back up into the birth canal. This retraction is normal. With each push, the baby comes down a little farther and recedes a little less afterward.

Getting an episiotomy

Just before it's born, the baby's head distends the *perineum* (the area between the vagina and the rectum) and stretches the skin around the vagina. As the baby's head comes through the opening of the vagina, it may tear the tissues in the back, or *posterior,* part of the vaginal opening, sometimes even to the point that the tear extends into the rectum. To minimize tearing of the surrounding skin and perineal muscles, your practitioner may make an *episiotomy* — a cut in the posterior part of the vaginal opening large enough to allow the baby's head to come through with minimal tearing or to provide extra room for delivery. Although an episiotomy decreases the likelihood of a severe tear, it doesn't guarantee that you won't get one (that is, the cut made for the episiotomy may tear open even further as the baby's head is delivered).

Whether you need an episiotomy can't be known until the head is almost out. Some doctors routinely make episiotomies, and others wait to see whether it's definitely necessary. Episiotomies are more common in women having their first baby than in those who have delivered before.

The type of episiotomy made may depend on your body, on the position of the baby's head, or on the judgment of your practitioner. Two main types of episiotomy are used — *median* and *mediolateral* (see Figure 9-3). A local anesthetic can be used to numb the area if you haven't had an epidural.

A median episiotomy may be less uncomfortable later on, and it may heal more easily. (See Chapter 10 for more coverage of the care and healing of episiotomy repairs.) However, this kind of episiotomy has a slightly greater chance of extending to the rectum. A mediolateral episiotomy, on the other hand, may be more uncomfortable, but it has less chance of extending to the rectum when the baby's head passes through.

Prolonged second stage

If you are having your first child and you remain in the second stage of labor for more than 2 hours (or 3 hours if you have an epidural), the labor is

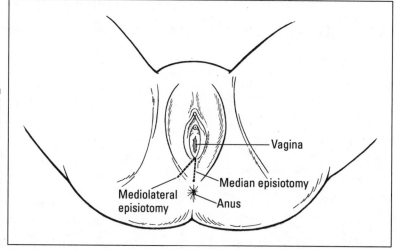

Figure 9-3:
The two
types of epi-
siotomies
most often
used are
known as
median and
mediolateral.

Vagina

Median episiotomy

Mediolateral
episiotomy

Anus

considered prolonged. If you are having your second or subsequent child, a second stage nearing 1 hour (or 2 hours if you have an epidural) is also considered prolonged.

A prolonged second stage may be due to inadequate contractions or to cephalopelvic disproportion (see Chapter 8). Sometimes, the baby's head is in a position that blocks further descent. Oxytocin (Pitocin) may help, or your practitioner may try to rotate the baby's head. You may also try changing your position to push more effectively. Sometimes forceps do the trick (see "Having an Operative Vaginal Delivery," later in this chapter) if the baby's head is low enough in the birth canal. If all else fails, your doctor may recommend a cesarean delivery.

Delivery at last!

When the baby's head remains visible between contractions, your nurse helps get you into position to deliver. If you're laboring in a birthing room, all that needs to be done is to remove the platform at the foot of your bed and set up padded leg supports. If you need to be moved to a delivery room (more like an operating room), your nurse moves you and all your monitors to a stretcher. Whether you deliver in a birthing room or a delivery room depends both on the facility where you have your baby and on any risk factors you may have.

After you're in position to deliver, you still have to keep pushing with each of your contractions. Your doctor or nurse cleans your perineum, usually with an iodine solution, and places drapes over your legs to keep the area as clean as possible for the newborn. As you are pushing, your perineum is getting

Our patients want to know . . .

Q: "Do I really need an episiotomy?"

A: The answer to this question depends on many factors, including the point of view of your practitioner. It's an issue of frequent debate among people who deliver babies. And, as you may already know, it's also a big topic of discussion among pregnant women. Many practitioners believe that repairing a controlled cut in the perineum is easier than repairing any uncontrolled tear through the skin and perineal muscles that may occur without an episiotomy. The same people usually contend that episiotomies heal better, too. It's true that it's usually easier to see the layers of tissue in a cut than in a tear, but whether that makes any difference is the point of contention. Compounding the issue is the fact that it's difficult to tell *before* labor whether the patient will need an episiotomy.

As we've said, the baby's head stretches the opening to the vagina when the mother pushes. Many times the birth canal stretches enough that the baby's head doesn't need the extra room that an episiotomy provides. Then again, sometimes it doesn't. If you are able to "hold" the head at the perineum to let additional stretching occur, you may help matters. But holding the head there is easier said than done because of the incredible pressure that the baby's head exerts. One potential advantage of epidurals is that they allow for a slower delivery of the head and therefore reduces the chances that you'll need an episiotomy.

In some special situations, the extra room that an episiotomy provides is crucial — especially for delivery of a very large infant or for *operative* deliveries (ones that use forceps or vacuum), where there may not be enough time for the perineum to stretch adequately.

more and more stretched out. Whether or not you need an episiotomy is usually determined at the final moments. If it seems that you will otherwise tear the perineum or rectal area, your practitioner will probably decide to make an episiotomy. For more information about episiotomies, see the preceding section of this chapter.

With each push, the baby's head descends farther and farther until finally, it comes out of the birth canal. After the baby's head delivers, your practitioner tells you to stop pushing so that he or she can suction secretions from the baby's mouth and nose before the rest of the body comes out.

To stop pushing at this point can be difficult because of the intense pressure in your perineal area; panting may make it a little easier not to push. If you have an epidural, you may not feel this intense pressure.

Your practitioner also checks at this point to see whether the umbilical cord is wrapped around the baby's neck. A *nuchal cord,* as it's called, is actually quite common and almost always no need to worry. Your practitioner simply removes the loop from around the baby's neck before delivering the rest of the baby.

After suctioning the mouth and checking for a nuchal cord, your practitioner instructs you to push again to deliver the baby's body. Because the head is typically the widest part, delivery of the body is usually easier. When the whole body is out, the baby's mouth and nose are suctioned again.

Your baby's first cry

Shortly after delivery, the baby takes its first breath and begins to cry. This crying is what expands the baby's lungs and helps clear deeper secretions. In contrast to stereotype, most practitioners do not spank a baby after it's born, but instead use some other method to stimulate crying and breathing — rubbing the baby's back vigorously, for example, or tapping the bottom of the feet. Don't be surprised if your baby doesn't cry the very second after it's born. Often, several seconds, if not minutes, pass before the baby starts making that lovely sound!

Cutting the cord

The next step is to clamp and cut the umbilical cord. Some practitioners may offer your labor coach the opportunity to cut the cord — but your partner certainly doesn't have to and shouldn't if he or she doesn't want to. If having the opportunity to cut the cord is something you feel strongly about, let your practitioner know ahead of time.

After cutting the cord, your practitioner either lays your baby on your abdomen or hands the baby to your labor nurse to put under an infant warmer. The choice depends on your baby's condition, your doctor's or nurse's standard practice, and on the institutional policy where you're delivering. (See more on newborn care in Chapter 10.)

Appearance of the baby

Often a baby comes out covered with some blood or *vernix* (a thick, white substance). The nurse cleans the baby so that it looks more like what you might expect.

Depending on how your labor progressed and on how long you pushed, the baby may have a bit of a conehead (see Chapter 10 for an illustration). This conehead shape is very normal and goes away in one to two days. It happens as the baby's head molds to fit through the birth canal. The little knit caps that most babies wear to prevent heat loss often make the shape unnoticeable.

You can read more about the appearance of your new baby in Chapter 10.

Delivering the placenta

After the baby is born, the third stage of delivery begins — the delivery of the placenta, also known as the *afterbirth* (refer to Figure 9-1d). This stage lasts only about 5 to 15 minutes. You still have contractions, but they are much less intense. These contractions help separate the placenta from the wall of the uterus. After this separation occurs and the placenta reaches the opening of the vagina, you may be asked to give one more gentle push. Many women, exhilarated by and exhausted from the delivery, pay little attention to this part of the process and later on don't even remember it.

After the placenta is out, your practitioner inspects your cervix, vagina, and perineum for tears or damage and then repairs (with stitches) the episiotomy or any tears. (If you didn't have an epidural and you have sensation in your perineum, your practitioner may use a local anesthetic to numb the area before repairing it.)

These tears are graded, according to the degree of severity, from first- to fourth-degree:

- A *first-degree tear* involves only the skin and topmost tissue layers.

- A *second-degree tear* involves the same layers as in a first-degree plus the muscle layer below. This is the most common tear and almost always heals without a problem. When an episiotomy is done, the layers cut usually correspond to a second-degree tear.

- A *third-degree tear* includes all the layers in a second-degree tear and also indicates a tear into the *sphincter* muscle (a circular muscle that helps maintain rectal continence) surrounding the anus.

- A *fourth-degree tear* includes all the lower-degree tears but also indicates that the tear extends into the lining of the rectum.

Third- and fourth-degree tears are more uncomfortable during the healing process and may take longer to heal but usually leave no long-term problems. All perineal tears are sewn up in layers by your practitioner. If you need extra pain relief during the repair, he or she can give you a local anesthetic.

After the repair is done, your perineal area is cleaned, your legs are taken out of the leg supports, and you are given warm blankets. You may also continue to feel mild contractions; these contractions are normal and actually help to minimize bleeding.

Shaking after delivery

Almost immediately after delivery, most women start to shake uncontrollably. Your partner may think that you are cold and offer you a blanket. Blankets do help some women, but you really are not shivering because you're cold. The cause of this phenomenon is unclear, but it is nearly universal — even among women who have cesarean deliveries. Some women feel nervous about holding their babies because they are shaking so much. If you feel this way, let your partner or your nurse hold your baby until you feel up to it.

Our patients want to know . . .

Q: "Should I save my baby's umbilical cord blood?"

A: Umbilical cord blood is sometimes saved because it contains the kind of cells that can be used in a bone marrow transfusion. Bone marrow transfusions are performed to treat a variety of blood disorders, such as leukemia and some forms of severe anemia. The bone marrow cells that are actually needed are the so-called *stem cells.* When someone needs a bone marrow transfusion, finding a donor whose stem cells are compatible with those of the person needing the transplant is necessary. Because umbilical cord blood is a rich source of stem cells, saving this blood by freezing it has become a popular practice — for its future use for someone in the baby's family or anyone else who may need it.

Many people considering cord blood banking think that the potential benefit is for the child whose blood is banked — that is, the child may someday be able to use his or her own cells. However, it isn't clear at this time whether giving someone his or her own stem cells if he or she develops a problem requiring bone marrow transplantation is a good idea. The problem may have a genetic component that is present in the stem cells also.

Two kinds of agencies collect umbilical cord blood: large, nonprofit blood banking agencies such as the American Red Cross, and private corporations that specialize in storing cord blood for the use of individual families. The nonprofit agencies collect blood from as many deliveries as they can and store it so that anyone who needs a transplant has a greater likelihood of finding a match. In such cases, the donor (that is, the baby) has no absolute claim to the stored cells.

Companies that store cord blood for a profit, on the other hand, charge the parents a fee (currently around $1,500 at the time of delivery and then about $100 a year thereafter) to keep the blood until such time as someone chosen by the donor or the parents may need it. In these cases, the cord blood is considered the donor's property.

The advantage to the first approach is that enormous numbers of samples can be banked for anyone needing a transplant. The downside of donating to one of these agencies is that the blood may not be available should the donor or some other member of the donor's family need it later on. (Of course, you may be able to use other matching samples at the bank.) The advantage of the second approach is that the cells are available to your family at any time. The downside is the cost — especially when you consider that the likelihood that any of the donor's relatives will need such a transplant in their lifetimes is quite low. Also, no good evidence is available to suggest that stem cells still function well after they're stored (frozen) for many years. Many parents feel that the money can be invested more wisely in other ways.

The decision about cord blood banking is a personal one. If you plan to use a commercial for-profit agency, you should make plans well in advance of delivery. However, do not let advertisements aimed at persuading you to store your baby's cord blood make you feel guilty for not doing so.

You need not be concerned at all about this shaking. It usually goes away within a few hours after delivery.

Having an Operative Vaginal Delivery

If the baby's head is low enough in the birth canal and your practitioner feels that the baby needs to be delivered immediately or that you won't be able to deliver the baby vaginally without some added help, he or she may recommend the use of forceps or a vacuum extractor to assist the delivery. Using either of these instruments is called an *operative vaginal delivery*. Such a delivery may be appropriate to use when

- You've pushed for a long time, and you're too tired to continue pushing hard enough to deliver.

- You've pushed for some time, and your practitioner thinks you won't deliver vaginally unless you have this type of help.

- The baby's heart rate pattern indicates a need to deliver the baby quickly.

- The baby's position is making it very difficult for you to push it out on your own.

As shown in Figure 9-4, *forceps* are two curved, spatula-like instruments that are placed on the sides of the baby's head to help guide it through the outer part of the birth canal. The *vacuum extractor* is a suction cup that is placed on the top of the baby's head, to which suction is applied to allow your practitioner to gently pull the baby through the birth canal.

Either technique is safe for both you and the baby if the baby is far enough down in the birth canal and the instruments are used appropriately. In fact, these techniques can often help women avoid cesarean delivery (but not always — see the next section). The decision to use forceps or vacuum often depends upon the judgment and experience of your practitioner and the position and station of the baby.

You may need extra local anesthesia, if you haven't had an epidural, for a forceps or vacuum delivery, and most practitioners perform an episiotomy to make extra room. After the forceps or vacuum are applied, you are asked to continue to push until the head emerges. The forceps or vacuum extractor are then removed, and the rest of the baby is delivered with your pushing.

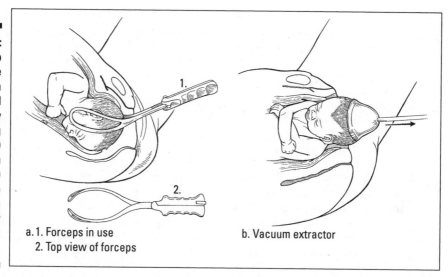

Figure 9-4:
Two ways to help the process of a vaginal delivery along: using forceps (a) or a vacuum extractor (b) to help guide the baby through the birth canal.

a. 1. Forceps in use
2. Top view of forceps

b. Vacuum extractor

If forceps are used, very often the baby is born with marks on his or her head where the forceps were applied. If this happens to your baby, remember that it's quite typical, and the marks disappear within a few days. A vacuum extractor may cause the baby to be born with a round, raised area on the top of the head where the extractor was applied. This mark, too, goes away in a few days.

Having a Cesarean Delivery

Many patients wonder whether they'll need a cesarean. Sometimes your doctor knows the answer before labor even begins — if you have placenta previa (see Chapter 14), for example, or if the baby is in a *transverse lie* (that is, the baby is lying sideways within the uterus rather than head-down). But most of the time, neither you nor your doctor can know whether you'll need a cesarean until you see how your labor progresses and how your baby tolerates labor.

Because a cesarean is a surgical procedure, it's always performed by a doctor. All nurse-midwives and many family-practice doctors work with an obstetrician trained to perform cesarean deliveries in case any of their patients need one. Some family-practice physicians have had the special training needed to perform cesarean deliveries.

A cesarean delivery is performed in an operating room under sterile conditions. An intravenous line must be in place and a catheter put in the bladder. After the patient's abdomen is scrubbed with antiseptic solution, sterile sheets are placed over her belly. One of the sheets is elevated to create a screen so that the expectant parents don't have to watch the procedure. (Although childbirth is usually an experience shared by both parents, a cesarean delivery is still a surgical operation. Most doctors feel that the procedure is not something that expectant parents should watch, because it involves scalpels, bleeding, and exposure of internal body tissue that's normally not seen, which is disturbing to many people.)

Many hospitals allow the coach or partner to stay in the operating room during a cesarean delivery, but this decision depends on the nature of the delivery and on hospital policy. If the cesarean is an emergency, the doctors and nurses are moving quickly to ensure the safety of both the mother and the baby, which may make it necessary for the partner or coach to wait elsewhere.

The exact place on the woman's abdomen where the incision is made depends on the reason she's having the cesarean. Most often, it is low, just above the pubic bone, in a transverse direction (perpendicular to the torso). This cut is known as a *Pfannensteil incision* or, more commonly, a *bikini cut* (see Chapter 11 for an illustration). Less often, the incision is vertical, along the midline of the abdomen.

After the skin incision is made, the abdominal muscles are separated and the inner lining of the abdominal cavity, also called the *peritoneal cavity,* is opened to expose the uterus. An incision is then made in the uterus itself, through which the infant and placenta are delivered. The incision on the uterus can also be either transverse (most common) or vertical (sometimes called a *classical* incision), depending again on the reason for the cesarean and previous abdominal surgery. After delivery, the uterus and abdominal wall are closed with sutures, layer by layer. A cesarean delivery takes 30 to 90 minutes to perform.

Anesthesia for a cesarean delivery

The most common forms of anesthesia used for cesarean deliveries are epidural and spinal (see Chapter 8 for more information on anesthesia). Both kinds of anesthesia numb you from mid-chest to toes but also allow you to remain awake so that you can experience the birth of your child. You may feel some tugging and pulling during the operation, but you do not feel pain. Sometimes the anesthesiologist injects a slow-release pain medication into the epidural or spinal catheter before removing it in order to prevent or greatly minimize pain *after* the operation.

Why they call it *cesarean*

Cesarean delivery, in which the baby is born through an incision in the mother's abdomen, is hardly a new medical innovation. Cases have been documented since the beginning of recorded history. In fact, many famous works of medieval and Renaissance art depict abdominal deliveries.

The origin of the term *cesarean section* is a subject of some controversy. Julius Caesar, it turns out, was probably not delivered this way, according to *Cesarean Delivery*, a history written by physicians Steve Clark and Jeffrey Phelan. In those days, it was rare for the mother to survive the procedure. Yet Caesar's mother survived her delivery and was depicted in Renaissance art recounting the life of Caesar as an adult.

One theory is that the name comes from the *Lex Cesare*, the laws of the ancient Roman emperors. One of those laws mandated that any woman who died while she was pregnant be delivered by an abdominal incision so that the infant could be baptized. This rule later became canon law of the Catholic church. A third possible explanation for the term *cesarean* is its relationship to the Latin term *cadere*, which means *to cut*. The term *section* also implies surgical cutting, so if *cadere* is indeed the origin of *cesarean*, then *cesarean section* is redundant. In modern obstetrics, we prefer the phrase *cesarean delivery* or *cesarean birth*. Still, many people continue to call the operation a *cesarean section* or *C-section*.

If the baby has to be delivered in an emergency and there's no time to place an epidural or spinal, general anesthesia may be needed. In that case, you are asleep during the cesarean and totally unaware of the procedure. Also, general anesthesia may be needed in some cases because of complications in pregnancy that make it unwise to place epidurals or spinals.

Reasons for a cesarean delivery

The reasons your doctor may perform a cesarean delivery are many (see the list later in this section), but all are about delivering the infant in the safest, healthiest way possible while also maintaining the mother's well-being. A cesarean delivery can be either planned ahead of labor *(elective)*, unplanned during labor (when the doctor determines that delivering the baby vaginally isn't safe), or done as an emergency (if the mother's or the baby's health is in immediate jeopardy).

All surgical procedures involve risks, and cesarean delivery is no exception. Fortunately, these problems are not common. The main risks of cesarean delivery are

✔ Excessive bleeding, rarely to the point of needing a blood transfusion

✔ Development of an infection in the uterus, bladder, or skin incision

✔ Injury to the bladder, bowel, or adjacent organs

✔ Development of blood clots in the legs or pelvis after the operation

If your practitioner feels that you need a cesarean delivery, he or she will discuss with you why it is needed. If your cesarean is elective or it's done because your labor isn't progressing normally, you and your partner have time to ask questions. In cases in which the baby is in a breech position, you and your practitioner may consider together the pros and cons of having either an elective cesarean delivery or a vaginal breech delivery (see Chapter 7). Both carry some risks, and often your practitioner asks you which risks are most acceptable to you. If the decision to perform a cesarean is due to a last-minute emergency, the discussion between you and your doctor may happen quickly, while you're being wheeled to the operating room.

If things seem hurried or rushed when you're on your way to the operating room for an emergency cesarean, don't panic. Doctors and nurses are trained to handle these kinds of emergencies.

Your practitioner may suggest that you have a cesarean delivery for one of many different reasons. This list describes the most common ones.

Reasons for elective cesarean delivery:

✔ The baby is in an abnormal position (breech or transverse).

✔ Placenta previa (see Chapter 14).

✔ You've had extensive prior surgery on the uterus, including previous cesarean deliveries or removal of uterine fibroids. (See Chapter 13 for more information on vaginal births after cesarean delivery.)

✔ Delivery of triplets or more.

Reasons for unplanned but nonemergency cesarean delivery:

✔ The baby is too large in relation to the woman's pelvis to be delivered safely through the vagina — a condition known as *cephalopelvic disproportion* (CPD) — or the position of the baby's head makes vaginal delivery unlikely.

✔ Signs indicate that the baby is not tolerating labor.

✔ Maternal medical conditions preclude safe vaginal delivery, such as severe cardiac disease.

✔ Normal labor comes to a standstill.

Reasons for emergency cesarean delivery:

- ✔ Bleeding is excessive.
- ✔ The baby's umbilical cord pushes through the cervix when the membranes rupture.
- ✔ Prolonged slowing of the baby's heart rate.

Other than the fact that the baby and placenta are delivered through an incision in the uterus rather than through the vagina, a cesarean delivery for the baby is of little difference. Babies delivered by a cesarean before labor usually don't have the coneheads that we mention earlier in this chapter, but they may if you are in labor for a long time before having a cesarean.

Recovery from a cesarean delivery

After the surgery is finished, you are taken to a recovery area, where you stay for a few hours, until the hospital staff can make sure that your condition is stable. Often, you can see and hold your baby during this time.

During the first day after a cesarean, you need to spend most of the time in bed. After that, you need to gradually increase your activity, so that you can build the strength you need to take care of yourself and the baby at home. (If you have a cesarean, follow your practitioner's instructions on this subject.) The recovery time from a cesarean delivery is usually longer than from a vaginal delivery, because the procedure is a surgical one. Typically, you stay in the hospital for two to four days — sometimes longer, if complications arise.

After you have a cesarean, you may feel pain where the incisions were made through your skin and uterus. Ask your nurse for pain medication if you need it. Your doctor usually leaves orders for pain medications, but they aren't automatically given unless you ask for them. (We discuss breast-feeding and pain medications in Chapter 12.) The anesthesia needed to perform a cesarean delivery also tends to slow the bowels and to cause some bloating and abdominal discomfort. Again, medications can help. Prune juice and other juices also can help.

After a cesarean, *lochia* (bleeding) may come from the vagina, just like in a vaginal delivery. This discharge gradually decreases and eventually disappears.

A few words about cesarean rates

Some women choose their practitioner or the hospital where they are going to deliver based on the number of cesarean deliveries (as a percentage of total deliveries) that the practitioner, group, or hospital has done. That number is meaningless, however, unless you also know the demographics of the practice or hospital. For example, a maternal-fetal medicine specialist who predominantly cares for older women, women with many medical problems, or women carrying twins or more is expected to have a higher cesarean rate than a doctor or midwife who takes care of young, healthy women. The important issue is not the cesarean delivery rate, but whether or not the cesareans were done for appropriate reasons.

Women who have labored for a long time only to find that they need a cesarean delivery are sometimes, understandably, disappointed. This reaction is natural. If it happens to you, keep in mind that what is ultimately most important is your safety and the safety of your baby. Having a cesarean delivery doesn't mean that you are, in any way, a failure or that you didn't try hard enough. Practitioners stick to basic guidelines when monitoring progress through labor, and those guidelines are all about giving you and your baby the best chance for a normal, healthy outcome.

Congratulations! You Did It!

After their babies are born, women may experience any and every kind of emotion. The spectrum of feelings is truly infinite. Most of the time, you are completely overcome with joy when your long-awaited baby finally is born. You may be incredibly relieved to see that your baby appears healthy and obviously okay. If your baby requires extra medical attention for some reason and you can't hold him or her right away, you may be upset or, at the very least, disappointed. Just remember that very soon you'll have him or her to hold and enjoy for the rest of your life. Some women feel too scared or overwhelmed to care for their baby right away. Don't feel guilty about any such feelings — they, and most others, are completely normal. Just take one moment at a time. You've come through a phenomenal event.

Causes for Concern

Childbirth may not be the easiest thing a woman ever does in her life, but in the vast majority of cases, it occurs in a fairly predictable way that causes no problems for the mother or the baby. However, in some cases, things can get complicated. In this section, we cover three problems that occur in a minority of pregnancies.

Lacerations to the birth canal

Most tears or lacerations that occur during delivery are in the perineum (the area between the vagina and rectum) or are extensions of an episiotomy, which is also in that area (see the description earlier in this chapter). Occasionally, especially when the baby is exceptionally large or you have an operative vaginal delivery, lacerations can occur in other areas, such as the cervix, the walls of the vagina, the labia, or the tissue around the urethra. Your practitioner examines the birth canal carefully after delivery and sews up any lacerations that need to be repaired. These lacerations usually heal very quickly and almost never cause long-term problems.

Postpartum bleeding

After delivery — either vaginal or cesarean — your uterus begins to contract in order to squeeze the blood vessels closed and thus slow down bleeding. If the uterus doesn't contract normally, excessive bleeding may occur. This condition is known as _uterine atony_. It can happen when you have multiple babies (twins or more), if you have some infection in the uterus, or if some placental tissue remains inside the uterus after the placenta is delivered. Then again, in some cases, excessive bleeding happens for no apparent cause. If it happens to you, your doctor or nurse may first massage your uterus to get it to contract. If massage doesn't solve the problem, you may be given one of several medications that promotes contracting, like oxytocin, methergine, or Hemabate.

If you have some placental material remaining in your uterus, it may need to be removed by reaching inside the uterus or by a _D&C_ (dilation and curettage), which involves scraping the lining of the uterus with an instrument. The vast majority of the time, the bleeding stops without a problem. However, if it doesn't stop with the medications and procedures we just mentioned, your doctor will discuss other forms of treatment with you.

Shoulder dystocia

Normally, after the baby's head delivers, the shoulders and body follow easily. Occasionally, though, the baby's shoulders may be stuck behind the mother's pubic bone, which makes delivery of the rest of the baby more difficult. This situation is known as _shoulder dystocia_. If you have this problem, your practitioner can perform various maneuvers designed to dislodge the shoulders and deliver the baby. These methods include

  - Applying pressure directly above your pubic bone to push away the entrapped shoulder
  - Flexing your knees back to allow more room for delivery
  - Rotating the baby's shoulders manually
  - Delivering the posterior arm of the baby first

Women who are most at risk for shoulder dystocia are those who have any of the following conditions:

  - Very large babies
  - Gestational diabetes
  - In labor a very long time
  - Had previous large babies or babies with shoulder dystocia

However, shoulder dystocia can also occur in women with no risk factors.

Chapter 10

Hello, World! The Newborn

• •

In This Chapter

▶ Making first impressions

▶ Adjusting to the first days of life in the hospital

▶ Coming home

▶ Getting your baby medical care when there are problems

• •

For 40 weeks, you and your baby have been in one body, and if you're like most women, you've focused on staying healthy to help your baby grow — and on preparing to deliver your baby safely. Now suddenly, your baby is out on its own, and you finally get to take your first real look at it. You may find that in some ways, your baby's appearance surprises you. Newborns typically look a little funny. It helps to know ahead of time that many superficial aspects of your baby's appearance — the cone-shaped head, the blotches, and especially the white, pasty goo — will soon disappear.

In this chapter, we let you know what you can expect your baby to look like and also how he or she is cared for in the hospital. Medical tests are conducted (usually nothing too strenuous), your baby is cleaned up, and you make your first efforts at breast-feeding, if you so choose. We go over various minor health problems the baby may have and how the hospital's medical staff deals with them. And we give you an idea of how to manage those first days with your new baby at home.

Love at First Sight

Immediately after delivery, your practitioner either puts your baby on your belly or hands him or her over to your nurse for some judicious cleansing and toweling off before putting the baby in your arms.

In the first moments after your baby is born, you may be overwhelmed by feelings of love. You may also be dazed by the shock and relief of it all. Most likely, you also think that your baby is the most beautiful thing you've ever seen. But contrary to the fairy tales you see on TV soap operas, *I Love Lucy* reruns, and cartoons, babies don't always come out clean and smelling like a spring shower. Your baby is far more likely to be covered with some of your blood, amniotic fluid, and a white goo known as *vernix*. His or her skin may be blotchy, and he or she may even have suffered a few bruises during delivery. So you may need to keep an open mind when assessing his or her appearance right off the bat.

It is not uncommon for some women to feel a little hesitant at first or overwhelmed at the sight of their new baby. Often it takes a few days before you establish a true connection or bond with your baby. If you are feeling like this, don't worry. As reality sets in and you get to know your baby, you feel much better.

You notice many other things about your new baby's appearance — from his or her little stump of an umbilical cord to the amazingly long finger- and toenails. And you observe his or her first behaviors — from the initial cry to the way he or she startles at loud noises. In this section, we go over many of the characteristics you're likely to notice in your newborn.

Vernix caseosa

A thick, white, waxy substance typically covers a newborn baby from head to toe. The formal name for this substance is *vernix caseosa,* a phrase with Latin roots meaning "cheesy varnish." Vernix is a mixture of cells that have sloughed off from the outer layer of the baby's skin and of debris from the amniotic fluid. Experts have several theories about the function of this substance. Some doctors believe that vernix acts as an emollient to protect the tender fetal skin from the dryness that may result from living within a bag of amniotic fluid. Others believe that the vernix acts as a lubricant to help the baby slide through the birth canal. Some babies have more vernix than others; some have none at all. The amount isn't significant. If your baby passed meconium while inside the uterus (see Chapter 8), the vernix may look a little greenish.

Regardless of what it looks like, most of the vernix probably comes off when the nurses dry off your baby, which is fine. There's no reason to leave the vernix on the baby's skin. Whatever vernix doesn't come off in the drying process is probably absorbed within the first 24 hours.

Caput and molding

Caput succedaneum — more commonly called *caput* — refers to a circular area of swelling on the baby's head, located at the spot that pushed against the opening to the cervix during delivery. The exact location of the swelling varies, depending on the position that the baby's head was in. The swollen area can range in size from only a few millimeters in diameter to several centimeters (a few inches). Caput generally disappears within 24 to 48 hours after birth.

Babies who are born head-first *(vertex)* often go through a process known as *molding.* This molding occurs because throughout the process of labor, as the baby descends gradually through the birth canal, it "fits" its way along (see Figure 10-1). In fact, sometimes your practitioner may tell you that he or she can feel the baby's head molding to the canal even before the baby is born. Molding doesn't cause any harm. The bones and soft tissues in the baby's head are designed to allow this molding to happen. The result is often a baby with a cone-shaped head (see Figure 10-2). By 24 hours after delivery, the molding is usually gone, and the baby's head appears round and smooth.

Some women, particularly those who have had children before or who had rapid labor, have babies with no molding whatsoever. Also, babies born in the breech presentation or by cesarean may not have molding.

Sometimes, during the passage through the birth canal, a baby's ears can also fold down into strange positions. The same thing can happen with the baby's nose, so that at first, it may appear *asymmetric,* or pushed to one side.

Figure 10-1:
A baby's head is often molded as it descends through the birth canal.

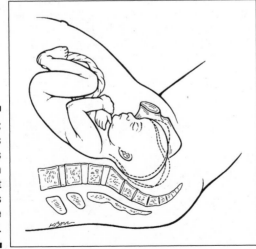

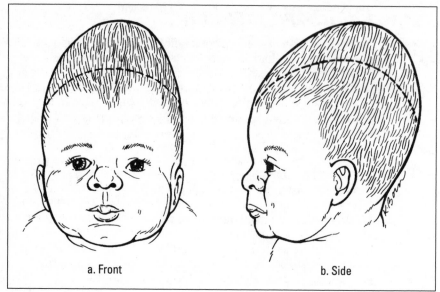

Figure 10-2:
The cone
shape often
goes away
after about
24 hours.

a. Front

b. Side

But these features are no reason to rush your baby to a plastic surgeon.
These minor oddities are temporary and disappear during the first few days.

Black and blue marks

Quite often, babies are born with black-and-blue marks on their heads from
the labor and delivery process. These marks may happen because the forces
of labor put so much pressure on the baby's scalp, or as a result of a forceps
or vacuum delivery. A bruise doesn't indicate that anything harmful has
occurred; it's merely a reflection of how vigorous the labor process can be.
Most black-and-blue marks go away within the first few days of life.

Blotches, patches and other skin-deep characteristics

Most people think of newborn skin as blemish-free — the very definition of
perfection. But at first, babies have all kinds of spots and markings — most of
which disappear within a matter of days or weeks. Some of the most common
skin conditions that affect newborns are described in the following list:

- **Neonatal acne:** Some babies are born with tiny white or red pimples around the nose, lips, and cheeks, and some develop them weeks or months later. These bumps are completely normal and are sometimes called *neonatal acne* or, in some cases, *milia*. No need to rush to the dermatologist, though. The little bumps disappear in time.

- **Stork bites:** You may notice small ruptured blood vessels around your baby's nose and eyes or on the back of the neck. These marks are commonly known as *stork bites* and *angel kisses*. They're common in newborns, and they also disappear after a while, although it sometimes takes weeks or months.

- **Red spots:** Reddish discoloration on the skin, whether very deep and dark or light and hardly noticeable, is very common in newborns. Most of these discolorations go away or fade, but some may persist as birthmarks. One type in particular, *erythema taxicum,* can be extensive. It looks like bad hives, and it comes and goes over the baby's first few days of life.

- **Hemangiomas:** Another type of reddish spot, known as a *hemangioma,* may not appear until a week or so after delivery. It can be almost any size, large or small, and can occur anywhere on the infant's body. While the majority go away in early childhood, some persist. Those that become bothersome (because of their appearance) can be treated. You can discuss treatment options, if needed, with your pediatrician.

- **Mongolian spots:** Bluish-gray patches of skin on the lower back, buttocks, and thighs are especially common in Asian, Southern European, and African-American infants. These patches are sometimes called *mongolian spots.* They often disappear in early childhood.

- **Dry skin:** Some babies, particularly those who are born late, have an outer layer of skin that looks shriveled like a raisin and peels off easily shortly after birth. You can use lotion or oil, if needed, as a moisturizer.

Baby hair

Some babies enter the world totally bald, while others come out looking as though they already need a haircut. The amount of hair present at birth often reflects the hair pattern of the parents, but it doesn't necessarily predict what the baby's hair will look like later on. Most typically, newborn hair thins out and is replaced by new hair. Different babies grow hair at different rates; some have relatively little hair even at a year of age, while others already need a trip to the beauty salon.

Often, babies' bodies are covered by a soft, fine layer of dark hair that can be especially prominent on the forehead, shoulders, and back. This hair is called *lanugo,* and like so many aspects of a newborn's appearance, is quite normal. Lanugo is most common in preterm babies and in infants of mothers who have diabetes. It falls out within several weeks of life.

Newborn extremities

Newborn babies often assume a position similar to the one that they became familiar with inside the uterus, the so-called *fetal position*. You may notice that your baby likes to be curled up a bit, with his or her arms and legs bent and fingers balled into a fist.

Watch out for those nails, though! Newborn fingernails and toenails may be surprisingly long and sharp. Many hospitals dress newborn babies in little shirts with mitten-like attachments to cover the hands so that the babies can't scratch themselves. Because babies can easily scratch themselves, it is important that you keep the nails relatively short. Pick up a pair of baby nail scissors or clippers from your local drug store.

A good time to trim fingernails and toenails is when your baby is fast asleep and oblivious to what you're doing.

Newborn eyes and ears

At birth, a baby's vision is quite limited. Newborns can see only objects that are close-up and see things best at a distance of about 7 to 8 inches away. They also respond to light and appear to be interested in bright objects.

All newborn babies have dark blue or brown eyes, regardless of what color eyes the parents have. By the age of four months, baby eye color changes to the permanent hue. When your baby is first born, the whites of his or her eyes may have a bluish tint. This tint is normal and disappears in time.

Often, a newborn's eyes may appear a little swollen or puffy. This puffiness is caused by the whole delivery process; it is perfectly normal, and it quickly subsides. Some puffiness may also be due to antibiotic put in the eyes after birth (see the "Eye care" section later in this chapter).

Babies are fully able to hear from the moment they are born, which is why you may notice that your baby reacts with a startled motion to loud or sudden noises. Newborns also can distinguish various tastes and smells.

Newborn external genitalia and breasts

Babies are often born with a swollen or puffy scrotum or labia. The breasts also may appear slightly enlarged. This swelling is caused by maternal hormones that cross the placenta. Sometimes, high maternal hormone levels may even cause the baby to secrete whitish or pinkish discharge from the breasts (known as *witch's milk*) or from the vagina (like a period) in female babies. Like so many newborn characteristics, these secretions are both normal and transient; they go away within a few weeks after birth.

Umbilical cord

The stump of your baby's umbilical cord probably has a little piece of plastic attached to it. After delivery, the cord is closed with a small plastic clamp and then cut. Usually, this clamp is removed before you take the baby home. Then the umbilical cord stump quickly dries up and shrivels so that it looks like a hard, dark cord. Within one to three weeks, the stump usually falls off on its own. It's not a good idea to try to pull it off yourself.

To keep the stump clean, you can dip a cotton swab in water, alcohol, or peroxide and clean around the base. However, some pediatricians think this cleaning is unnecessary — unless a lot of goopy stuff is around the base.

Newborn size

In general, newborn babies weigh anywhere from about 6 to 8 pounds (about 2,700 to 3,600 grams) and measure 18 to 22 inches (46 to 56 centimeters) long. The exact size depends on the baby's gestational age (basically, the number of weeks the pregnancy lasted), genetics, and factors such as whether the mother had diabetes, whether she smoked, how healthy her diet was during pregnancy, and many other factors.

You may notice that your baby's head seems disproportionately large compared to his or her body. This is true of all newborns. Your baby is not immediately able to hold up his or her head. It takes time to develop muscles strong enough to support the head and hold it up without assistance. You also may notice soft spots on the back and top of your baby's head. These are fontanelles, areas where the baby's skull bones meet. Fontanelles serve an important purpose — they allow for the rapid growth of the baby's brain. The back spot (posterior fontanelle) usually closes within a few months, but the anterior or top fontanelle (the one most typically called the soft spot) usually remains until the baby is ten months to one year old.

Baby's first cry

Often, the baby starts to cry spontaneously shortly after delivery, but not every baby cries right away. A full-throated cry is music to the ears of everyone on the hospital staff because they know that the cry triggers the baby's first breathing efforts. Healthy breathing can begin without a loud cry, however, and some babies give only a little whimper. Some babies have normal respiration even if they don't wail at high decibels. If your baby passed meconium during labor, your practitioner suctions out the baby's lungs before he even has a chance to cry, in order to prevent the baby from breathing meconium into the lungs. If your baby is slow to start breathing spontaneously, you may notice the doctor, nurse, or midwife stimulating your baby by rubbing her back, by drying him off, or by tapping her feet.

Contrary to the stereotype portrayed in old movies, your practitioner is unlikely to turn your baby upside down and give him or her a little spank on the behind to elicit that first cry.

During pregnancy, a fetus's lungs develop and mature in preparation for life outside the uterus. A fetus receives oxygen through the placenta. After delivery, the baby takes over respiratory function by using his or her own lungs. A baby's lungs are bathed in special fluid, and this fluid is often pushed out during delivery. Sometimes, however, a baby needs extra time and help — in the form of suctioning or stimuli — to expel all the fluid in the lungs.

You may notice that your baby breathes differently than you do. Most babies breathe 30 to 40 times a minute. A newborn's respiratory rate also can increase with physical activity. Newborns breathe through their noses rather than their mouths. This great natural adaptation enables them to breathe while nursing or bottle-feeding.

You may also think that your baby's belly looks unusually large and protuberant, but it is just a normal new baby's belly. The fact that the belly rises up and down quite noticeably during breathing and gets somewhat distended as the baby starts to swallow some air only enhances the effect. This movement is also normal and is due to the fact that babies use their diaphragms to breathe, not their chest muscles, as older children and adults usually do.

Baby's First Test

All babies are evaluated by the Apgar score, named for Dr. Virginia Apgar, who devised it in 1952. This score is a useful way of quickly assessing the baby's initial condition to see whether he or she needs special medical attention. Five factors are measured: heart rate, respiratory effort, muscle tone, presence of reflexes, and color, each of which can be given a score of 0, 1, or 2, with 2 being the highest score. The Apgar scores are calculated at both one and five minutes. An Apgar score of 6 or above is perfectly fine. Because some of the characteristics are partially dependent on the infant's gestational age, premature babies frequently get lower scores. Factors such as maternal sedation also can affect a baby's score.

Many new parents anxiously await the results of their child's Apgar score. In fact, an Apgar score taken one minute after the baby is born indicates whether the baby needs some resuscitative measures but is not useful in predicting long-term health. An Apgar score taken five minutes later can indicate whether resuscitative measures have been effective. Occasionally, a very low five-minute Apgar score may reflect decreased oxygenation to the baby, but it correlates poorly with future health. The purpose of the Apgar score is merely to help your doctor or pediatrician identify babies who may need a little extra attention in the very early newborn period.

Newborn Care in the Hospital

After your nurse and practitioner are assured that your baby is fine, the hospital staff start cleaning up the baby and helping him or her make a comfortable transition to life outside the womb. Like butterflies emerging from their cocoons, newborns must adjust to a new state of being in various ways. Suddenly, and for the first time, they are able to breathe on their own and to see the wide world around them.

Keeping the baby warm and dry

Because body temperature drops rapidly after birth, it's important that your new baby be kept warm and dry. If newborns become cold, their oxygen requirements increase. For this reason, a nurse dries the baby off, places him or her in a warmer or warmed bassinet, and then watches the baby's temperature closely. Often the nurse wraps or swaddles the baby in a blanket and puts a little hat on him or her to reduce the loss of heat from the head — the site of most heat loss (just as your mother told you). When the baby gets to the nursery, he or she is usually dressed in a little shirt and then wrapped up again in a blanket.

Eye care

The staff at most hospitals routinely place an antibiotic ointment into a newborn's eyes to lower the chance that the baby may develop an infection from passage through the vagina of a mother who has chlamydia or gonorrhea. The ointment doesn't appear to be bothersome to babies and is completely absorbed within a few hours.

Some parents worry that the ointment may blur the baby's vision and thus hinder parent-child bonding. You don't have any reason to be concerned about possible blurring, however. Babies don't see clearly in any case (see the "Newborn eyes and ears" section earlier).

Vitamin K

Most hospitals routinely give newborns an injection of vitamin K to decrease the risk of serious bleeding. Vitamin K is important in the body's production of *clotting factors* — substances that help the blood clot. This nutrient doesn't pass through the placenta to a baby very easily, however, and newborn livers, because they are immature, produce very little of it. So babies are typically low in this nutrient. Giving the baby vitamin K is an important preventive measure.

ID bracelets for Baby, Mom, and Dad

At the hospital, your baby gets an identification bracelet to identify him or her as yours. All hospitals also require that the mother wear a bracelet with the baby's ID number on it. Each time the baby is brought to the mother, the numbers are read off to ensure that the right baby is given to the right mother. Most hospitals also take additional security measures to prevent any mix-ups and to prevent unauthorized individuals from gaining access to the nursery. Many nurseries are locked and all are closely supervised.

Many hospitals now also require every new father to wear an ID band to identify you as the proud and rightful father.

Footprints

Most likely, footprints are taken shortly after your baby is born to make a permanent record of his or her identity. (The unique ridges that form on a baby's feet are actually present several months before birth.) Some hospitals give you a copy of your baby's footprints for your scrapbook. Although most hospitals still use this technique of identification, not all do.

Hepatitis B vaccine

Many hospitals now routinely start the vaccination process against hepatitis B for newborn babies, while others prefer that a pediatrician administer the first of the three shots after the baby is discharged from the hospital. (The last two are given over the course of the next six months.) Wherever it is given, this shot is an important tool to reduce the baby's chance of contracting hepatitis B later in life.

Baby's first doctor visit

Before or after delivery, someone from the hospital asks you the name of the pediatrician you have chosen to care for your baby. This doctor should be someone who is authorized to work at the hospital where you have delivered but may or may not be the same pediatrician you plan to use after you leave the hospital. If you live some distance from the hospital and have selected a pediatrician close to your home who doesn't have privileges at the hospital where you deliver, you still need another pediatrician to care for your baby during the hospital stay. Depending on the time you deliver, the pediatrician may see the baby on the same day, or he or she may see the baby the next day.

When the pediatrician examines your baby, he or she checks the baby's general appearance, listens for heart murmurs, feels the fontanelles (the openings in the baby's skull where the various bones come together), looks at the extremities, checks the hips, and just generally makes sure that the baby is in good condition. The pediatrician orders a variety of standard blood tests and newborn screening tests. The specific screens that are required vary from state to state but often include tests for thyroid disease, PKU (a condition in which a person has trouble metabolizing some amino acids), and other inherited metabolic disorders. The results of these screening tests probably don't come back until after you take your baby home. The pediatrician gives you the results at your baby's first office visit. If any of the tests come back positive, the state also notifies you by mail. Be sure to ask the pediatrician upon discharge when your baby should be seen again.

Newborn heart rate and circulatory changes

Remember how your practitioner checked the fetal heart rate during prenatal visits? You may have noticed then how fast the beat was. In utero, the baby's heart rate is, on average, 120 to 160 beats per minute, and this heart rate pattern continues during the newborn period. Your baby's heart rate also can increase with physical activity and slow down when he or she sleeps.

After your baby is born, important changes in circulation occur. In utero, because a fetus doesn't use its lungs to breathe, much of the blood is shunted away from the lungs through a structure called the *ductus arteriosus*. Normally, this shunt closes on the first day of life. Sometimes, a murmur is heard in the first days after the baby is born, which indicates changes in blood flow. This murmur, called a PDA for *patent ductus arteriosus,* may be perfectly normal and nothing to worry about. However, some heart murmurs may require further investigation — specifically, a special sonogram of the baby's heart, called an *echocardiogram*. Even when murmurs due to small structural problems are found (like a small hole in the septum of the heart), many go away on their own. If your baby is diagnosed with a murmur, you should discuss it thoroughly with the baby's pediatrician or a pediatric cardiologist who specializes in these conditions.

Newborn weight changes

Most newborns lose weight during their first few days of life — usually about 10 percent of their body weight — which, of course, if you weigh only 7 or 8 pounds (3,200 or 3,600 grams), doesn't amount to more than a pound (454 grams). This phenomenon is completely normal and is usually caused by fluid loss from urine, feces, and sweat. During the first few days of life, the typical infant takes in very little food or water to replace this weight loss. Preterm babies lose relatively more weight than full-term babies, and it may take them longer to regain their weight. In contrast, babies who are small for their gestational age may gain weight more rapidly. Generally, most newborns regain their birthweight by the tenth day of life. By the age of five months, they're likely to double their birthweight. By the end of the first year, they triple it.

Urinating and bowel movements

Most babies wet their diapers six to ten times a day by the time they're one week old. The frequency of bowel movements depends on whether you are bottle- or breast-feeding. Typically, a breast-fed baby has two or more bowel movements per day, whereas a formula-fed baby has only one or two per day.

Don't be surprised if your baby's first stool looks like thick, sticky, black tar — that's normal. It's called *meconium*. Ninety percent of newborns pass their first stool within the first 24 hours, and almost all the rest do so by 36 hours. Later on, the color of the stools lightens, and the texture becomes more normal. A formula-fed baby typically has semi-formed, yellow-green stools, whereas a breast-fed baby has looser, more granular, and more yellowish stools.

Most newborns urinate within the first few hours after birth, but some don't urinate until the second day. The passage of meconium and urine is an important sign that your baby's gastrointestinal and urinary tracts are functioning well.

Circumcision

Circumcision is the surgical removal of the foreskin on the penis of a male infant. Parents of boy babies must decide whether they want their child to have this procedure performed. The decision to have a circumcision may involve cultural and religious considerations, as well as personal preferences. Circumcision is performed on more than half of newborn boys in the United States. But in many other countries, it's rarely performed. The frequency of circumcision in the U.S. is on the decline, as new information emerges that challenges the medical arguments for performing the procedure.

Doctors once thought that circumcision helped reduce the incidence of penile cancer, that it prevented infections, and that it reduced the incidence of changes in the appearance of a penis related to a tight foreskin. However, these advantages have not proved to be true. In fact, the American Academy of Pediatrics has issued a formal statement that there is currently no absolute medical indication for routine circumcision. Circumcision based on cultural or religious views is still relatively common. The decision, of course, is one that both parents should be comfortable with.

If you decide that you do want your baby to be circumcised, your obstetrician performs the procedure within a day or two after your baby is born — as long as the baby is healthy, full-term or nearly full-term, and without any congenital abnormalities that would cause your doctor not to do the procedure. Some Jewish families have a ceremonial circumcision after the baby is discharged from the hospital, performed by a *mohel.*

Until several years ago, circumcisions were done with no anesthesia whatso-ever. But these days, many hospitals offer an anesthetic cream that doctors can apply to the baby's penis prior to the procedure. The new emphasis on pain medication is a humane and important medical advance, prompted by studies that show that newborns do indeed react to the pain and stress asso-ciated with circumcision. Still, some doctors prefer not to use pain medi-cation because it prolongs the procedure, which in itself can increase the baby's discomfort.

After circumcision, the baby's penis is wrapped in a petroleum jelly-soaked gauze for about four hours. When this gauze falls off, the top of the penis may look reddish and slightly swollen.

If the gauze doesn't fall off, don't pull hard at it. Squeeze warm water over the gauze to help it loosen. In the first few days, clean the area with warm water and keep it dry. After each diaper change, apply ointment — an antibacterial ointment, for example, or petroleum jelly — until the penis is well healed.

The penis is usually completely healed within one week. During this time, you may notice a crusty substance at the tip; this substance is normal and goes away with time. But if the penis looks unusually swollen and discolored or if your baby has a fever, give your pediatrician a call.

Newborn jaundice

When your baby is two to five days old, his or her skin may take on a yellow-orange tint. This condition is known as *physiological jaundice of the newborn*, and it develops in about one-third of all babies. Jaundice is caused by an increase in the concentration of bilirubin in the baby's blood. *Bilirubin* consists of byproducts of hemoglobin from the baby's red blood cells, byproducts that are normally disposed of through the liver and kidneys. Elevated bilirubin levels may occur because a baby's liver is not yet fully mature. (Significant jaundice is most common in preterm babies, whose livers are especially immature.) Feeding the newborn early in his or her life may help to decrease the risk of jaundice, because feeding causes the baby to stay well hydrated and stimulates the digestive tract.

If jaundice occurs very early or lasts longer than usual, the pediatrician may want to keep a close eye on your baby, checking his or her bilirubin levels daily. If bilirubin levels are high enough, the pediatrician may want to start therapy, which involves placing the baby under special phototherapy lights. This lighting helps to break up the bilirubin and causes the baby to excrete it more quickly. Keeping the baby's skin exposed to sunlight — through a window, for example — may also help to break down the bilirubin.

Bringing baby home

Finally, the day comes when you are discharged from the hospital and are able to bring your baby home with you. You need to bring a change of clothes for your baby to wear home. Of course, the best choice of clothes depends on whether it's summer or winter, fall or spring, and on whether you live in San Diego, New York City, Miami, or Minneapolis. You can buy many beautiful clothes for newborns. But keep in mind that babies need frequent diaper changes, so choose clothes that you can easily open, close, put on, and take off.

Most important is that you have an infant car seat to carry your baby home. They are eminently useful in preventing injuries to babies, and we cannot recommend them highly enough. In many states, they are also a legal requirement prior to the hospital discharging the baby.

In some cases, the mother is ready to leave the hospital before her baby. This can happen, for example, when a baby is born prematurely and needs time to grow and mature before leaving the hospital. It can also happen when a baby has jaundice and needs phototherapy in the hospital. Whatever the reason, going home without their new baby can cause the parents to feel incredibly disappointed and empty. If this happens to you, keep in mind that your feelings are completely normal. It's hard to go home alone after all the time you spent anticipating bringing the baby with you. Just remember that your baby will be home soon, and then you'll forget all about the first few days of separation. Your baby will be with you for a lifetime, and that includes plenty of time to build a beautiful, loving relationship. What's most important is that your baby comes home healthy!

Neonatal Intensive Care Units

During the hospital stay after delivery, most newborns end up either rooming in with their mothers or staying at least part of the time in the regular hospital nursery — sometimes called the *well-baby nursery*. But sometimes newborns need the kind of extra attention they can get only in a *neonatal intensive care unit* — sometimes called a *special care nursery*. Within such a nursery, you may find a special area for critical care, where one-on-one nursing, sophisticated monitors, breathing machines, and so on are available. You may also find the so-called *step-down area*, for babies who aren't yet ready to go to the well-baby nursery but don't need critical, one-on-one care.

If your pediatrician thinks that your baby should be cared for in a neonatal intensive care unit, it doesn't automatically mean that something is wrong. Often, babies are brought to special care nurseries for a short while just for observation — for any number of reasons. These are some of the most common (this list is far from inclusive):

✔ The baby has been born prematurely.

✔ The baby may not weigh quite enough to make the birthweight cutoff established by your particular hospital.

✔ The baby may have to be given antibiotics — for example, because the mother had a fever during labor or because she had a prolonged rupture of membranes prior to delivery.

✔ The pediatrician may be concerned because the baby's breathing seems somewhat labored, or the baby appears to be exerting extra effort to breathe. This reason is a relatively common one for putting a baby under observation for a short period of time. One common condition is called *transient tachypnea of the newborn,* which goes away within a few days.

✔ The baby has a fever or a seizure.

✔ The baby is anemic.

✔ The baby is born with certain congenital abnormalities.

✔ The baby requires surgery.

Newborn Care at Home

On one hand, bringing your baby home is a great privilege. On the other, it is a huge responsibility. Suddenly, you and your partner are in charge of his or her care, without the benefit of the hospital nursing staff. You may have family members or even a baby nurse to help, but ultimately the responsibility is now yours! In this section, we go over many of the ways in which you take care of your newborn — everything except feeding, which we cover in Chapter 12.

Bathing

Until your baby's umbilical cord falls off, you should keep your baby clean with sponge baths only. Prepare a small container of warm water and lay your baby on the changing table or on a table or countertop padded with a towel or on one of those large sponges sold in some baby stores. With a clean washcloth, gently wash the baby from head to toe. Use a separate wet cotton ball for each eye. Make sure to dry your baby off right away so that he or she doesn't get cold. Some mothers find it helpful to wash the head first, dry it right away, and then wash the rest of the body. Because a great deal of heat is lost from the head, keeping the head dry while bathing the rest of the baby makes sense.

After your baby's umbilical cord stump falls off, you're free to give him or her a bath in a tub. Many baby stores sell small plastic tubs that are designed for newborns. Some parents find it convenient to place the tub in the kitchen sink or on the counter. See the nearby sidebar "Bath tips" for some hints on keeping your baby clean.

Hand-to-body contact is an easy way to transmit infections from one person to another, so make sure that people who come in contact with your baby have washed their hands well. Make sure that they wash with soap, not just water, so that their hands are as clean as possible.

Burping

Often babies swallow air when they're feeding, especially if they're bottle-feeding. The accumulation of air inside a baby's stomach may make him or her feel uncomfortable. The good news is that all the discomfort goes away with one big burp! See Chapter 12 for some techniques that you may find helpful for burping your baby.

Keep a cloth diaper or burp cloth over your shoulder while burping the baby. Babies often spit up some formula or milk when burping, and the cloth protects your clothes.

Sleeping

We could describe a host of philosophies about the sleeping patterns of babies. Some people say it's better for a baby to establish a distinct pattern of sleeping and eating. The advantage is that you, the parent, can then plan your life better and schedule your activities around the baby's needs. Others feel that it is better to simply be attentive to your baby's desires — to watch and listen for when your baby wants to eat or sleep. In case you have difficulty choosing a point of view on this subject, entire books are devoted to the topic that you may find helpful. If your baby's habits become a problem for you, you may want to consult your pediatrician.

Here are a few general pointers on dealing with your baby's sleeping habits:

✔ Pediatricians recommend that babies sleep on their backs — not on their stomachs — because sleeping prone has been associated with SIDS (sudden infant death syndrome). To keep your baby turned on his or her back, you can roll up a blanket and use it as a prop or wedge that prevents the baby from rolling over. Infant stores sell special small cushions designed for this purpose, too.

Bath tips

You may find that bathing your squirming baby can be a little difficult, but following these tips can help you both enjoy bath time:

✔ Using your elbow, test the water temperature to make sure that it isn't too hot. (Your hand may not be as sensitive to heat.)

✔ *Before* you put your baby in the bath, make sure that you have all your supplies: washcloth, cotton balls, mild soap if you like (washing with no soap is fine, too), mild shampoo, a dry towel, a clean diaper, and clean clothes.

✔ Be sure that your baby's head and body are securely supported during the bath. Remember, it will be a while before your baby can hold up his or her own head.

✔ Use plain water — no soap — to clean the baby's face.

✔ Use a washcloth to clean the outside part of the ears. It's not recommended that you use a cotton swab inside your baby's ears — or nose.

✔ Wash a baby girl's genitals from front to back (to avoid washing any stool forward). For boys, clean underneath the scrotum and wash the foreskin without pulling back strongly on it.

✔ If your baby has very dry skin or even *eczema* (a condition in which the skin is chronically dry and flaky), consider bathing your baby less frequently — every other day, perhaps — because too much water can promote dryness. If it doesn't improve, talk it over with your pediatrician.

✔ If your baby has trouble settling down to sleep at night, you may want to consider a bath before bedtime. Your baby may find it relaxing.

✔ If you have twins, try bathing one baby when the other one is sleeping, so that you don't get into a situation in which you have to attend to one crying baby while you're bathing the other one.

✔ You may want to keep bright pictures or hanging objects around the crib to give your baby something interesting to look at when he or she is lying awake. But be careful not to place pillows or stuffed toys inside the crib or bassinet, in order to minimize any risk of suffocation.

✔ Playing soft music before a nap may help your baby get into the mood for sleep.

✔ Some babies fall asleep more easily when they're rocked to sleep. Be aware, however, that you may end up establishing a pattern that's difficult to reverse.

✔ Don't put your baby to sleep with a formula- or milk-filled bottle. This habit can lead to teeth problems later on.

Some babies go through what's known as day-night reversal: They sleep during the day but are wide awake at night. If this behavior happens to your baby, you can try to keep him or her more awake during the daytime — by stimulating him or her with pictures, toys, or activities. But usually, if a baby wants to sleep, a baby wants to sleep, and there is very little you can do about it. The good news is that most babies outgrow this syndrome and suddenly reverse their habits.

Crying

You may as well face it — babies cry. It's their main way of expressing themselves. During the first week of life, some babies hardly cry at all; they seem so incredibly happy and peaceful. But by the second week they can turn into the loudest criers in the world. Many newborns develop a variety of crying patterns and sounds, each of which can mean a different thing. You soon learn to distinguish your baby's messages, but occasionally, a baby may cry for no apparent reason whatsoever. You can try any number of soothing techniques — walking the baby around a bit, rocking, talking, bouncing on your knee, whatever. If nothing works, and you really can't identify any problem, don't jump to the conclusion that you are a terrible parent. You aren't. Babies don't always cry for a reason, and maybe your baby just needs to cry a little!

C is for colic

Unfortunately, there is such a thing as colic. It is traditionally defined as a baby who cries for more than three hours a day, three days a week, for three consecutive weeks. Doctors don't know the exact cause, but some think it

---

Some reasons why babies cry

The sound of a crying baby is ingeniously designed to make parents pay attention. Very often, it's a cry for help, and you can do something — feed the baby, hold him or her, change the diaper — to make the baby stop crying. Sometimes, on the other hand, a baby seems to cry for no apparent reason, and you may just have to let it happen — and don't feel like a bad parent for doing so. Here is list of things that may cause babies to cry:

- They're hungry.
- They need a diaper change.
- They have gas pains and need to be burped.
- They're tired.
- They're uncomfortable — their clothes are too tight, they're too hot, or they don't like the position they're in, for example.
- They're scared.
- They're overstimulated.
- They want to be held.
- They want to suck on something.

TIP

What to try if your baby cries and cries

In most cases, you can use your own common sense to figure out how to calm your crying baby. But it may help at first to have a list of all the tried-and-true strategies:

✔ Feed the baby.

✔ Burp the baby, trying various techniques.

✔ Change the diaper.

✔ Hold the baby in a warm, supportive, loving manner.

✔ Rock the baby, walk around with the baby, or change his or her position.

✔ Take the baby for a walk in the stroller or a ride in the car.

✔ Put the baby in the infant car seat and set the car seat on top of a running washing machine, holding on to it to make absolutely sure that it doesn't fall off. Some babies find the gentle shaking motion soothing.

✔ Give the baby a pacifier.

✔ Entertain the baby with a toy.

✔ Play music.

✔ Give the baby a bath.

✔ Let the baby rest and relax in a quiet room (quiet except for the sound of his or her crying, that is).

✔ Put the baby down in his or her crib to rest.

✔ Rock the baby in a baby swing — making sure that he or she is carefully strapped in and never left unattended.

✔ If all else fails, and you're assured that your baby seems not to be suffering any real discomfort, you may need to just let him or her cry! Then the trick is to find a way not to let it bother you. (Hint: Try turning up the radio.)

may be related to intestinal discomfort. You may be lucky and never have this ugly creature rear its head. Or you may be like many of us, who can remember the days of colic as if they were yesterday. Colic often starts at about 4 to 6 weeks and ends by about 12 weeks. When your baby has colic, he or she cries and cries, with little that can be done to console him or her. Often it happens in the evening, around 6 o'clock to 10 o'clock. If you are working outside the home, and this is the time of day when you finally get to be with your baby, you may think that your baby doesn't like you. Be assured that the timing doesn't hinge on you — it's just that the evening hours are the bewitching hours. You can try the suggestions in the nearby sidebar to calm your baby's crying, but don't be frantic if nothing works. Thank goodness, colic almost always goes away on its own. If it doesn't, discuss it with your pediatrician.

Hiccups

You may recall from your pregnancy that a fetus can be prone to hiccups. You soon discover that newborns often get hiccups, too. Sometimes feeding the baby or giving him or her a little water (perhaps with a little sugar dissolved in it) can relieve hiccups.

Shopping for the baby

Newborn fashion is an industry all to itself. Many of the clothes made for babies today are lovely and cute and adorable — those for boys as well as for girls — and if you're tempted to buy things by the dozen, you're not alone. But be forewarned: You may end up using not even half the clothes you buy or receive as gifts. It's shocking how quickly newborns outgrow their clothes. Also, as you become accustomed to daily life with your new baby, the novelty of sweet little clothes wears off, and your appreciation for practicality takes over. Simple, sacklike gowns are easier to take on and off and to launder than fully coordinated baby outfits with matching booties and hats.

The following are some tips for shopping for baby clothes:

- ✔ Before your baby's umbilical cord stump falls off, dress your baby in long- or short-sleeved undershirts, so that no material irritates the stump. After the cord falls off, you may find that undershirts and one-piece underclothes that snap under the diaper are most convenient.

- ✔ Look for simple gowns with drawstring closings at the foot for the first several weeks of babyhood. They're comfortable and extremely easy to handle.

- ✔ Hats are a good idea, no matter what the season. In summer, they protect your baby's skin from the sun; in winter, they keep your baby warm.

- ✔ One-piece outfits of cotton or terry cloth are good for going out in.

- ✔ It goes without saying: Bibs are a must.

- ✔ Winter or summer, your baby needs a sweater or two.

- ✔ In winter, make sure that your baby has a one-piece bunting or a snowsuit (unless you live in a warm climate).

- ✔ Be sure you have a few pairs of socks to keep his or her feet warm.

- ✔ The most convenient baby clothes are those with snaps that open on bottom for easy diaper access.

- ✔ Snaps at the shoulder make it easier to get the clothes over your baby's arms and head.

In addition to clothing, your baby needs a full set of household supplies, collectively referred to as the *layette*. Here are some suggestions:

- Receiving blankets.

- Crib.

- Bassinet.

- Changing table.

- Crib and bassinet sheets.

- Crib bumpers (pads to put around the edges of the crib so that your baby doesn't bump his or her head on the bars).

- Two or three rubber pads that you can place under the crib sheet and on the bassinet and changing table.

- Cloth diapers to use for all kinds of things — as burping cloths, to protect your clothes when you're bathing your baby, to provide a clean surface on which to lay your baby, and so on.

- Baby towels and washcloths.

- Baby soap.

- Baby shampoo.

- Gentle detergent and fabric softener.

- Petroleum ointment, or some other ointment suitable for babies.

- Medicated cream for diaper rash.

- Infant medications (anti-pyretics and analgesics for fever and pain relief).

- Bandages.

- Antibiotic cream.

- Nasal aspirator (bulb syringe) for suctioning stuffy, congested noses.

- Rectal thermometer.

- Pacifiers, if you want. You may want to ask your pediatrician's opinion about using a pacifier. "Orthodontic" pacifiers are available, but some pediatricians don't advocate the use of pacifiers in general because of potential future orthodontic problems in children.

- Baby hairbrush.

- Baby nail clippers or scissors.

- Bottles for water, juice, or formula.

- Infant car seat.

- Stroller that goes back to let the baby lie down.

- A good reference book on baby care and baby health. Ask your pediatrician which one he or she recommends. (A reference book makes a great shower gift, because most people don't think of it.)

Causes for Concern

Like pregnant women, new parents are often easily worried and concerned by any possible signs that something may not be going perfectly with the new baby. If you haven't been around babies much, you may find that your own baby is a little hard to read, especially at first. Babies spit up all the time, and they develop little rashes and other problems. But when should you call the pediatrician? Here are some guidelines:

- ✔ If you notice a change in your baby's behavior — for example, if a baby who usually falls asleep easily suddenly begins to cry a lot, or if a baby who is usually a healthy eater suddenly won't eat at all.

- ✔ If your baby's breathing becomes labored or is extremely short, shallow, and rapid.

- ✔ If your baby has two to three episodes of diarrhea or vomiting in a day.

- ✔ If your baby has fewer than four wet diapers in a day.

- ✔ If your baby's temperature is higher than 100 degrees or less than 97.5 degrees Fahrenheit.

- ✔ If your baby develops a sudden rash or discoloration of his or her skin.

From Mary and John to Emily and Michael: The most popular baby names of the 20th century

In your local library or bookstore, you can find a wide selection of books that offer suggestions for what to name the baby. The lists that these books provide are far more extensive than anything we can offer without using up too many pages of this book. You may find it interesting to look back through the century and see how parents' name choices have changed, gradually, over the years — from John and Mary (in 1900 and most of the early years of the century) to Michael and Emily (in 1997). To find the ten top names of every year since the late 19th century on the Internet, go to www.babynames.com.

Chapter 11

Taking Care of Yourself after Delivery

· ·

In This Chapter

▶ Recovering in the hospital

▶ Recovering from cesarean delivery

▶ Knowing what's in store for you after you get home

▶ Getting back into shape with exercise and diet

▶ Thinking about having sex again (and maybe even actually having sex!)

▶ Going back for your postpartum doctor visit

▶ Dealing with the baby blues or postpartum depression

· ·

According to the old adage, it takes nine months for a woman to make a baby and nine months for her body to return to normal afterwards. In reality, the time it takes to recover from childbirth varies widely from woman to woman. But most of the changes that your body goes through during pregnancy revert to normal during the postpartum period — sometimes called the *puerperium* — which begins immediately after delivery of the placenta and lasts for six to eight weeks.

As you go through this period of change, you're likely to have many questions about what you can do to make the postpartum transition as easy as possible. In this chapter, we tell you what life may be like as your body gets back into its old shape, as you begin to have sex again, and as you deal with all the physical and psychological challenges of new motherhood.

Postpartum: In the Hospital

The average hospital stay after an uncomplicated vaginal delivery is 24 to 48 hours. After a cesarean, you may stay in the hospital for three to four days. In some hospitals, you spend this recovery period in the same room in which you delivered. In others, you move to a separate postpartum unit. The nurses continue to monitor your vital signs (blood pressure, pulse, temperature, and breathing) and check the position of your uterus to make sure that it is firm and well contracted (see later in this section). Nurses (often the same ones taking care of you) also monitor your baby's vital signs. Your nurses can provide you with pain medication that your practitioner has prescribed, if you need it, and help you care for your episiotomy or cesarean incision, if you have either one.

Bleeding

Experiencing vaginal bleeding after delivery is completely normal, even if you had a cesarean delivery. Average blood loss after a vaginal delivery is about 500 cc, or one pint. After a cesarean, the average blood loss is twice that — about a liter, or a quart. In order to minimize excessive blood loss, many practitioners give oxytocin (brand name Pitocin) through the mother's intravenous (IV) line or methylergonovine malleate (Methergine) as an intramuscular injection. These medications help keep the uterus contracted. When the uterus contracts, it squeezes shut the blood vessels from the placental bed to reduce bleeding. If your uterus doesn't seem to be contracting well, your doctor or nurse may massage your uterus, through your abdomen, to promote contractions.

The blood coming from your vagina, called *lochia*, may initially appear bright red and contain clots. Over time, it takes on a pinkish and later a brownish color. It gradually diminishes in volume, but the flow may persist for weeks after delivery. You may notice that the amount of bleeding increases each time you breast-feed. This increase happens because the hormones that help produce breast milk also cause your uterus to contract, and this contraction squeezes out any blood or lochia in the uterus. Many patients tell us that the bleeding is heavier when they stand up after being in bed for a while. This extra bleeding happens simply because the blood pools in the uterus and vagina while you're lying down, and when you stand up, gravity draws it out. It's perfectly normal.

If your lochia takes on a foul odor, let your nurse or practitioner know.

Perineal pain

The amount of pain or soreness you feel in your *perineum* (the area between the vagina and the rectum) depends largely on how difficult your delivery was. If your baby came out easily after only a couple of pushes and you have no episiotomy or lacerations, you probably feel little pain. If, on the other hand, you pushed for three hours and delivered a ten-pound budding linebacker, you're more likely to have perineal discomfort. (See tips for handling the pain in the nearby sidebar "Tips on perineal care after delivery.")

The pain you feel has several causes: The baby, as it comes through the birth canal, causes stretching and swelling of the surrounding tissues. Also, an episiotomy or tears in the perineum naturally hurt, just as an injury to any other part of your body would. The pain is worse during the first two days after delivery. After that, it rapidly improves and is usually nearly gone within a week.

Your perineum may be swollen, and if you had an episiotomy, you have stitches closing it up. Sometimes these stitches are visible on the outside, and sometimes they are buried underneath the skin.

Many women are concerned about the stitches used to sew up their episiotomy or lacerations. These sutures are not meant to be removed. They gradually dissolve over the next one to two weeks. They are strong enough to handle most activities, so don't worry that a sneeze, a difficult bowel movement, or lifting your 10-pound baby will cause the stitches to tear open.

Keeping the perineal area clean to prevent an infection from developing is important. Such an infection is a rare complication, but call your doctor if you notice a foul-smelling discharge or increasing pain and tenderness in the area.

Swelling

Immediately after delivery, especially after a vaginal delivery, you may discover that your entire body looks swollen. Don't freak out — it's normal. Many women develop swelling during the last few weeks of pregnancy, and this swelling often persists for a few days into the postpartum period. The intense pushing efforts required to deliver the baby may further cause your face and neck to swell, but this also goes away a few days after delivery. In general, it can take up to two weeks for the swelling to completely go away.

A little advice: Don't step on the scale the day after you deliver. You may find that you have actually gained weight from all the water you retain during delivery.

Tips on perineal care after delivery

Here are the best ways to care for your perineum (the area between the vagina and the rectum) as it recovers from your delivery:

✔ Keep the perineal area clean. You may want to use a squirt bottle filled with warm water to help clean places that are difficult to reach. Sometimes your nurse at the hospital can give you one to take home with you.

✔ Some women get relief from pain by taking a *sitz bath*. A sitz bath consists of soaking your bottom in a small amount of warm water. In the hospital, the nurses provide you with special basins for taking sitz baths. At home, you can sit in a few inches of warm water in the bathtub. If you have a lot of swelling in the area, putting Epsom salts in the water may give you added relief.

✔ You can buy various kinds of anesthetic sprays and pads that you can apply to the perineum to help ease the pain. Or you can soak gauze pads in witch hazel and apply them to the area. Some women find that chilling the witch hazel increases its effectiveness. (You can also buy little gauze pads that are presoaked in witch hazel — Tucks, for example.) Other women find that ointment or petroleum jelly is soothing, too. It keeps the skin moist and soft and prevents it from sticking to sanitary pads.

✔ An ice pack applied to the perineum during the first 24 hours after delivery helps minimize swelling and decreases your discomfort.

✔ Over-the-counter pain relievers — such as acetaminophen (Tylenol is a well-known example) or ibuprofen (such as Motrin or Advil) — or some prescribed pain medications further ease the pain. These medications are not a problem if you're breast-feeding.

✔ Avoid standing for long periods of time, which can make the pain worse.

✔ After a bowel movement, try not to contaminate the area with the toilet tissue you use to wipe yourself. Clean the area around the anus with a separate toilet tissue, and don't wipe from back to front. If the areas around the anus or the perineum are tender, try to just pat the area dry, instead of wiping. You may find that using baby wipes is really helpful, because they clean the area very well, don't shred, and are gentle on healing tissues.

✔ Do not insert anything into your vagina (such as a tampon), and do not douche for the first six weeks.

Many patients ask, "Isn't there something you can give me to help relieve the swelling, like a diuretic or something?" Prescribing medication is usually not necessary because the swelling goes away on its own in a few days, when you are back up and around. Just be patient. You *will* have ankles again.

Your feet may be so swollen that fitting into your normal shoes is difficult. Bring a large, comfortable pair (running shoes or sneakers are good) to wear home from the hospital.

Battle scars

You may find that after delivery, your face is not only swollen but also very red and possibly splotchy. Some women even have black eyes or broken blood vessels around their eyes and, all in all, look as though they've just been in a prize fight. All these characteristics are to be expected; they're caused by the rupture of tiny blood vessels in your face during pushing. Don't be alarmed. You'll look like your old self again in a few days.

Afterpains

The intense contractions that you experienced during labor and delivery that caused your cervix to dilate and helped to push your baby out gradually space out and fade away. But a few persist sporadically after delivery. These contractions are called *afterpains*. As we mention earlier, you may notice that the afterpains are worse or more noticeable while you are breast-feeding. These contractions are completely normal and gradually go away.

Your bladder function postpartum

You may find urinating difficult immediately after delivery, or you may feel discomfort when you do urinate. This discomfort is a result of the way the bladder and urethra are compressed when the baby's head and body come through the vagina. The tissues around the opening to the urethra are often swollen after delivery, and this swelling can add to the discomfort. Some women may need to be *catheterized* (a thin, flexible plastic tube is inserted through the urethra into the bladder) after delivery to help empty the bladder. The problem is sometimes worse in women who have an epidural, because the anesthesia can hang around in your system for several hours and temporarily make the bladder more difficult to empty. But your bladder regains its normal tone a few hours after delivery, so urinary discomfort is usually a short-lived problem.

If you feel primarily a burning sensation during urination, let your doctor or nurse know, because it may be a sign that you're developing a urinary tract infection.

Some women experience the opposite problem; they find that they don't have good control over their bladder function. Some women even find that they leak a little urine when they stand up or laugh, or that they have to run like a cheetah to make it to the john in time. If this incontinence happens to you, don't worry too much, because time usually solves the problem. In some cases, it may take a number of weeks to get things under control.

Kegel exercises (see the section later in this chapter) may be useful if the problem persists. Another good strategy is to make a conscious effort to go to the bathroom at regular intervals to empty your bladder before you absolutely have to.

The hemorrhoid blues

Most of your pushing efforts during delivery are focused toward the rectum, a fact that causes many women to develop *hemorrhoids* — dilated veins that pop out from the rectum. Unfortunately, having no problems with hemorrhoids before you go into labor is no guarantee that they won't appear after delivery. If you develop hemorrhoids during the last part of your pregnancy, they may get worse after delivery. At times, hemorrhoids can be more uncomfortable than an episiotomy, and they last a little longer.

In the past, it was thought that sitting on a rubber donut cushion was a good idea for dealing with hemorrhoids, because it supposedly took pressure off the swollen tissue. However, more recent information suggests that these cushions may actually increase pressure on the hemorrhoids and make matters worse.

Sometimes the pain associated with hemorrhoids is due to spasms of the *anal sphincter,* which is the muscle around the rectum. A warm sitz bath helps relax the sphincter and reduces the pain. You can take a sitz bath as often as three or four times a day. Pads soaked in witch hazel or local anesthetic creams also can help relieve pain.

The good news is that the problem is usually temporary. Postpartum hemorrhoids typically go away within a few weeks. Sometimes they don't go away completely, but for the most part they are not bothersome. You may not be troubled by them at all for a few months, and then they may be uncomfortable again for a few days, and then get better again.

Things you can do to help have a bowel movement after delivery

Making whatever efforts you can to promote having a bowel movement after your delivery pays off. Here are a few ways to help the process along:

✔ Walk around the postpartum ward as much as you can. Walking improves circulation to

the bowels and can help to eliminate any residual effects of the epidural.

✔ Try taking stool softeners such as Colace.

✔ Try not to think about it too much. Things happen in time.

Postpartum bowel function

Many women find that they do not have a bowel movement for a few days after delivery. This lack of bowel function happens for several reasons:

✔ You usually don't eat much food around the time of labor and delivery, so you may have very little waste in your system to get rid of.

✔ Epidurals and some other pain medications sometimes slow down the bowels a little, and your system may take a few days to return to normal.

✔ Many women are afraid of bearing down because they don't want to tear the stitches used to repair their episiotomy, so they avoid having a bowel movement altogether. But doing this is not a great idea. You have no reason to be afraid of tearing the stitches. Your episiotomy is repaired in several layers with strong sutures. Tearing the sutures is extremely difficult, especially by having a bowel movement.

If you have hemorrhoids or have a laceration that reaches back to the rectal area (see Chapter 9), a bowel movement may be painful. You can reduce the discomfort by using a local anesthetic cream and by using stool softeners. Also, you may want to take a pain reliever shortly before you anticipate having a bowel movement.

In-Hospital Recuperation after a Cesarean Delivery

As we mention earlier, the hospital stay after a cesarean delivery is generally a few days longer than after a vaginal delivery — usually on the order of three to four days in total. If you have a cesarean delivery, you're put on a stretcher immediately afterward and transported to the recovery room. You may be able to hold your baby in your arms during the trip.

Going to the recovery room

When you're in the recovery room, your nurse and anesthesiologist monitor your vital signs. The nurse periodically checks your abdomen to make sure that the uterus is firm and that the dressing over the incision is dry. Your nurse also checks for signs of excessive bleeding from the uterus. More than likely, you have a catheter in your bladder, and it stays in place for the first night so that you don't have to worry about getting up to go to the bathroom. You also have an intravenous (IV) line in place to receive fluids and any medications your doctor prescribes. If you had an epidural or spinal anesthetic, your legs may still seem a little numb or heavy. This feeling wears off in a few hours. If you had general anesthesia (that is, if you were "put to sleep"), you may feel a little groggy when you get to the recovery room. Just as with a vaginal delivery, you may experience some shaking (see Chapter 9). If you're up to it and if you want to, you can breast-feed your baby while you're in the recovery room.

Most likely, you receive pain medication in the operating room, and you don't need any more while you're in the recovery room. In some hospitals, if you have an epidural or spinal, your anesthesiologist injects a long-lasting medication into the catheter that keeps you almost pain-free for about 24 hours. If, however, your pain medication doesn't seem to be working, by all means let your nurse know.

When your nurse and anesthesiologist are confident that your vital signs are stable and that you're recovering normally from the anesthesia, you're discharged from the recovery room — generally about two or three hours after delivery. You're transported on a stretcher to a hospital room, where you spend the rest of your recovery time.

The day of delivery

The day of your cesarean, you should pretty much plan on just staying in bed. Thanks to your catheter, you don't need to worry about getting up to go to the bathroom. If your surgery took place early in the morning, you may feel like getting up later in the evening. At least, you may feel like getting out of bed and sitting in a chair. Just be sure to check with your nurse first to see whether getting up is okay. When you get up the first time, make sure that someone is there to help you.

Although some doctors still prefer that patients not have any food immediately after a cesarean, many doctors now allow women to eat and drink shortly after the surgery. Often, we find that the patient is the best judge of what she should and should not do: If you feel queasy and nauseous, you're better off not eating. But if you feel hungry, drinking liquids and having small amounts of solid food is probably fine.

Day one after delivery

The first day after your surgery, your doctor is likely to encourage you to get out of bed and start to walk around. The first couple of times you get up to walk may be pretty uncomfortable — you may feel pain around the incision in your abdomen — so you may want to ask for a so-called *top up* dose of pain medication 20 minutes or so before getting up.

You should have someone with you the first few times you get up to make sure that you don't fall.

Depending on your fluid needs, your doctor may also discontinue your IV line. Most of the time, you're able to drink liquids on the first day, and many doctors also let you eat solid food.

Most likely, you have a bandage over your abdominal incision. Sometimes this bandage comes off on day one, but sometimes doctors prefer to leave it on longer.

Dealing with post-op pain

Like women who have had a vaginal delivery, you should expect some vaginal bleeding *(lochia)* after a cesarean. The bleeding may be quite heavy during the first few days after your surgery. The amount of pain or discomfort experienced after a cesarean delivery varies from woman to woman, depending on the circumstances of her delivery and on her tolerance for pain. Your practitioner can prescribe pain medication, but he or she probably will specify that the medication should not be given unless you ask for it. (Sometimes this is hospital policy.) So if you want the pain relief, ask for it — before your pain intensifies to the point of being excruciating. Ask for the medication when you anticipate getting out of bed or just before your next dose of medication is due (usually after three or four hours), so that you give your nurse enough time to get it for you.

Your final days in the hospital

Most women who have a cesarean delivery and have staples in their skin (see Figure 11-1) worry that removing the staples will hurt. But don't worry. Staple removal is a quick and painless procedure.

Many women ask about "rooming in" — that is, having the baby stay in the room with them — after a cesarean delivery, especially after they've had a day or so to recover a bit from the procedure. Having the baby in the room with you is certainly fine if you feel up to it. But by no means feel that you have to. Keep in mind that you just had abdominal surgery, and you may not be physically able to attend to every single one of your baby's needs during the first few days afterward. The hospital nurses are there to help, so during this time devote as much energy as possible to your own recovery. You'll be that much better able to care for your baby after you get home.

After surgery, you'll find that each day is noticeably easier and more comfortable than the one before. Over the course of three days, you will gradually find it easier to get out of bed and walk around. You will start to eat normally again. You will also be able to shower — and many women find that first

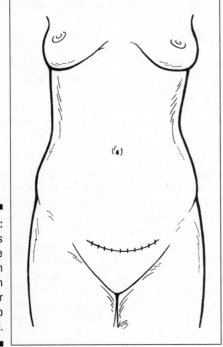

Figure 11-1:
Staples
hold the
cesarean
incision
together
and help
it heal.

shower a truly big relief. But please keep in mind that you have just been through not only major surgery but also nine months of pregnancy! And you must recover from both. Some women really do recover quickly and feel like going home after only a couple of days. But many women need more time to feel strong enough to leave the hospital. As you probably know already, the length of your stay may be determined to some extent by what your insurance plan allows and what is mandated by individual state laws. And occasionally, a post-operative infection or some other complication necessitates a longer than usual hospital stay. But typically you're ready to go home after about three days.

Here are some indications that you may be ready to go home:

✔ You tolerate food and liquids without any problem.

✔ You urinate normally and without difficulty.

✔ Your bowels are on their way to recovering normal function.

✔ You have no signs of infection.

Causes of post-cesarean pain

You may feel a kind of burning pain at the site of your abdominal skin incision. This pain is worse when you get out of bed or change positions. Eventually, the burning diminishes to a sort of tingling sensation. It is much improved within a week or two after surgery.

You may also feel pain from post-delivery uterine contractions — just as women who deliver vaginally do. Your doctor is likely to give you oxytocin (Pitocin) for the first few hours after your surgery to encourage contractions and thus minimize blood loss. Pain from contractions diminishes by the second day, although it may recur when you breast-feed, because breast-feeding can trigger more contractions.

You may feel pain in tissues deep beneath your skin. A cesarean is not a simple slit through the surface of a woman's belly. The physician must cut through several layers of tissue in order to reach the uterus. Each layer must then be repaired. And every one of the repaired incisions can generate pain. That's why women often feel pain deep in their abdomen after a cesarean. This pain usually takes one to two weeks to fade away. Many women tell us that they feel more pain on one side or the other, possibly because the stitches are a little tighter on one side. Whatever the reason, uneven pain is very common and nothing to worry about.

Many women say the worst pain of all is gas pain. The intestines accumulate a large amount of gas after a cesarean delivery, in part because of the way the intestines are manipulated during the surgery but also as a result of the medications — the anesthetics used during the operation and the painkillers given afterward. Gas pains typically begin on the second or third day after delivery and improve when you start to pass gas. It pays to get up and walk around as much as possible, because doing so gets the gastrointestinal tract moving again.

If you have a cesarean delivery after going through labor for hours, you may have perineal pain — from pushing and from any number of internal exams — on top of everything else. This pain disappears soon after delivery.

Postpartum: At Home

You may wonder why this book — or any pregnancy book — covers the time after the baby is born, after you return home from the hospital. It's not just to help you get started with newborn care — although we try to help get you going on that, too (see Chapters 10 and 12). But it takes six to eight weeks for your body to return to anything like normal after pregnancy (no more swelling or bleeding, your skin may be better, and most of your clothes fit again), and much longer to be fully back to your old size and shape (getting back to your pre-pregnancy weight, having your cesarean delivery scar heal completely, and having your stretched-out skin return to normal). And the transition from pregnant to nonpregnant comes with a few side effects.

Recovering from a vaginal birth

By the time you're discharged from the hospital after a vaginal delivery, most of the acute pain is gone. After you get home, however, you can still expect some soreness. The main area of discomfort is around your perineum. No matter how easy your delivery may have been, this part of your body has undergone some real trauma, and it simply needs time to heal. Try not to let the lingering discomfort associated with having just given birth frustrate you. Keep in mind what an amazing thing your body has just been through. In addition to dealing with the soreness from delivery, you need to adjust to a new lifestyle — getting up at all hours of the night, changing diapers, and feeding your new baby.

Perineal care

If you have an episiotomy or any lacerations in your perineum that have to be repaired after your delivery, you probably continue to feel discomfort or pain after you return home from the hospital. You can continue to take sitz baths three to four times a day. Just put a few inches of warm water in the tub and soak your bottom for 10 to 15 minutes. You can also continue to use pads soaked in witch hazel or topical anesthetic sprays, if they work for you. As we mention previously, petroleum jelly or ointment is helpful in keeping the healing tissue smooth and soft.

Relieving the gravitational pressure on your perineum from time to time by getting off your feet and lying down for a short while is important. Finding the time may be hard — given that you're incredibly busy caring for a new baby — but make it a priority. And take heart — usually in a week and certainly by two weeks, most of your discomfort is gone.

If you're extremely uncomfortable, you may want to ask your doctor to prescribe pain medications. If you notice that your perineal area is very red or purple and tender, if you run a fever, or if you notice a foul-smelling discharge, let your practitioner know.

If you had any lacerations that extended near your rectum, you may want to take a stool softener (such as Colace), *not* a laxative, so that bowel movements aren't too terribly painful. At least make sure that you drink extra fluids and consume extra fiber in your diet so that your stool is soft. When you anticipate having a bowel movement, you may want to take a pain reliever ahead of time — acetaminophen (Tylenol), perhaps, or some other so-called *nonsteroidal anti-inflammatory agent* such as ibuprofen (Motrin or Advil).

Hemorrhoids

If you develop hemorrhoids during delivery or if you have hemorrhoids that become worse during labor, you may also benefit from taking frequent sitz baths. In this case, too, try to lie down several times a day to take some of the pressure off. You may find some over-the-counter anesthetic creams that help in easing the pain. Witch hazel pads are also very helpful in relieving some of the discomfort of hemorrhoids. Consider taking a stool softener (such as Colace), as we mention earlier, and make sure that you consume plenty of fluids and fiber. This way, bowel movements won't hurt so much and you won't have to push too hard (which makes hemorrhoids worse). Your hemorrhoids are likely to go away within one to two weeks.

Recovering from a cesarean birth

When you're discharged from the hospital after a cesarean delivery, you're well on your way down the road to recovery. However, it takes a little longer to get back on your feet than it does after a vaginal delivery, and for the first week or two after you return home, you should take it easy.

Get the help you need from family and friends, if possible. If you can afford it, consider hiring professional help — a baby nurse — for the first few weeks. (A baby nurse can be quite helpful for women who've had vaginal births, too.) Try to keep the household chores you do to a minimum. Avoid running up and down stairs a lot. Devote your energy to taking care of your new baby and taking care of yourself. Pay attention, and your body will clearly let you know how much activity you can handle.

Most doctors recommend that you not drive a car yourself for the first week or two. This restriction is not because of the anesthesia you may have had; it really doesn't affect your reflexes for more than a day or two after delivery. The problem is simply that any leftover pain you may be experiencing after delivery may make it difficult for you to quickly move your foot from the gas pedal to the brake if you need to stop suddenly. When your pain is gone, it's safe to resume driving.

Most doctors also advise you to postpone any abdominal exercises until after your six-week checkup, so that the incisions in all the layers of your abdomen have time to heal completely.

Most women feel pretty much back to normal by the six-week point. But some need as long as three months to fully recover.

Taking extra iron

By the time you're home from the hospital, you should be able to eat normally. If you lost a great deal of blood during your surgery, however, you may want to ask your doctor whether you should take extra iron supplements.

Your scar

At first, the scar from your cesarean delivery looks reddish or pinkish. In time, it may turn a darker shade of purple or brown, depending to some extent on the color of your skin. Over the course of a year, the scar will fade and, eventually, assume a very pale color. If you have dark skin, it may be brownish. Most of the time, a cesarean scar is pencil thin or even thinner. A scar from a cesarean delivery may look prominent immediately after the procedure, when the staples are still in place, but after they're removed and the scar has several weeks to heal, you'll observe how it begins to fade into something far less obvious.

Many factors can affect the healing process and thus determine what the scar ultimately looks like. Some women naturally are prone to form a thick type of scar, called a *keloid*. In these cases, little can be done to change the situation.

You may notice that the area around your incision becomes numb. This numbness occurs because in making the incision, your doctor cut through some of the nerves that transmit sensation in that area. The nerves do grow back, however, and in time the numbness turns into a mild tingling sensation and then returns to normal.

Some women notice a blood-tinged fluid discharge coming from the center or side of their incision. This drainage sometimes happens when blood and other fluids accumulate under the incision and then seep out. If only a small amount oozes out and then stops, it's okay. But if you notice persistent blood-tinged or yellowish discharge from your incision, let your doctor know. Occasionally, the incision may open at the point where the drainage occurs. If so, your doctor may want you to take special measures to keep the opening clean so that it heals on its own.

Concerning all new moms

Many aspects of postpartum life are the same whether you had a vaginal or a cesarean delivery. Now that you're no longer pregnant, your body begins shifting back to its prepregnancy state, and you're in for a number of changes.

Night sweats and perspiration

If you're managing to get any sleep at night despite having a new baby in the house, you may find that you wake up drenched in sweat. Even during the daytime, you may notice that you perspire significantly more than usual. This sweating is very common and is thought to have something to do with fluctuations in hormone levels that occur as your body returns to a nonpregnant state. It is very similar to the night sweats and hot flashes that menopausal women get, due to a drop in estrogen levels. As long as the sweating is not associated with any fever, it's not a problem. It goes away over the course of the next month or so.

When to call your doctor after a cesarean birth

Most women who have cesarean deliveries recover without any problems. In some cases, however, you may not heal quickly and smoothly. Call your doctor if you notice any of the following:

✔ If you notice that pain from your incision or from your abdomen increases, rather than decreases

✔ If large amounts of blood or blood-tinged fluid drain from your incision

✔ If you have a fever higher than 100.4 degrees Fahrenheit

✔ If your incision begins to open up

Bathing

Traditionally, doctors told women not to take deep tub baths after delivery if they were still bleeding. Today, many practitioners say that tub baths are okay, and most feel that shallow sitz baths, at least, are perfectly acceptable. If your practitioner feels that it's better for you to wait until your bleeding has subsided, it is due to the concern that full baths may increase the chance that you may develop some infection inside your uterus. The trouble is that doctors really have no data on this topic — no studies demonstrate a risk from taking full baths. You should ask your practitioner what he or she thinks you should do.

Breast engorgement

A woman's breasts typically begin to *engorge* — fill with milk — three to five days after she delivers her baby. You may be amazed to see how huge your breasts can really be! If you're breast-feeding, your baby lessens the problem for you as he or she gets the hang of nursing, learns to take in more milk, and establishes a pattern of feeding. At the same time, you also get the hang of breast-feeding, and your nipples stop feeling sore, especially when your baby first latches on. (See Chapter 12 for more information about breast-feeding.)

If you're not breast-feeding, you may find that your breasts stay engorged for 24 to 48 hours (which can be quite painful) and then you begin to feel better. Wearing a tight-fitting supportive bra may make the process a little less uncomfortable. Applying ice packs or bags of frozen peas to your breasts helps the milk to "dry up," as does taking cold showers. Cold temperature causes the blood vessels in the breasts to constrict, lessening milk production, while warmth causes the blood vessels to dilate, promoting milk production. (Doctors no longer prescribe a medication to help a woman's milk dry up, because the drug they once used has been associated with some significant complications.)

Bleeding long after delivery is over

Lochia starts off bright red and then gradually lightens in both color and quantity. It usually stops sometime between three to six weeks after delivery, but in some women it continues for as long as eight weeks.

Some women worry if they find that clots of blood come out when they get up from lying down, just as they did in the hospital. But these clots are very normal during the first week after delivery. Blood accumulates in the uterus or vagina, it clots, and it finally comes out when you stand up. It may be more noticeable if you're breast-feeding because breast-feeding causes the uterus to contract and thus squeeze blood out.

If you have very heavy bleeding with clots that lasts for several weeks after your delivery, let your practitioner know.

The best way to deal with postpartum bleeding is to use sanitary napkins. Pads in varying thicknesses, to accommodate whatever amount of bleeding you have, are available. Tampons are not advised because they may promote infection during the time that your uterus is still recovering. Although the bleeding usually subsides tremendously after two weeks, some women experience bleeding for six to eight weeks. Occasionally, fragments of placental tissue stay within the uterus, and this condition can lead to extensive bleeding.

Stretch marks

The majority of women develop some stretch marks during pregnancy. If you don't, you're one of the lucky few. Whether you have them and the extent to which you have them depends in part on how much weight you gain, the type of skin you have, and your basic genetic propensity to develop stretch marks. The marks usually fade over the course of several months after delivery. In light-skinned women, stretch marks become silvery white; in dark-skinned women, they turn lighter brown. Many women apply vitamin E, creams, lotions, and other concoctions to their stretch marks, but these products are generally not effective. Indeed, we know of no cure for stretch marks, although some dermatologists are trained in laser techniques that may reduce the extent of the stretch marks considerably.

Hair loss

One of the stranger aspects of the postpartum return to normalcy is hair loss. A few weeks or months after delivery, most women notice that they're shedding like crazy. This shedding is normal. It is one of the effects that estrogen has on your body during pregnancy. This common problem doesn't last long. Your hair is usually back to normal by nine months after delivery.

All hair follicles go through three phases of development: a *resting* phase, a so-called *transitional* phase, and a *shedding* phase. The elevated levels of estrogen that are present during pregnancy essentially freeze your hair in the resting phase. Within a few months after delivery, all that hair proceeds on to the shedding phase. Suddenly, you notice large amounts of hair sticking in your brush or washing down the drain.

Getting Back to Exercise

It typically takes six to eight weeks for the changes that your body experiences during pregnancy to disappear — which means that, after delivery, your body needs some time to get back in shape for vigorous exercise. Resume your sports and workouts gradually. Naturally, the amount of exercise you can handle depends on what kind of shape you've been in before and during your pregnancy. Whatever your condition, you're well advised to make exercise a priority. Fitness has many important benefits for both your physical and emotional well-being. It can help your body recover from the stress of pregnancy, and it helps you feel more even-tempered and better about yourself.

Kegel exercises

Kegel exercises are squeezing motions aimed at strengthening the muscles of the pelvic floor that surround the vagina and rectum. These muscles give support to the bladder, rectum, uterus, and vagina. Keeping them strong is key to reducing the adverse effects that pregnancy and delivery can have on this part of the body. If the pelvic floor muscles are very weak, the chances are greater that you will develop *urinary stress incontinence* — a leakage of urine when you cough, sneeze, laugh, or jump — or *prolapse* or *protrusion* of the rectum, vagina, and uterus — in which these organs begin to sag below the pelvic floor. Pregnancy places extra weight on the pelvic floor muscles, and vaginal delivery stretches and puts added pressure on them. The net result is a general weakening. Some women seem to naturally maintain excellent muscle tone in the pelvic floor after delivery. But others notice symptoms of weakness: a little urinary incontinence, the feeling that their vagina is loose, or pressure on their pelvic floor from a sagging uterus, vagina, or rectum. The way to strengthen the pelvic floor muscles — to avoid or diminish these symptoms — is to perform Kegel exercises.

To perform these exercises, you tighten the muscles around your vagina and rectum. Here's a simple way to find out what it feels like to do the exercises correctly: Sometime when you're urinating, try to stop the flow of urine midstream. Or insert a finger in your vagina and try to tighten the muscles around your finger. If you're doing Kegels correctly, your finger feels the squeeze. (Both of these techniques are simply ways of figuring out how to squeeze the muscles, not the way you normally practice the exercise.)

When you're first doing Kegels, squeeze the muscles for only a few seconds and then release. Squeeze five to ten times per session, and try to do three to four sessions a day. Ultimately, you can build up to the point where you hold each squeeze for ten seconds and do 25 squeezes per session. You should continue to do the Kegels four times a day. You can do them while you're sitting, standing or lying down, and you can do them while you're also doing something else — bathing, cooking, talking on the phone, watching television, driving your car, or standing in line at the grocery store.

Abdominal exercises

After pregnancy, restoring strength to your abdominal muscles is especially important. In some women, pregnancy causes the abdominal or *rectus* muscles to separate a little, as shown in Figure 11-2. The medical term for this separation is *diastasis*. Doing abdominal exercises to restore their strength and draw them together is important.

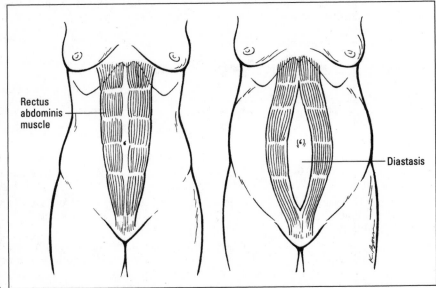

Figure 11-2:
After pregnancy, your abdominal muscles may be separated a bit, one side from the other.

Rectus abdominis muscle

Diastasis

The thing you must do to restore strength to your abdominal muscles is contract them. Any number of styles of abdominal exercises called *crunches* work fine.

A good abdominal exercise is the most basic, simple one: Lie on your back with your knees bent and feet flat on the floor a few inches apart. Raise your head and shoulders three to six inches above floor level. When you do this exercise correctly, you can literally feel your abdominal muscles tightening. Start with three sets of 8 or 10, and see whether you can work up to doing three sets of 16.

Working your lower abdominals is also important. One good exercise is to lie on the floor with your legs lifted up in the air at about a 90-degree angle. Slowly lift your bottom an inch or two off the floor, breathing out as you do. Try doing 8 to 10 repetitions, rest for a while, and then repeat — and repeat again. After a while, you can work yourself up to doing 15, 20, or even 30 in a row.

You can also do some exercises with your baby — and get the most out of playtime. Lying on your back, lift your legs up and bend your knees at a 90-degree angle. Then you can lay your baby stomach-down on your lower legs and lift your head and shoulders upward, reaching your face toward your baby's. Start with three sets of 5.

You can also do push-ups while playing with your baby. Just lay the baby on the floor and position your hands on either side, with your body stretched out away from the baby. Start with your arms straight and then slowly bend your elbows to lower your body until you're close enough to touch your nose to your baby's. Straighten your arms to raise your body; repeat. If you're not strong enough to do a standard push-up, keep your knees on the floor. Try to start with two sets of 10 and work your way up to two sets of 15 or 20 (on the toes).

When your baby is old enough to hold up his or her head, you can try the simple — and fairly self-explanatory — baby bench press: Lie flat on your back, hold your baby to your chest, and simply (and gently) lift him or her straight up in the air — again and again. Start with two sets of 10. Later on, try for three sets.

Over the course of two weeks, depending on how you feel, you can gradually increase your exercising until you're fully active again. Finding the time may be a problem, of course. But fitting exercise into your schedule is worth every effort. Taking care of a newborn can make you feel as though you've just run a marathon, but real exercise is what your body needs. In fact, by improving your overall sense of well-being, exercise can make the whole challenge of caring for a new baby much easier.

Walking is great exercise for just about everyone. During the first two weeks after delivery, take it slow. But after that, you may find that long or brisk walks are enjoyable for both you and your baby — and a great form of exercise.

Pondering Your Postpartum Diet

Any woman who's just had a baby needs to once again examine her diet. If you're breast-feeding, you want to ensure, as you did when you were pregnant, that you're eating a healthy combination of foods that provide both you and your baby with good nutrition and also getting enough fluid. (For more information about how to follow a balanced, nutritious diet, see Chapter 4.) What's more, many women who have just delivered babies are eager to return to their prepregnancy weight.

Losing the weight

You may feel like jumping onto a scale right after delivery to see how much weight you've lost. But take caution. Some women do lose a lot of weight quickly after delivery, but some actually gain weight from all the fluid retention. Rest assured that you will soon weigh less than you did before you delivered, probably about 15 pounds less, but the loss may not register until a week or two after delivery.

Here's what accounts for the initial weight loss:

Baby	6 to 9 pounds
Placenta	1 to 2 pounds
Amniotic fluid	1 to 2 pounds
Maternal fluids	4 to 8 pounds
Shrinking uterus	1 pound

Your uterus continues shrinking for several weeks. Immediately after you deliver, it still extends up to about the level of your navel — about the same point as when you were 20 weeks pregnant. However, because of the excess skin you now have, you probably still look pregnant when you stand up. Don't let your appearance get you down! Your uterus keeps contracting and your skin regains much of its tone until, by about two months after delivery, your belly is down to its prepregnancy size.

Most women need two to three months to get back to their normal weight, but, of course, the time varies according to how much weight you gain during pregnancy. If you gain 50 pounds (and had just one baby), don't expect to look fabulous in a bikini six weeks after you deliver. Sometimes it takes a woman an entire year to get back into shape. A healthy diet and regular exercise help the weight come off.

Try to get as close to your prepregnancy weight — or your ideal body weight (see Chapter 4) — as soon as is reasonably possible. You don't have to let a pregnancy turn into a permanent weight gain. If you let each successive pregnancy cause a little more accumulation, your health may suffer in the long run.

Taking your vitamins

Whether or not you breast-feed, continue taking your prenatal vitamins for at least six to eight weeks after you deliver. If you do breast-feed, keep taking vitamins until you stop breast-feeding. If you lost a particularly large amount of blood during your delivery, your practitioner may suggest that you take iron supplements to help restore your blood count. Calcium is also very important for any woman, especially if you're breast-feeding, in order to keep your bones strong. A calcium supplement or extra calcium in your diet is a good idea.

Having Sex Again

If you're like most women postpartum, sex is the last thing you want to think about. Many women find that their interest in sex declines considerably during the first weeks and months after pregnancy. But at some point, the fatigue and emotional stress of childbirth ease up, and your thoughts are likely to be more amorous again. For some lucky women, the rebound occurs fairly quickly. For others, it may take 6 to 12 months.

The drastic hormonal shifts that occur after delivery directly affect your sex organs. The precipitous drop in estrogen leads to a loss of lubrication for your vagina, and less engorgement of blood vessels, as well. (Increased blood flow to the vagina is a key aspect of sexual arousal and orgasm.) For these reasons, intercourse after childbirth can be painful and sometimes not all that satisfying. With time, as hormone levels return to their prepregnancy norm, the problem tends to correct itself. In the meantime, using petroleum jelly or some other lubricant sold specifically for this purpose helps.

The exhaustion and stress of caring for an infant further reduces the desire for sex in some women. Your attention, and your partner's, too, is likely to be focused more on the baby than on the relationship between the parents. It may help to set aside some time for the two of you to be alone together, to be intimate. This time together need not even include sex — just holding, hugging, and expressing feelings for each other.

Giving your body time to heal

Most doctors recommend that women refrain from intercourse for four to six weeks after the baby is born in order to give the vagina, uterus, and perineum time to heal and for the bleeding to subside. At your six-week follow-up doctor visit, you can ask your practitioner about various methods of birth control (see the next section).

Choosing contraception

Many people believe that breast-feeding prevents a woman from becoming pregnant. But while it is true that breast-feeding *usually* delays the return of ovulation (and, thus, periods), some women who are nursing do ovulate — and do conceive again (see Chapter 12). You may not ovulate the entire time that you breast-feed, or you may start again as early as two months after delivery. And if you don't breast-feed, ovulation begins, on the average, ten weeks after delivery, although it has been reported to occur as early as four weeks. If you breast-feed for less than 28 days, your ovulation will return at the same time as it does for non-nursing women. So considering your options for birth control before you have sex again is important. Most women have a wide range of birth control options. But some women have medical conditions that prevent them from using certain methods. Obviously, you should discuss your options with your practitioner at a postpartum visit. Following is a list of some potential options:

- ✓ **Condoms and contraceptive foam.**

- ✓ **Depo-Provera.** This progesterone-based injection is administered every three months.

- ✓ **Diaphragm.** If you already have a diaphragm, bring it along to your postpartum checkup so that your practitioner can make sure it's still the right size. Some women need a different size after delivering a baby.

- ✓ **IUD (intrauterine device).** An IUD is a good form of birth control for women who don't want to conceive for at least a few years after delivery and who are in a stable, monogamous relationship. An IUD can be placed six to eight weeks after delivery.

- ✓ **Norplant.** This form of contraception consists of five tiny capsules that are implanted just under the skin inside a woman's upper arm. Each capsule contains a slow-release form of progesterone. The capsules last, on average, five years. If you want to get pregnant before they're used up, your doctor can easily remove the implants.

✔ **Oral contraceptives.** If you're not breast-feeding, you can start taking birth control pills about six weeks after you deliver. If you are breast-feeding, your practitioner may advise against starting the Pill until breast-feeding is firmly established, because of concerns that the estrogen it contains may reduce your milk supply (at least at first). But after breast-feeding is well under way, most feel that taking the Pill is fine. An alternative is the progesterone-only pill, which is slightly less effective but has no effect on milk production.

✔ **Permanent forms of sterilization.** If you and your partner are certain that you're finished with childbearing, you may want to consider permanent sterilization. This form of birth control may be be performed immediately after delivery — or during a cesarean delivery — or as an outpatient procedure a few months later. When a tubal ligation is performed immediately after delivery, it involves tying a knot around a loop of fallopian tube, and then cutting off the loop above the knot. The procedure is repeated on the other fallopian tube. When a tubal ligation is performed six weeks later, it is most commonly performed by a laparoscopic technique that involves inserting a telescope-like device through the navel. Each tube is grasped and then cauterized, clipped, or banded. Some states require that special forms be signed for a specific number of days or weeks in advance of a tubal ligation, so if you're interested in having the procedure done at the time of delivery, discuss it with your practitioner during your pregnancy. Another way of managing permanent sterilization is for your partner to have a vasectomy. This is also an outpatient procedure, usually performed by a urologist.

Postpartum Doctor Visits

Most practitioners ask their patients to come in for a checkup about six weeks after delivery if both the pregnancy and the birth were uncomplicated. If you had a cesarean or some complication, you may be asked to come in earlier.

During a postpartum checkup, your practitioner performs a complete exam (including a breast and vaginal exam) and obtains a Pap smear. In most cases, the six-week checkup suffices for your annual gynecological exam. Your practitioner probably also talks with you about your birth control options. This is a good time to discuss the "spacing" of future children (see Chapter 13) and other things you should do before conceiving again — such as take folic acid a few months beforehand and, if this pregnancy had complications, getting whatever special blood tests your practitioner may advise.

The Baby Blues

The vast majority of women — as many as 80 percent, studies show — suffer a bout of the blues during the first days and weeks after they deliver. Typically, you begin to feel a little down a few days after the birth, and you may continue to feel vague sadness, uncertainty, disappointment, and emotional discontent for a few weeks. Many women are surprised at the feeling — after all, they've looked forward to motherhood, and they feel sure that they're really thrilled about it. No one knows for sure *why* women get the blues postpartum, but a few explanations are plausible. First, the shift in hormone levels that comes after delivery can affect mood. Also, when pregnancy ends, a mother must change her whole focus. After focusing on the birth for so many months, she suddenly finds that the big event is over, and she may feel almost a sense of loss. And let's face it — parenthood brings tremendous anxiety, especially for a first-time mother. Feeling overwhelmed by all the responsibility and all she needs to learn about caring for a baby is not unusual for a woman. Add in the physical discomfort — episiotomy repair, breast tenderness, hemorrhoids, fatigue, and the rest — and you begin to wonder how any new mother can avoid feeling a little blue.

Fortunately, postpartum blues tend to fade away rather quickly, usually by about two to four weeks after the birth. Keep in mind that what you're feeling is extremely common and that it doesn't mean you don't love your child or that you won't be a fabulous parent. Be open about it; let your spouse, family members, and friends know how you feel, because you need love and support at this time. Try to get as much sleep as possible, because fatigue only makes matters worse.

Coping with the blues

If you find yourself suffering from the baby blues, remember that you're not the first woman to feel this way. The feeling is as normal as pregnancy itself. And take heart: Those who have already grappled with the problem have found a number of ways to ease the blues. Here is a list of some of the best strategies:

- Lack of sleep compounds the problem of the baby blues. Everything is worse when you're physically fatigued. The amount of stress that you can handle when you've had your rest is much greater than if you haven't slept enough. So try to get more sleep. If the baby is napping, try to lie down and nod off yourself.

- Accept other people's offers of help. In most cases, there's no reason you should have to take care of your baby entirely by yourself. You're a great mom, even if you do let Aunt Suzie or Grandma Melba change a diaper or burp the baby.

✔ Talk about how you feel with other mothers, close family members, and friends. You're likely to find that they felt exactly as you do now. They can empathize with you and offer suggestions for how to cope.

✔ If possible, try to get some time to yourself. Often, new parents are overwhelmed by the realization that their time is no longer their own. Get out of the house for a while, if you can. Take a walk, read, watch a movie. Often the blues are exacerbated by the fact that your body is still not back to what it used to be, and now you no longer have the excuse of being pregnant. So pamper yourself with a manicure or pedicure, a trip to the hair salon, or a massage. Have dinner with your husband or with a friend.

If you do not begin to feel better in three or four weeks, let your practitioner know. Some women go beyond the blues into full-blown postpartum depression.

Postpartum depression

True *postpartum depression* is not nearly as common as the blues, but it does affect more women than you might imagine. Between 10 and 15 percent of women develop depression within six months after they deliver. Symptoms include severe unhappiness, an inability to enjoy being with the baby (or life in general), lack of interest in caring for the baby, insomnia, weak appetite, inability to function day to day, extreme anxiety or panic attacks, and even thoughts of harming the baby or yourself. While postpartum blues are usually mild and transient, full-blown depression can be severe and lasting. Despite the severity of the symptoms, postpartum depression often goes unrecognized, or the mother may attribute the problem to something else.

No one knows exactly why postpartum depression occurs, but certain characteristics put a woman at higher than normal risk. These risk factors include:

✔ History of postpartum depression

✔ History of depression in general

✔ Experience of anxiety before the birth

✔ Life stress

✔ Lack of good support systems

✔ Marital dissatisfaction

✔ An unplanned pregnancy

✔ Unhappiness about the labor and delivery process

If you have postpartum blues and they don't go away after three or four weeks, if the feeling seems to be getting worse, or if you develop the blues more than two months after your delivery, discuss the situation with your doctor. Your blues may have blossomed into full-fledged postpartum depression.

Treatment for postpartum depression includes counseling (group or individual psychotherapy), antidepressant medications, and, rarely, hospitalization. Recent studies have suggested that in some cases, taking small doses of estrogen under the tongue can help. This treatment, of course, should only be done under your doctor's supervision. Your doctor may want to check to see whether you have *postpartum thyroid disease,* which can mask itself as depression or make your depression worse. These are all details that you should discuss with your doctor.

To get further information about how to handle postpartum depression, you may want to get in touch with one of the following resources:

✔ Postpartum Support International; phone (805) 967-7636

✔ Depression After Delivery, Inc.; phone (800) 944-4PPD; Web site www.behavenet.com/dadinc

Chapter 12

Feeding the Baby

● ●

In This Chapter

▶ Breast or bottle — making the decision that's right for you

▶ Getting into the breast-feeding routine

▶ The basics of formula-feeding

● ●

*O*ne of the first big decisions any new parents make is whether to breast-feed their infant or use formula and bottles. Although the majority of parents these days choose to breast-feed, the decision is by no means always an easy one. If you find it difficult to decide, take comfort in the fact that both choices are sound and legitimate. In this chapter, we lay out the basic first steps you need, no matter which way you go.

Deciding between Breast and Bottle

Ask almost anyone — your obstetrician, your pediatrician, your friends, total strangers — and they will advise you to breast-feed. This opinion represents, in part, a return to early 19th-century values but also incorporates recent medical knowledge. Bottle-feeding became all the rage in the 1950s, during the peak of the baby boom, when techniques were developed to pasteurize and store cow's milk in formulas appropriate for infant nutrition. Breast-feeding has regained popularity largely because people and organizations (including the American College of Obstetrics and Gynecology and the American Academy of Pediatrics) have come to recognize the many good medical reasons to do it. It strengthens the baby's immune system and helps prevent allergies, asthma, and sudden infant death syndrome. (See the sidebar later in the chapter for more details about the reasons to breast-feed.)

However, the decision whether or not to breast-feed isn't always simply a medical one. It also involves issues of convenience, aesthetics, body image, and even conditions surrounding delivery (see the upcoming sidebar, "The bottle versus the breast"). Some women find that they are uncomfortable with the whole physical concept of breast-feeding. Others want to bottle-feed so that they aren't the only one who can feed the baby. Still others have work or time pressures that make bottle-feeding more convenient. In the final analysis, the decision about how to feed the baby is a personal one that every mother has a right to decide for herself. Learning to breast-feed takes an incredible commitment, and you shouldn't feel pressured to do it if your heart isn't in it. If you have decided that bottle-feeding is the best decision for you and your baby, don't feel guilty about it.

You may hear that breast-feeding offers the best opportunity for a mother to bond with her baby. But in fact, bottle-feeding can also be a very warm and loving way to interact with your baby — and not only for the mother but also for the father and whoever else may be helping care for the baby. And while breast-feeding offers certain undeniable benefits, the vast majority of bottle-fed babies are — and remain — perfectly healthy.

Whatever your decision, make it *before* you deliver, so that you have adequate time to prepare for the moment when your baby starts feeding. Some women elect to try out breast-feeding for a little while to see how they like it. Some decide from the beginning to use a combination of both breast and bottle (filling the bottle with either formula or breast milk that has been pumped and refrigerated).

The bottle versus the breast

Both bottle-feeding and breast-feeding have their benefits. The following two lists give you food for thought when making your feeding decision.

Reasons to breast-feed:

✔ Human breast milk can strengthen the baby's immune system and help prevent allergies, asthma, and sudden infant death syndrome. It can also decrease the number of upper respiratory infections in the baby's first year of life.

✔ Mother's milk contains nutrients that are ideally suited to a baby's digestive system. Cow's milk is not as easily digested, and the nutrients it contains are not as readily used by the baby.

✔ Human milk also contains substances that help protect a baby from infections until his or her own immune system matures. These substances are especially plentiful in the *colostrum* — the premilk substance that mothers' breasts secrete during the first few days after the baby is born.

✔ Babies are more likely to have an allergic reaction to cow's milk than to mother's milk.

✔ Breast-feeding is emotionally rewarding. Many women feel that they develop a special bond with their baby when they breast-feed, and they enjoy the closeness surrounding the whole experience.

✔ Breast-feeding is convenient. You can't leave home without it. You never have to carry bottles or formula with you.

✔ Mother's milk is cheaper than formula and bottles.

✔ You don't have to warm up breast milk; it's always the perfect temperature.

✔ Breast-feeding provides some form of birth control (though it's not totally reliable — see the section "Birth control for nursing mothers").

✔ *Lactation* (milk production) causes you to burn extra calories, which may help you lose some of the weight you gained during pregnancy.

✔ A breast-fed baby's bowel movements don't have as strong an odor as those babies who formula-feed.

✔ Breast milk is organic — no additives, no preservatives.

✔ Some studies suggest that women who breast-feed may reduce their lifetime risk of breast cancer.

Reasons to bottle-feed:

✔ You don't want to breast-feed. If your heart's not in it, it ain't gonna happen. Too much trial and error is involved in making breast-feeding work for someone who's not truly committed to succeed.

✔ If you've tried breast-feeding and your breasts don't produce enough milk to feed your baby (or babies!).

✔ Bottle-feeding may better fit your lifestyle. Although many working mothers are able to breast-feed, many feel that juggling the requirements of their job with those of breast-feeding is just too difficult. Bottle-feeding is one solution.

✔ Some women find the whole concept of feeding their baby a "bodily secretion" unpleasant.

✔ Bottle-feeding enables other family members (or caregivers) to feed the baby.

✔ If you have a chronic infection — HIV, for example — bottle-feeding helps ensure that it's not passed to the baby (it can be passed to the baby via breast milk). Women who carry the hepatitis B virus are able to breast-feed as long as the baby has received HBIG and the hepatitis B vaccine.

✔ If you or your baby is very sick after delivery, bottle-feeding may be your only option. A mother or baby who's in the intensive care unit (ICU) because of a complicated delivery often can't initiate breast-feeding. The mother can use a mechanical pump to empty the milk from her breasts and freeze the milk to feed to the baby later (up to six months), when the baby's condition improves. Even if the baby can't use the pumped milk at this time, pumping at least keeps the supply of milk flowing. Occasionally, a mother can start lactating later on, when she or the baby recovers, but this option isn't always possible. Restarting the flow of milk often requires the assistance and advice of a lactation specialist.

✔ If you've had previous surgery on your breasts, bottle-feeding may be your best bet (you may not be able to lactate). No medical evidence indicates that lactation has any effect on the progression of breast cancer after it has already been diagnosed, but some women who have had surgery or other treatment for breast cancer are unable to lactate. Also, there is some evidence that women who have had breast implants produce less milk. However, many of these women produce some milk and can still breast-feed.

✔ If you take certain medications, bottle-feeding may be best. Some women take medications that could pass through the breast milk and affect the baby adversely. Such drugs include anticancer and antileukemia drugs (such as cyclophosphamide, doxorubacin, methotrexate, and cyclosporin), Parlodel, (bromocriptine), lithium, and some migraine treatments (ergotamine, specifically). Ask your doctor about any medications you take regularly.

In any case, if you have made an informed choice about whether to breast-feed or bottle-feed, don't let anyone change your mind or make you feel guilty about your decision.

The Basics of Lactation

The flood of estrogen and progesterone that your body experiences during pregnancy causes your breasts to grow — sometimes to astonishing size. This growth starts early, within three to four weeks of conception, which is why the first sign of pregnancy for many women is breast tenderness. As pregnancy goes on, small amounts of serum-like fluid can leak from the nipples. But serious milk production doesn't start until after the baby is born.

During the first days after delivery, the breasts secrete only a yellowish fluid known as *colostrum,* which doesn't contain much milk but is rich in antibodies and protective cells from the mother's bloodstream. These substances help the newborn fight off infections until his or her own immune system matures and can take over. Colostrum lasts for about five days. Gradually, it turns to milk.

Don't be alarmed if your baby doesn't seem to get much milk during the first few days. The colostrum is very beneficial on its own. Your baby probably doesn't even have much of an appetite until he or she is three to four days old. And he or she is likely to need the first few days to practice sucking movements.

The action of your baby beginning to suck on your breasts signals your brain to have the breasts start producing milk. About three or four days after delivery, milk production sets in. When milk enters the ducts, the breasts become engorged with milk (see Figure 12-1). The engorgement can be so great that your breasts feel rock-hard and sometimes very tender. Don't worry, though. When your baby starts feeding regularly and your milk starts flowing, the engorgement is no longer so intense. The *letdown reflex* (milk entering the ducts) occurs each time your baby feeds. After you have been nursing for a while, you may find that the mere sound of your baby crying or the feel of your baby cuddling next to you can trigger the reflex.

Lactating women typically produce about 600 milliliters (10 ounces) of milk per day by the end of the first postpartum week. This increases to about 800 milliliters (14 ounces) by the end of the third week and peaks at 1½ to 2 liters (25 to 35 ounces).

The protein content of human milk and formula is less than that of cow's milk, but human milk and, to a lesser extent, formula, have a greater proportion of whey protein, which is the most beneficial kind. Human milk doesn't contain appreciable amounts of vitamin K, which is why newborns usually get a shot of vitamin K at delivery (to help prevent problems with blood clotting). Formula contains the most iron, but substances in human milk enhance the absorption of iron, so babies who breast-feed actually end up getting more of it. Human milk is highest in saturated fats, which are important for the growth and maturation of the baby's nervous system.

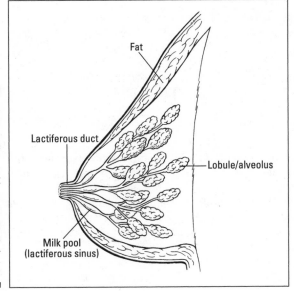

Figure 12-1:
Your breasts
contain a
network of
milk ducts,
which start
delivering
colostrum
during the
first days
after
delivery.

Fat

Lactiferous duct

Lobule/alveolus

Milk pool
(lactiferous sinus)

All You Ever Wanted to Know about Breast-Feeding

Pregnancy goes a long way toward preparing your body for breast-feeding. The key pregnancy hormones cause the breasts to enlarge and prepare the glands inside the breasts to lactate. But you can do a few things for yourself to prepare for day-to-day nursing. You can, for example, toughen your nipples a bit — and thus minimize soreness later on — in a few different ways.

✔ You can wear a nursing bra with the flaps down (allowing your clothing to rub against your nipples).

✔ You can roll your nipples between your thumb and forefinger for a minute or so each day.

✔ You can rub your nipples briskly with a terry washcloth after bathing or showering.

Be aware, however, that stimulating your nipples late in your pregnancy can elicit uterine contractions. When you near the end of your pregnancy, you should ask your practitioner before doing this kind of stimulation. One way to get around this problem is to avoid the nipple itself and just rub petroleum jelly, an antibacterial ointment, or baby oil over the areola.

Some women have inverted nipples and worry during pregnancy that their nipples will make breast-feeding difficult. Usually, the problem corrects itself before the baby is born, but a few techniques can help things along:

✔ Use the thumb and forefinger on one hand to push back the skin around the areola. If this doesn't bring the nipple out, use your other thumb and forefinger to gently grasp your nipple, pull it outward, and hold it for a few minutes, as shown in Figure 12-2. You can do this exercise several times a day.

✔ You can also try wearing special plastic breast cups (available at most drug stores) designed to help draw out the nipple over time.

The best idea is to start one of these preparation techniques for short sessions during the second trimester and then gradually increase the amount of time you work your nipples or wear the cups until your nipples stay out on their own.

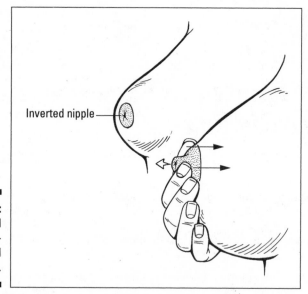

Inverted nipple

Figure 12-2:
One method
of correct-
ing inverted
nipples.

Breast-feeding positions

You can breast-feed in one of three basic positions, as shown in Figure 12-3. Use whichever position works and is comfortable for you and your baby. Most women alternate among the positions according to where they are when they're breast-feeding.

✔ **Cradling:** The simplest way is to cradle your baby in your arms with his head next to the bend in your elbow and tilted a bit in toward your breast. (See Figure 12-3a.)

✔ **Lying down:** In the lying down position, you lie on your side in bed with the baby next to you. Support the baby with either your lower arm or pillows so that her mouth is next to your lower breast, and use your other arm to guide your baby's mouth to the nipple. This position is best for middle-of-the-night feedings or after a cesarean delivery when sitting up is still uncomfortable. (See Figure 12-3b.)

✔ **Football hold:** Another common position is known as the *football hold:* You cradle your baby's head in the palm of your hand and support the body with your forearm. You may find that placing a pillow underneath your arm for extra support helps in this position. You can use your free hand to hold your breast close to the baby's mouth. (See Figure 12-3c.)

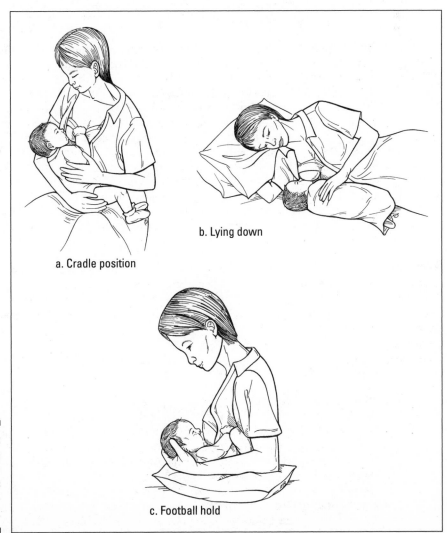

a. Cradle position

b. Lying down

c. Football hold

Figure 12-3: The three basic positions for breast-feeding.

You may find that you need to try different combinations of these basic positions to find the one that works best for you.

Getting the baby to latch on

If you choose to breast-feed, there's no reason why you can't get started immediately after delivery, wherever you happen to be — the birthing room, the delivery room, or the recovery room. As soon as the nurses have checked your baby's health and your baby has settled down a bit from the delivery, you can begin. Things are likely to be a little awkward at first, and you may as well anticipate this situation and try not to get too frustrated. Many babies don't want to breast-feed immediately. Have patience — you and your baby will eventually get the hang of it.

Babies are born with a suckling reflex, but many of them don't follow it enthusiastically right off the bat. Sometimes babies need some coaxing to latch onto the breast. After you have your baby in one of the basic breast-feeding positions (see the preceding section), use your nipple to gently stroke the baby's lips or cheek. This action probably causes the baby to open his mouth. If your baby doesn't seem to want to open his mouth, try *expressing* (gently pressing out) a little milk — colostrum, really — and rubbing some on the baby's lips. When the mouth is wide open, bring the baby's head to your breast and gently place the baby's mouth over your entire nipple. This prodding usually causes the baby to start sucking. Make sure that the entire areola is inside the baby's mouth, because if it isn't, he doesn't get enough milk and you get sore nipples. However, don't stuff your breast into your baby's mouth. Rather, bring the mouth to your nipple, and let the infant take in the breast.

The tip of the baby's nose should be barely touching the skin around your breast. The only way the baby can breathe is through her nose, so be careful not to completely cover the baby's nose with your breast. If your breast obstructs the baby's nose, use your free hand to depress your breast in front of the nose to let some air in.

Feeding sessions

After your baby latches on, you know that she is sucking when you see regular, rhythmic movements of the cheeks and chin. Several minutes of sucking may go by before your milk letdown occurs. In the beginning, let your baby feed for about five minutes on each breast per nursing session. Over the course of the first three or four days, increase the amount of time on each breast to 10 to 15 minutes. Don't get too hung up about timing the feedings, though; your baby lets you know when she has had enough by not sucking and letting the nipple slip away.

If your baby stops sucking without letting go of the nipple, insert your finger into the corner of his mouth to break the suction. (If you just pull your breast straight out, you'll end up with sore nipples.)

When switching from one breast to the other, stop to burp your baby by laying her either over your shoulder or your lap and gently patting her back. Figure 12-4 shows you some of the various burping positions. You should burp her again when the feeding is finished.

Typically, mothers breast-feed about eight to twelve times a day (averaging ten). This pattern enables your body to produce an optimal amount of milk, and it allows your baby to get the proper amount of nutrition for healthy growth and development. Try to space the feedings fairly evenly throughout the day; of course, your baby has some influence on the schedule. You don't have to wake your baby for a feeding — unless your pediatrician specifically advises you to do so. You especially don't have to wake your baby at night; if the baby's willing to sleep through, just count yourself lucky. Nor do you have any reason to withhold a feeding if your baby is hungry — even if only an hour or so has passed since the last feeding. (Also keep in mind that the number of feedings in a day may be less than average if you supplement breast-feeding with some formula feedings.)

You can tell whether your baby is getting enough milk by watching for the following indications:

✔ Your baby nurses ten times a day on average.

✔ Your baby gains weight.

✔ Your baby has six to eight wet diapers a day.

✔ Your baby has two to three bowel movements a day.

✔ Your baby's urine is pale yellow (not dark and concentrated).

If your baby is not meeting these criteria or if you have *any* concern that your baby is not getting enough milk, call your pediatrician. Some women, no matter how diligent they are, just can't produce enough breast milk to totally meet the needs of their baby and need to supplement breast milk with formula.

Breast-feeding diet

During breast-feeding, as during pregnancy, your nutrition is largely a matter of educated common sense. The quality of your breast milk isn't significantly affected by your diet unless your eating habits are truly inadequate. However, if you don't take in enough calories, your body has a difficult time producing adequate milk. You may also find that your baby reacts a different way to certain foods. For example, he may be extra gassy if you've eaten particular foods. If you can pay attention to how your baby seems to respond to different foods, it will help you figure out what foods you might want to avoid.

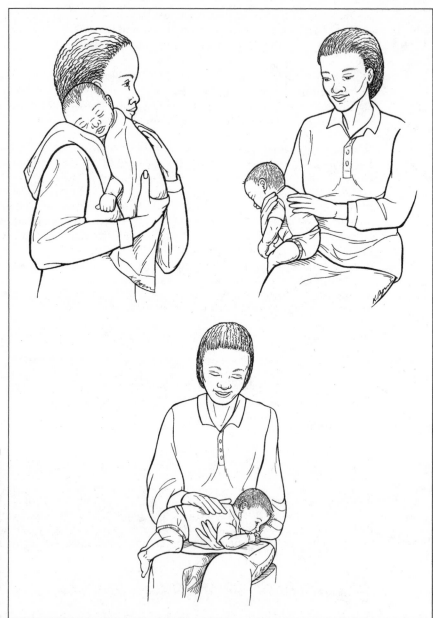

Figure 12-4:
There's more than one way to burp a baby. Here are a few of the tried-and-true positions.

Women who are breast-feeding should take in an extra 400 to 600 calories a day over and above what they would normally eat. The exact amount varies, of course, according to how much you weigh and how much fat you gained during pregnancy. Because lactating does burn fat, breast-feeding is a good way to help get rid of some of the extra fat stores you may have. But avoid losing weight too fast, or your milk production will suffer. Also, avoid gaining weight while you're breast-feeding. If you find that you're putting on more pounds, you're most likely taking in too many calories.

In addition to calories, you also need extra vitamins and minerals — especially vitamin D, calcium, and iron. Keep taking your prenatal vitamins or some other balanced supplement while you're nursing. Also consume extra calcium — either a supplement or extra servings of milk, yogurt, and other dairy products.

Breast milk is mainly water (87 percent). To produce plenty of breast milk, you must take in at least 72 extra ounces of fluid per day, which is about nine extra glasses of milk, juice, or water. Don't go overboard, however, because if you drink too many fluids, your milk production may actually decrease. A good way to tell whether you're getting the right amount of fluid is to monitor your urine output. If you urinate infrequently or if the color is a deep yellow, you are probably not getting enough. If you constantly run to the bathroom, you may be drinking too much.

Birth control for nursing mothers

Although breast-feeding does decrease the likelihood of ovulation, it by no means guarantees that you won't become pregnant again. For a woman who chooses *not* to breast-feed, it takes an average of 10 weeks after the birth to resume ovulation — that is, to become fertile again. About 10 percent of women who *do* breast-feed also begin ovulating again after 10 weeks, and about 50 percent are fertile again by 25 weeks postpartum — about six months after their babies are born. Clearly, breast-feeding is not a great form of birth control.

After you resume intercourse, consider using some effective form of birth control, because chances are you don't want to become pregnant again right away (see Chapter 11). You can use birth control pills (see the nearby sidebar "Our patients want to know . . ."), barrier methods (condoms, diaphragm, and so on), or long-acting progesterone shots (such as Depo-Provera). Discuss your options with your practitioner at your six-week checkup.

Medications and breast-feeding

Just about any medication you take gets into your breast milk, but usually only in tiny amounts. If you need to take a medication while breast-feeding, try taking the lowest dose possible and, as a rule, take it just *after* you finish a breast-feeding session. That way, much of the medication is broken down by the time you need to breast-feed again. In general, don't deprive yourself of medications that you really need just because you're afraid that some of it may get to the baby and cause harm. You should check with your doctor about medications to be sure that they're fine to take while breast-feeding.

The following medications are okay to take while breast-feeding:

- Acetaminophen (such as Tylenol)
- Antacids
- Most antibiotics
- Most antidepressants
- Antihistamines
- Aspirin
- Most asthma medications
- Decongestants
- Most high blood pressure medications
- Ibuprofen (such as Advil or Motrin)
- Insulin
- Most seizure medications
- Most thyroid medications

Problems that breast-feeding mothers may face

One of the greatest misconceptions about breast-feeding is that it comes easily and naturally to everyone. In fact, breast-feeding takes learning and practice. Problems can range from a little nipple soreness to, in rare cases, infections in the milk ducts. In this section, we discuss breast-feeding problems that some women experience.

Sore nipples

Many women experience some temporary nipple soreness during the first few days that they breast-feed. Fortunately, for most women, the pain is usually mild, and it goes away on its own. For some women, however, the soreness gets progressively worse and can lead to chapped or cracked nipples and moderate-to-severe pain. If your breasts are heading in this direction, take action before your suffering gets out of hand. The following list outlines some remedies.

- Review your breast-feeding technique to make sure that your baby is positioned correctly. If the baby isn't getting the entire nipple and areola in his or her mouth, the soreness is likely to continue. Try changing the baby's position slightly with each feeding.

Our patients want to know . . .

Q: "Can I breast-feed while I am on the Pill?"

A: It's fine, though it may, to some extent, affect the amount of milk you produce. Pills that contain estrogen decrease the amount of milk that you produce, and if you take them too soon after giving birth, they may make it difficult for your body to start milk production. However, after breast-feeding is well established, they are fine. Some women find that the newer progestin-only pills are a better alternative, because they have less effect on milk production, although they are slightly less effective.

✔ Increase the number of feedings and feed for less time at each feeding. This way, your baby won't be as hungry and may not suck as hard.

✔ Definitely continue to feed on the sore breast, even if only for a few minutes. This feeding is important to keep the nipple conditioned to nursing. If you let it heal completely, the soreness will only start all over again when you feed from that nipple again. We suggest that you feed on the least sore breast first, because that's when your baby's sucking is most vigorous.

✔ Express a little breast milk manually before you put the baby to the breast. This action helps initiate the letdown reflex so that the baby doesn't have to suck as long and hard to achieve letdown.

✔ Don't use any irritating chemicals or soaps on your nipples.

✔ After your baby finishes feeding, don't wipe off your nipples. Let them air-dry for as long as possible. Wiping them with a cloth may cause needless irritation.

✔ Exposing the nipples to air helps to toughen the skin, so try to walk around the house with your nipples exposed as much as possible. Also, if you wear a nursing bra, try leaving the flaps down as you go about your business at your house. As the fabric from your clothes rubs against them, your nipples toughen.

✔ If you're using pads to soak up leakage from your breasts, change them as soon as they get moist, or they may chafe your nipples.

✔ Try massaging vitamin E oil, ointment, olive oil, or lanolin into sore nipples and then let them air dry. It may sound kind of silly, but an old product called Udder Cream or Bag Balm, which was developed to treat chapped teats on milk cows, has found new popularity among some breast-feeding women. In fact, many drug stores and cosmetics stores now sell the cream. It contains lanolin and may be of help, if you can deal with the bovine name.

✔ Apply dry (not moist) and warm (not hot) heat to the nipples several times a day. You can use a hot water bottle filled with warm water.

Engorgement

As we mention earlier, when the breasts become engorged with milk, they can hurt. One way to avoid painful engorgement is to begin breast-feeding right after the baby is born. Other strategies that help include wearing a firm but not tight bra and massaging the breasts before feeding. Massaging facilitates letdown and relieves some of the engorgement. You can also try placing warm compresses on your breasts. (Some women feel that ice packs work better — try both and see which works best for you.)

Clogged ducts

Sometimes, some of the milk ducts in the breast may become clogged with debris. If this happens, a small, firm, red lump may form inside the breast. The lump may be tender, but it's usually not associated with a fever or excruciating pain. The best way to treat a clogged breast duct is to try to completely empty that breast after each feeding. Start the baby out on that breast when he or she is most hungry. If the baby doesn't completely empty the breast, use a breast pump on that side until all the milk is drained. Also, applying heat to the lump and massaging it manually is helpful. Most important, keep feeding!

If the lump persists for more than a few days, call your doctor to make sure that you're not developing an abscess.

Mastitis (breast infection)

Breast infections (mastitis) are reasonably common — occurring in about 2 percent of all breast-feeding women. They are usually caused by bacteria that come from the baby's mouth. They are most likely to happen two to four weeks after delivery, but they can occur earlier or later than that. Infections are more common in women who are breast-feeding for the first time, who have chapped nipples with cracks or fissures, and who do not empty the breasts completely at feedings.

The symptoms of mastitis include a warm, hard, red breast; high fever (usually over 101 degrees Fahrenheit); and malaise (like when you have the flu and your whole body feels achy). The infection in the breast may be diffused, or it may be localized to a particular segment of the breast (known as a *lobule*). If the infection is localized, the redness may appear as a wedge-shaped area over the infected portion of the breast, as shown in Figure 12-5. If these symptoms develop, call your doctor immediately. More than likely, he or she will prescribe an antibiotic and may even want you to come into the office for an examination.

You should continue to breast-feed your baby while you have the infection. It is not harmful to the baby; after all, the bacteria probably came from the baby's mouth. If you stop breast-feeding, the breast becomes engorged, making your discomfort even worse. Acetaminophen (such as Tylenol), ibuprofen, or warm compresses may help relieve the pain from mastitis while you give the antibiotics time to take effect. Drink plenty of fluids as you should when you have any illness — and get as much rest as you can, so that you allow your body's natural healing powers to work. Mastitis usually goes away about two days after you start taking antibiotics. However, continue your medication for the fully prescribed amount of time, to help make sure that the infection doesn't recur.

Breast abscess

If mastitis is not treated aggressively or if a clogged milk duct remains clogged, a *breast abscess* can develop. In fact, breast abscesses form in as many as 10 percent of all cases of mastitis. Symptoms of a breast abscess are extreme pain, heat and swelling over the area of the abscess, and high fevers (over 101 degrees Fahrenheit). Sometimes doctors can treat abscesses with antibiotics, but often the abscess needs to be drained surgically.

If you develop a breast abscess, you can continue to breast-feed on the other side, but you should stop feeding on the side of the abscess until the problem starts to resolve. Check with your doctor before resuming feedings on that side.

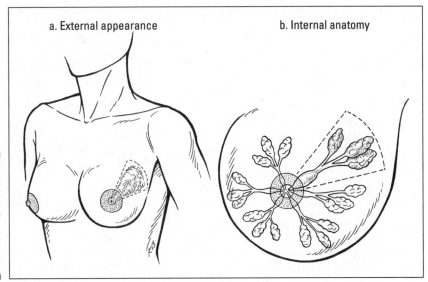

a. External appearance   b. Internal anatomy

Figure 12-5:
An outer view and an inner view of a wedge-shaped mastitis.

Breast-feeding twins

Even though it may seem daunting, some women with twins successfully breast-feed. Your body can make enough milk for two babies at once, especially if you're persistent and work up your milk production to a high level. But even if you have adequate milk, arriving at a system that works for you takes some experimentation. You may breast-feed both babies at once, or each one separately. Obviously, the advantage to the first alternative is that you don't have to spend all your time breast-feeding. The advantage to the second method is that it's easier. You don't have to deal with one baby finishing first and needing to be burped while the other one is still sucking. (Holding one baby over your shoulder and keeping another one at your breast can be very tricky, no matter how many pillows and props you use.) You may breast-feed one baby, bottle-feed the other, and then alternate at the next feeding. You may breast-feed each baby a little at each feeding and then supplement with the bottle. Or you may breast-feed both babies for most of the day and then supplement with a bottle before bedtime when your milk supply is low.

Women who breast-feed twins need to take in even more extra calories and fluids. You need about 400 to 600 extra calories per day for *each* baby you are breast-feeding. (Imagine how much you'd have to consume to breast-feed triplets!) Also, you need to increase your fluid intake from eight to ten glasses per day to about ten to twelve glasses per day.

Breast-feeding resources

If you have special problems or if you want more in-depth information about breast-feeding, contact one of the following organizations:

✔ The La Leche League International, 1400 N. Meacham Rd., Schaumburg, IL 60173-4048; phone 800-LA-LECHE; Web site www.lalecheleague.org.

✔ American College of Obstetricians and Gynecologists, 409 Twelfth St. SW, Washington, D.C. 20024; phone 800-673-8444; Web site www.acog.org.

✔ American Academy of Pediatrics, 141 Northwest Point Rd., Elk Grove Village, IL 60007; phone 800-433-9016; Web site www.aap.org.

✔ American Academy of Family Physicians, 8880 Ward Parkway, Kansas City, MO 64114; phone 816-333-9700; Web site www.aafp.org.

✔ American College of Nurse-Midwives, 818 Connecticut Ave. NW, Suite 900, Washington, D.C. 20006; phone 202-728-9860; Web site www.acnm.org.

✔ International Lactation Consultant Association, 4101 Lake Boone Trail, Raleigh, NC 27607; phone 919-787-5181; Web site www.ilca.com.

Or you can try one of the following approaches to get information and assistance with breast-feeding:

✔ Call the hospital where you intend to deliver or hospitals in the area where you live and ask to speak with a lactation consultant or lactation specialist.

✔ Ask your practitioner for breast-feeding information.

✔ Talk to friends and family members who have breast-fed their babies.

If you do decide to try breast-feeding twins, count on needing help from other family members and friends. Don't be afraid to ask for it. Good luck!

Bottle-Feeding for Beginners

Suppose you've decided to forego breast-feeding in favor of formula. Or you've been breast-feeding for a number of weeks or months, and you want to switch. In this section, we go over what you need to know to get your baby started on bottles.

Stopping milk production

If you do decide to formula-feed, you need to stop the process of milk production in your breasts. Milk production is triggered by warmth and breast stimulation. So to stop the production of milk, you want create the opposite environment. Here are some suggestions:

- ✔ Wear a tight-fitting bra.

- ✔ Apply ice packs to your breasts when they become engorged. This engorgement generally happens around the third or fourth day after your baby is born.

- ✔ Keep ice packs inside your bra, or use small packages of frozen vegetables, like peas or corn, which you can easily fold to fit within a bra. (We don't recommend going out in public this way, though.)

- ✔ Place cold cabbage leaves inside your bra. Cabbage works chemically to reduce the production of milk.

- ✔ Let cold water run over your breasts during a shower.

If you are going to breast-feed for a short period of time (6 to 12 weeks), consider giving your baby one bottle of formula per day while you are nursing to help make the transition easier.

Engorged breasts can be very uncomfortable. If you're in a great deal of discomfort, you may want to ask your doctor about pain medication. Fortunately, the engorgement usually lasts only 36 to 48 hours.

Choosing the best bottles and nipples

TIP

You won't have any trouble finding a wide choice of bottles and nipples, as shown in Figure 12-6. Some babies definitely demonstrate a preference for one type of bottle or nipple over another. Sometimes trial and error are the best tools for sorting out what works best for you and your baby. Four-ounce bottles are good for the first few weeks or months. Later, when your baby drinks a larger amount, you can switch to the larger eight-ounce bottles.

✔ Some bottles are actually plastic holders in which you insert little transparent plastic bags that hold the milk or formula. The advantage of this type, obviously, is that you can throw away the empty milk bag, and you don't have to worry about sterilizing the plastic container. Also, because the plastic bag is designed to collapse, less air gets into the bag and into the baby's stomach.

✔ Some bottles are angled, which also helps to allow less air to be taken in by the baby, leading to less gas.

✔ Nipples come in a wide variety. Orthodontic nipples are designed for a more natural fit. Some nipples have a flat surface, and others are more pointed. Some nipples are made out of latex, and others of silicone, which are clear and have less odor. Your baby may demonstrate a strong preference for one type over another, or may not notice much of a difference. The newborn nipples have a smaller hole, and the size of the hole increases with the age of the baby (nipples generally come in newborn, 3- and 6-month sizes, and then larger ones for older babies).

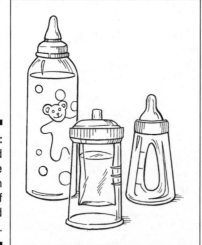

Figure 12-6:
Bottles and nipples are available in a range of sizes and shapes.

Bottle-feeding basics

Many parents are told to sterilize bottles by boiling them in water. But we and most pediatricians think that this step is unnecessary. After all, a mother who breast-feeds doesn't have to boil her nipples!

Many parents choose to warm their baby's bottle, but heating it isn't necessary. You can warm a bottle in different ways. You can place the bottle in a container filled with hot water or use a bottle warmer.

If you use the microwave to heat your baby's bottle, be careful. The formula may heat unevenly, and some parts of it may be too hot for the baby. However, if you shake the bottle after warming it, it may be okay. Just make sure you shake some onto your wrist to check the temperature first.

Saving leftover formula is generally not a good idea. However, some pediatricians say that reusing a bottle once is okay, so talk it over with your baby's doctor. In any case, don't leave a bottle filled with formula sitting outside the refrigerator for very long, because warmth encourages the growth of bacteria that can upset your baby's stomach.

Many formulas come premixed, but some come in either a powder or concentrated liquid form, both of which require you to add water. The powder and concentrated liquid forms cost less, but they may not be available in as wide a variety of formulas. (For example, some of the hypoallergenic formulas only come in the more expensive, premixed forms.)

Some babies develop an allergic reaction to their formula; they may have an upset stomach or get a skin rash. If your baby becomes allergic, talk with your pediatrician. He or she may want to switch your baby to a soy-based formula or some other hypoallergenic formula.

Pediatricians generally recommend against propping up a baby's bottle by laying it on a pillow next to the baby's mouth, because propping implies that the baby is being left unattended. Also, a baby lying flat on his or her back with the bottle propped creates more potential for choking. Propping a bottle may also promote tooth decay.

The most common position for bottle-feeding your baby is to hold the baby cradled in one arm, close to your body. You will find it most comfortable to put a pillow on your lap, which eases the strain on your arms and neck. Most women find it easier to always hold the baby in the same arm and in the same direction. For example, if you are right-handed, you may want to hold your baby in your left arm, and the bottle in the right. When the baby is a little older and has better control of his or her head and neck muscles, you may want to lay the baby in front of you vertically along your legs for a change of pace. This way, the baby can look straight ahead at you, and you both can make eye contact.

Here are some other tips for bottle-feeding moms:

- ✔ **Don't swaddle the baby too much or keep him too warm during feeding.** The baby may get so comfortable that he falls asleep instead of feeding.

- ✔ **Change the baby's diaper in the middle of a feeding.** This may help to wake her up, so that she can finish the rest of the bottle.

- ✔ **If your baby has trouble finding the nipple to put in his mouth, stroke his cheek, and he will turn in that direction.**

- ✔ **To check to see whether the baby is hungry, put the tip of your finger (a clean finger) into her mouth to see whether she starts to suck.**

- ✔ **Keep the bottle tilted in such a way as to completely fill the nipple with the formula, thereby minimizing the amount of air that gets into the baby.**

Burp your baby at least once midway through a feeding and again at the end of a feeding. (Refer to Figure 12-4 for various burping positions.) Babies often take in air along with the milk or formula they drink, and burping helps them to get rid of it. It makes them more comfortable and able to eat more.

Spitting Up

Whether they're breast-fed or bottle-fed, newborn babies have a tendency to spit up a little. Here are a few suggestions for dealing with this phenomenon:

- ✔ Keep a cloth over your shoulder when burping or holding your baby so that you don't have to constantly change, or ruin, your clothes.

- ✔ Keep a small bib on your baby during and after feeding so that you don't have to constantly change, or ruin, all the baby's clothes.

- ✔ Burp your baby after each feeding. Refer to Figure 12-4 to see some of the most common positions.

- ✔ If you're bottle-feeding, stop partway through the bottle to burp the baby, rather than allowing the baby to drink the entire bottle in one shot.

- ✔ Don't play with the baby too much after feeding. Jiggling the baby or moving the baby around a lot can lead to more spitting up.

- ✔ If your baby seems to be spitting up large quantities or if the spitting up is very forceful, let your pediatrician know.

Part IV
Special Concerns

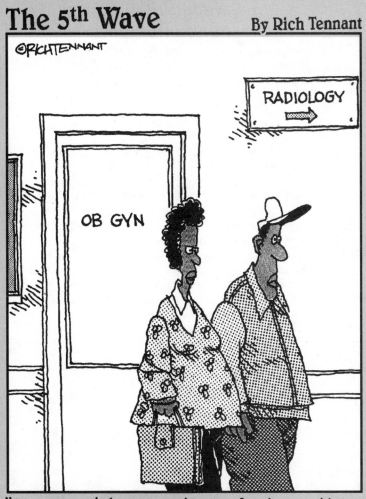

"I may not know anything about genetics, but I know that I'm overdue and it's your side of the family that's always late for family functions."

In this part . . .

You could actually go all the way through pregnancy without ever reading this part, especially if you're having your first child, you're not having twins (or more), and nothing — not even one tiny little thing — ever goes wrong or makes you uncomfortable. But very often, little things do come up. You get a cold and wonder how it affects your pregnancy. You develop an annoying rash. You're having twins or more. Or you have a significant medical problem or complication to deal with. We gather all these concerns into this part. More than any other part of the book, this one is designed to be read in pieces, depending on what particular situation you're in.

Chapter 13

Pregnancies with Special Considerations

• •

In This Chapter

▶ Starting parenthood later

▶ Meeting the challenge of multiple births

▶ Having second babies — and third, fourth, fifth . . .

▶ Being part of a thoroughly modern family

▶ Preparing older children for the new arrival

• •

*N*o two pregnancies are exactly alike. If you're like most women, you figure out pretty early in the game that your experience is different in some way from every friend and relative you talk to. You're not as nauseous as they were during the first three months — or your morning sickness is the worst you've ever heard of. You feel comfortable exercising throughout your pregnancy, while your sister was put on bed rest. Plenty of variation occurs within the boundaries of what is considered to be a normal, "average" pregnancy. But some special kinds of pregnancies come with their own particular characteristics and challenges. In this chapter, we describe the unique challenges that come along with older parenthood, having twins or more, and other unique situations.

Age Matters

Whether you're a prospective father or a prospective mother, age can make a difference — as many Baby Boomers are now finding out. In this section, we go over the special problems and issues that arise for men and women in their late 30s and older who are preparing to have children. We also touch on the teen mom and the challenges that can come with that situation.

The over-30 (or older) mom

Long gone are the days when almost all pregnant women were in their early 20s — and many were in their teens. Now, a greater number of women postpone having families until they've not only finished their education, but also have had a least a decade to become established in their careers. These days, too, divorce is far more common than ever before, and many women find themselves having children with a second husband — often when they're well into their 30s or 40s (and sometimes 50s). For these reasons, the age at which women have children has steadily increased.

How old is too old? The answer used to be when you reach menopause. Or in many cases, some years earlier, when your body no longer produces healthy eggs that can be fertilized to become embryos. But today, because of advances in assisted reproductive technologies — in vitro fertilization (IVF), using eggs donated from another woman — even women who are past the age of menopause can become pregnant.

Today, a more useful question is "At what age do you need to watch out for special problems?" And here, the answer is more specific. Any woman who is at least 35 years old during her pregnancy falls into the medical definition of *advanced maternal age,* or AMA. (An impersonal term, to be sure, but perhaps less insulting than the alternatives that are also used: *older gravida, mature gravida,* and the particularly unfortunate *elderly gravida.*) The reason for singling out older mothers with any special term at all is that the incidence of certain chromosomal abnormalities increases with advancing maternal age. At age 35, the risks begin to increase significantly, as shown in Figure 13-1.

At age 35, the risk that the fetus carries some chromosomal abnormality is great enough that it equals the risk of pregnancy loss after undergoing amniocentesis. Genetic testing — either amniocentesis or chorionic villus sampling (see descriptions of both in Chapters 6 and 5, respectively) — is routinely offered for pregnant women over the age of 35 in the United States. In other countries, the age may be different. (In England, for instance, the age is 37.)

The good news is that except for this increase in certain chromosomal abnormalities, babies born to women over 35, or even over 40, are as likely as any other babies to be healthy. The moms themselves do stand a higher than average risk of developing preeclampsia or gestational diabetes (see Chapters 14 and 15), and they stand an increased risk of needing a cesarean delivery. But these risks are not terribly high, and in most cases, any problems that result are minor. Naturally, an older woman's experience with pregnancy depends to a large extent on her underlying health. If a woman is 48 years old or even 50, but she is in excellent health, she is likely to do extremely well.

Maternal Age and Chromosomal Abnormalities (Live Births)		
MATERNAL AGE	RISK FOR DOWN SYNDROME	TOTAL RISK FOR CHROMOSOME ABNORMALITIES*
20	1/1667	1/526*
21	1/1667	1/526*
22	1/1429	1/500*
23	1/1429	1/500*
24	1/1250	1/476*
25	1/1250	1/476*
26	1/1176	1/476*
27	1/1111	1/455*
28	1/1053	1/435*
29	1/1000	1/417*
30	1/952	1/384*
31	1/909	1/384*
32	1/769	1/322*
33	1/602	1/286
34	1/485	1/238
35	1/378	1/192
36	1/289	1/156
37	1/224	1/127
38	1/173	1/102
39	1/136	1/83
40	1/106	1/66
41	1/82	1/53
42	1/63	1/42
43	1/49	1/33
44	1/38	1/26
45	1/30	1/21
46	1/23	1/16
47	1/18	1/13
48	1/14	1/10
49	1/11	1/8

Figure 13-1: As maternal age rises, so does the risk of chromosomal abnormalities.

Data of Hook (1981) and Hook et al. (1983). Because sample size for some intervals is relatively small, confidence limits are sometimes relatively large. Nonetheless, these figures are suitable for genetic counseling.*47.XXX excluded for ages 20-32 (data not available).

The not-so-young dad

As we mention earlier, pregnancies in older women call for some special scrutiny because of the increased risk of genetic complications. To some extent, pregnancies involving older dads should likewise be singled out for observation. There is no absolute age cutoff for "advanced paternal age," but many people use 45 or 50 (although some argue that it should be 35, just like for women).

A word about alternative conceptions

Thanks to assisted reproductive technologies, more and more women over 40 are becoming pregnant, some even with twins or triplets. While many of these women conceive with their own eggs, as we mention previously, many others conceive with someone else's. These women have unique issues to deal with — what to tell their future children, friends, and family. Some, when they are pregnant, experience internal conflicts about the baby's genetic identity; they worry what it will mean that the baby is biologically related to someone else. But often, these concerns disappear when the woman begins to feel her baby moving around inside her, and if not then, as soon as the baby is born.

Parents — even parents of children conceived the old-fashioned way — often discover after they meet their new baby in person that each child's identity is so unique that the exact genetic ancestry doesn't matter nearly as much as they may have thought it would. So it makes sense that women who have had children conceived with donor eggs typically find that, after only a few days of caring for the new baby, they feel every bit as maternal as any "biological" mother would. The same is true of fathers of children who have been conceived with donor sperm. As the number of people having children with donated eggs or sperm grows, the whole experience is likely to become more comfortable for everyone involved.

Whereas for women the main genetic risk is having a fetus with a chromosomal abnormality (most commonly an extra chromosome), for dads the risk is spontaneous gene mutations in the sperm that can lead to a child with an *autosomal dominant disorder.* This kind of problem, put in simplest terms, is one that can be caused by only one copy of an abnormal gene, such as *achondroplasia* (a type of dwarfism) or Huntington's disease. (In so-called *recessive genetic disorders* — cystic fibrosis and sickle-cell anemia, for example — two copies of the abnormal gene are required for the problem to occur.) Autosomal dominant disorders are very rare, however, and many are impossible to test for, which is why no routine testing exists for advanced paternal age.

The very young mom

Just as pregnancy can occur at an older age, it also occurs in teenage women. While this age group does not sustain any increase in chromosomal abnormalities, these women may experience a higher incidence of some birth defects. Because teenage moms tend to have less-than-optimal nutritional habits, they also experience a higher incidence of low-birthweight babies. Teenage moms are also at a higher risk of developing preeclampsia, are more likely to deliver by cesarean delivery, and are less likely to breast-feed. Due to their unique situation, these young moms need special guidance and counseling. If you are a teenage mom, we encourage you to receive adequate prenatal care, to follow a healthy diet, and to consider the benefits of breast-feeding.

Having Twins or More

The thought of having twins may seem simple — to someone who's never faced the reality of it. It's either "double the pleasure" or a living nightmare (twice the work and only half the sleep). In fact, twins *are* more complicated, as any mother of twins can tell you — for hours and hours, if you're willing to listen. Indeed, you could fill an entire book with advice for parents of twins, triplets, and more. And if such a book were written, a sizable first part of it would have to be about the experience of pregnancy for women carrying twins or more.

Keep in mind that if you are having triplets or more, what applies to twins generally applies to triplets (and more), only to a much greater extent.

Although the vast majority of twin pregnancies proceed smoothly and result in the birth of two beautiful, healthy babies, some risks are involved for both the fetuses and the mom. This is why most practitioners want women who are pregnant with twins to have checkups more frequently than other moms, and why they schedule plenty of extra ultrasound exams.

The number of twins that are conceived is much larger than the number that are actually born. Many pregnancies that begin as twin pregnancies end as single births because one of the fetuses never develops. In many cases, it seems, one of the fetuses disappears before the pregnancy is even diagnosed (the so-called *vanishing twin*). The incidence of twin births is usually estimated to be about 1 percent of all births. However, the incidence is rising, mainly due to the increasing use of fertility techniques.

Ethnic background and family history can, in some women, increase the chance of having twins. Such women are constitutionally more likely to ovulate more than one egg in a cycle. If twins occur in your family, let your practitioner know.

The incidence of spontaneous triplets is much more rare — about 1 in 7,000. For spontaneous quadruplets or more, it is exceedingly rare. However, with the increasing use of infertility treatments, the incidence of triplets has increased tenfold over the past few years.

Types of multiples

Twins can be either identical or fraternal. These old-fashioned terms do not completely describe how twins occur. *Identical* twins look very much alike and are always the same sex. They come from a single embryo, meaning that they are a product of the same union of one egg and one sperm. (In other words, they are *monozygotic* — they come from the same zygote.) They have exactly the same genes as each other, which explains their resemblance. In the United States, roughly one-third of all twins are identical. While it can happen that an egg splits into three, leading to identical triplets, it is very unusual.

Fraternal twins are conceived when a woman ovulates more than one egg, and the two eggs are fertilized by different sperm and implant in her uterus at the same time. These *dizygotic* twins — arising from two *zygotes* — do not share an identical set of genes. Instead, their genetic makeup is as similar as that of any pair of children born of the same parents. They're just born at the same time. They can be the same sex, or they can be of opposite sexes. Roughly two-thirds of all twins conceived spontaneously in the U.S. are this type. The incidence of "double ovulation" (and therefore fraternal twins, triplets, and so on) is higher in some African countries and lower in Japan than in the U.S. If three eggs are fertilized, the result is fraternal triplets. It is also possible that a triplet pregnancy consists of two fetuses that are monozygotic (from one egg that split) and one is from a second fertilized egg — leading to two babies that are identical and one that is fraternal.

The chances that a woman will have identical twins increases after she reaches the age of 35. The chances that a woman will have fraternal twins (because she ovulates more than one egg in any given month), on the other hand, rises until about the age of 35 and then drops off. Some families have more than their statistical share of fraternal twins. Fraternal twinning becomes more likely when a woman takes fertility drugs because these medications boost the chance that she ovulates more than one egg. Of course, the possibility still exists that a woman who takes fertility drugs produces an egg that gets fertilized and then splits in two to form identical twins.

Determining whether multiples are identical or fraternal

Many women who are pregnant with twins ask their doctor or ultrasonographer during an ultrasound exam if he or she can tell whether her twins are fraternal or identical. In some cases it is possible to tell; if you can see that the babies are two different sexes, you know they're fraternal. If they're the same sex, they may be either fraternal or identical. If they are the same sex, or if the sex of the fetuses is not yet visible, other findings on ultrasound can suggest whether the twins are identical.

- ✔ An egg that splits very early after fertilization, within the first two or three days, results in two embryos that have separate placentas and separate amniotic sacs. This situation is called *diamniotic dichorionic* (see Figure 13-2a). On ultrasound, they look no different from fraternal twins that came from two separately fertilized eggs.

- ✔ If an egg splits between the third and eighth day after fertilization, the resulting twins are in two separate amniotic sacs but share a single placenta (see Figure 13-2b). Your doctor may use the term *diamniotic/monochorionic* to describe this situation. If, on ultrasound, your doctor or ultrasonographer can see that a set of twins shares a single placenta, chances are that they are identical. (Keep in mind, though, that sometimes determining whether there is one placenta or two that are just very close together is difficult on ultrasound.) However, the thickness of the membrane separating the sacs gives another clue — with two separate placentas, a thick membrane is seen separating the two sacs, whereas with one placenta, the membrane is very thin.

✔ An egg that splits sometime between 8 and 13 days after fertilization results in twins that not only share a placenta but also are in a single amniotic sac (see Figure 13-2c). Twins like these are called *mono-amniotic/monochorionic*. If your doctor does an ultrasound examination and sees twins sharing the same amniotic sac, he or she can be sure that they are identical. This is pretty rare (1 percent of all twins, or 1 in 60,000 pregnancies).

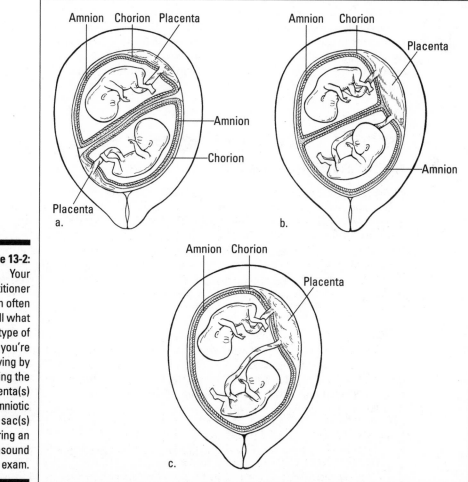

Figure 13-2:
Your practitioner can often tell what type of twins you're having by viewing the placenta(s) and amniotic sac(s) during an ultrasound exam.

✔ An egg that splits after the 13th day of gestation results in *conjoined* or "Siamese" twins. This is exceedingly rare.

The significance of these types of multiples becomes obvious when we talk later about problems that can arise with twin pregnancies.

An expert ultrasonographer can use subtle signs to help differentiate the various types of twins, although these signs are most often, although not always, definitive. It is most important to establish whether or not the twins have two separate placentas and less important to establish whether they are actually fraternal or identical. Establishing the type of placentation (monochorionic or dichorionic) is easier in the first trimester and harder in the second and third trimester.

Because different types of twins are associated with different problems and risks, trying to figure out what type of twinning is present is important. If the ultrasound signs are ambiguous and the medical situation suggests that determining the type of twinning is especially important, genetic tests can be used (these tests are called *zygosity studies*). These tests require some sort of invasive test, such as amniocentesis, chorionic villus sampling (CVS), or fetal blood sampling (see Chapters 5 and 6).

Genetic testing in pregnancies with twins or more

Chorionic villus sampling and amniocentesis are a little trickier with twins or more. The two main challenges are to make sure that each fetus is sampled separately and that none of the tissue taken from one fetus contaminates the tissue taken from the other. In the case of identical twins, this issue isn't as critical, because in this case, the fetuses have the same genetic makeup, and if you find a genetic abnormality (or lack of any genetic abnormalities) in one, the same is almost always true for the other. But with fraternal (dizygotic) twins, triplets, or more, testing each one separately is critical.

Amniocentesis

Amniocentesis (see Chapter 6) is the most common way of doing genetic testing in multifetal pregnancies. This method requires inserting a separate needle into the uterus for each fetus being tested. The amniocentesis is, of course, done under ultrasound guidance. After some fluid is taken from the first fetus, the needle is left in place so that the doctor can inject a harmless organic blue dye (called *indigo carmine*) into that fetus's amniotic sac. (This blue dye is absorbed over time. Don't worry — the baby won't be born with blue skin.) Then, if the fluid from the second needle comes out clear (not blue), the doctor knows that he or she has sampled the second sac. If there are more than two fetuses, a few drops of blue dye can be added to each consecutive sac as it's tapped.

CVS

Chorionic villus sampling, or CVS (see Chapter 5), can be somewhat complicated in multifetal pregnancies, but experienced doctors can usually handle the job. In some cases, the placentas are positioned in such a way that CVS is technically impossible. In these cases, the mother has the option of having an amniocentesis a little later in pregnancy (at about 15 to 18 weeks, rather than 12 weeks for CVS).

Keeping track of which baby is which

Your doctor designates your babies before birth as Twin A and Twin B (or Triplets A, B, and C). These designations enable your doctor to communicate to you and others (nurses and other medical personnel) which baby is which and to follow the progress of each baby separately and consistently throughout the pregnancy. By convention, the fetus closest to the cervix (the opening to the womb) is designated as Twin A (or Triplet A). This baby is usually born first. In a triplet pregnancy, the highest triplet (closest to your chest) is designated as Triplet C. (Some patients come up with their own clever names. We had one patient with triplets who named her babies Itsy, Bitsy, and Ditsy before birth so she could keep track of them.)

Day-to-day life during a multiple pregnancy

If you're pregnant with multiples, there's no reason to ignore everything else we've written in this book. In many ways, your pregnancy proceeds like any other. The difference, as you may already know, is that your experience is more intense in various ways: You grow a larger belly, your nausea may be

Our patients want to know . . .

Q: "Is doing an amniocentesis or CVS for twin or triplet pregnancies riskier than for singleton pregnancies?"

A: Although little scientific research has been done on this question, it appears that the chances of complications are not substantially greater in multifetal pregnancies, if the procedure is done by someone experienced in performing it in mothers carrying twins or more.

worse, your amniocentesis (if you have one) is a bit more complicated (as we describe earlier in this chapter), and the birth may take longer. With triplets or more, these physical changes and symptoms are even more exaggerated. In addition, certain complications are more frequent in multiples than in singletons. In the next sections, we describe many of the ways that your experience may be somewhat different.

Weight gain

The average weight gain for a twin pregnancy is 35 to 45 pounds (15 to 20 kg). But the exact amount that you gain depends on your prepregnancy weight. The Institute of Medicine recommends that mothers with twin pregnancies gain about one pound per week during the second and third trimesters. Others recommend weight gains of 45 to 50 pounds (20 to 23 kg) by 34 weeks for triplets and more than 50 pounds (23 kg) for quadruplets.

Diet

Many experts recommend that women carrying twins consume an extra 300 calories a day above what is required for a singleton (in other words, an extra 600 calories per day above their prepregnancy intake). For triplets and more there is no general consensus, but obviously your food intake should be somewhat greater.

Nausea

Most women carrying two or more fetuses definitely have more nausea and vomiting in early pregnancy than those with only one. This nausea may be related to higher levels of hCG (a pregnancy hormone) circulating through the bloodstream. The amount is greater with two or more fetuses. The good news is that nausea and vomiting for mothers of multiples, as for mothers of single babies, usually goes away by the end of the first trimester.

Iron and folic acid

Women carrying twins, triplets, or more stand a greater chance of developing anemia. This is due to a dilutional anemia (see Chapter 4) as well as greater demands for iron and folic acid. Supplemental iron and folic acid are recommended for women carrying two or more fetuses.

Activity

In the old days, doctors used to recommend that women with twins be placed on bed rest beginning at 24 to 28 weeks. However, no data shows that bed rest makes a difference in the outcome. Women placed on bed rest appear to be no less likely than others to experience preterm delivery or have babies of low birthweight. Whether you need to reduce your activity depends upon your prior obstetrical history as well as how smoothly your pregnancy goes week to week. If you develop preterm labor or have problems with fetal growth, your doctor may recommend that you take it easy. With triplets or more, the benefit is unclear, but many obstetricians routinely recommend bed rest starting in the second trimester.

Prenatal doctor visits

Your practitioner is likely to follow pretty much the same routine he or she uses for mothers of single babies. That is, you have your blood pressure, weight, and urine checked at each visit. But because you have more than one fetus, you may be asked to come in more frequently. Some practitioners perform routine pelvic exams to make sure that your cervix is not dilating prematurely; others may suggest that your cervix be checked with an ultrasound exam. On the other hand, if you do not have any symptoms of preterm labor, your doctor may decide that you do not need to have these extra exams.

Ultrasound examinations

Most practitioners suggest that mothers of twins or more have periodic ultrasound examinations — every four to six weeks — throughout their pregnancy in order to check fetal growth. If there are any problems, these exams may need to be more frequent. With more than one fetus, your doctor can't use fundal height measurements to evaluate the growth. And because women with twins, triplets, or more are at a higher risk of having problems with fetal growth (see "Intrauterine growth restriction," later in this chapter), these periodic ultrasound exams are very important.

Labor and delivery in twin births

Almost always, women carrying triplets are delivered by cesarean. Recently, however, some studies have suggested that under very specific situations and with very strict criteria, delivery of a triplet pregnancy vaginally may be possible. At this time, because almost all triplets are delivered by cesarean, the following section on birth positions and delivery is really addressed to women carrying twins.

Often, pregnancy itself goes smoothly for mothers of twins, but labor and delivery can still be complex. For this reason, we recommend that women carrying more than one fetus deliver in a hospital, where extra personnel are present to handle any complications that may arise.

Assuming that the babies are full-term, much depends on what position the babies are in at the time of delivery. Basically, their positions fall into three possibilities:

✔ Both fetuses can be head-down *(vertex),* as they are in about 45 percent of twin pregnancies (see Figure 13-3a).

✔ The first fetus can be head-down and the second not, as is the case about 35 percent of the time.

✔ The first fetus can be breech or *transverse* (lying horizontal across the uterus), and the second can be breech, head-down, or transverse, as they are about 20 percent of the time (see Figures 13-3b and 13-3c).

If both fetuses are head-down, you often can deliver them vaginally. In fact, studies show that in such cases, vaginal delivery is successful 60 to 70 percent of the time. But if at least one baby is breech or transverse, a cesarean delivery is more likely.

Even if both babies are head-down, the labor and delivery process is usually more complicated with twins. One of the twins may not be able to move down the birth canal properly. If the second twin is not head-down, there is a good chance that he or she may be delivered as a breech unless your practitioner can turn the second baby to a head-down position. Whether trying to manipulate the baby in this way makes sense is a matter of some debate among practitioners. Your doctor's choice of whether to try turning the baby around or to deliver the baby breech depends on his or her training, experience, and professional bias.

You may end up having a cesarean delivery. If both twins are feet-down, most obstetricians and the American College of Obstetrics and Gynecology (ACOG) recommend that you have a cesarean. With any of these combinations of positions, if the babies are preterm, the options may be different. In any case, discuss the possibilities with your doctor before the time of delivery.

Special issues for moms with multiples

If you're pregnant with twins or triplets (or more), your doctor puts you under a little closer surveillance, because the risk of certain complications is greater in multifetal pregnancies. The following topics are some of the things he or she is watching out for.

Don't let this list scare you. The important thing is to be aware of potential problems so that if they develop, they can be recognized early and managed appropriately to give you the best outcome possible.

Preterm delivery

The biggest risk you face in carrying more than one baby is that you may have preterm labor and delivery. The average length of pregnancy for a singleton is 40 weeks, but for a twin pregnancy it's only about 36 weeks; for triplets, 33 to 34 weeks; and for quadruplets, about 31 weeks. A pregnancy is considered to have gone full term if it lasts 37 weeks or more. Preterm delivery is technically considered between 24 and 37 weeks, but most babies born at 35 or 36 weeks are generally as healthy as babies delivered after 37 weeks.

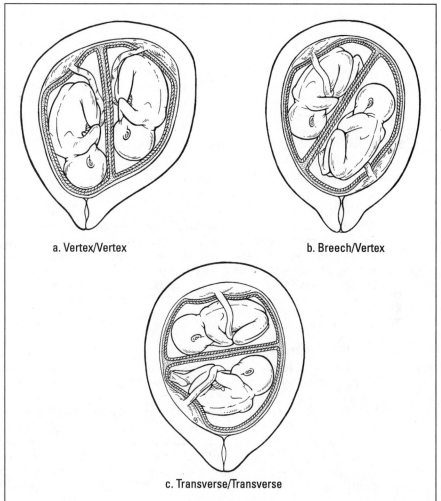

a. Vertex/Vertex   b. Breech/Vertex

c. Transverse/Transverse

Figure 13-3:
Three possible positions
of twins
before
delivery.

Many women go into preterm labor without actually delivering their babies early. About 80 percent of mothers carrying triplets and 40 percent of those with twins experience preterm labor, but not all deliver early. (See details about preterm labor and delivery in Chapter 14.)

Diabetes

Because the incidence of gestational diabetes is higher with twins or more, many practitioners recommend that all women carrying more than one fetus be screened for this condition. (See Chapter 15.)

Chromosomal abnormalities

When you have more than one fetus and they are *not* identical, the chance that either one of them has a genetic abnormality is somewhat higher. After all, with more than one baby, each has its own individual risk of some abnormality, and the risks add up. While mothers of single babies are considered to be of *advanced maternal age* (AMA) at 35, as we describe earlier in the chapter, in twin pregnancies derived from two separate eggs, AMA may be as early as 33, and for triplets, 31 or 32. This all becomes relevant for women considering the genetic testing we mention earlier.

Hypertension and preeclampsia

Hypertension — high blood pressure — is more common in multifetal pregnancies. The risk is proportional to the number of fetuses present. Some women develop hypertension alone, without other symptoms or other physical signs. Others develop a condition unique to pregnancy called *preeclampsia,* which involves high blood pressure in association with either edema (swelling) or spilling protein in the urine (see the description of preeclampsia in Chapter 14). Forty percent of mothers carrying twins and 60 percent or more with triplets develop some form of hypertension during pregnancy. For this reason, your practitioner keeps a close eye on your blood pressure.

Intrauterine growth restriction

Problems with fetal growth occur in anywhere from 15 to 50 percent of all twins. The problem is even more common in triplets and in fetuses who share the same placenta. In the case of a single placenta, the blood may not be distributed equally to both twins, which may cause one twin to get more nutrients than the other. In multiples who have different placentas, growth restriction can result when one placenta is implanted in a more favorable position within the uterus and therefore provides better nourishment than the other. Your doctor is likely to schedule periodic ultrasound exams during your pregnancy to check that both (or all three) fetuses are growing properly.

Twin-twin transfusion syndrome

Twin-twin transfusion syndrome is specific to twins who share a single placenta (monochorionic). In some cases, the single placenta contains blood vessels that interconnect between the two fetuses. This connection enables the two fetuses to exchange blood — and allows the blood to become distributed unequally. The fetus who gets more blood grows bigger and produces extra amniotic fluid, while the one who gets less blood may suffer impaired growth and have significantly decreased amniotic fluid in its sac. This situation can be very serious, but fortunately, it affects only 10 to 15 percent of monochorionic twins. If it happens in your pregnancy, your doctor may suggest one of several strategies to try to treat the problem:

✔ Performing an *amnioreduction,* which means doing an amniocentesis, but removing a much larger quantity of fluid. This may have to be done several times if excess fluid keeps accumulating in the sac of the larger fetus.

✔ Performing a *septostomy,* which refers to making a small hole in the membrane separating the two sacs, allowing extra fluid to flow from the larger fetus's sac to the smaller one's.

✔ Performing a special procedure that utilizes a laser to close up the connections between the two placental circulations or having a procedure whereby the umbilical cord of one fetus is tied off. This option results in the death of that fetus but is sometimes necessary to allow the other one to grow.

Multifetal pregnancy reduction

Some doctors perform the *multifetal pregnancy reduction* procedure to reduce the number of fetuses a woman is carrying in order to improve the chances that she delivers healthy babies. It is most commonly used in women who have at least three viable fetuses resulting from fertility treatments because of the high risk of preterm delivery if they try to carry all the fetuses. Also, some women carrying twins want to reduce their pregnancy to a singleton. A multifetal pregnancy reduction is done during the last weeks of the first trimester, between 9 and 13 weeks. The procedure is performed only in special centers. The risk involved is acceptably low when an experienced physician specifically trained in this procedure, usually a maternal-fetal medicine specialist, performs the procedure. The important thing is to find out about all possible options, so that you have as much information as possible to make the best decision for you.

Selective termination

A *selective termination* procedure can be used in a multifetal pregnancy to terminate one of the fetuses when that fetus has a significant abnormality. It can be performed only if the fetuses have separate placentas, so that the medication used can't cross over and affect the normal fetus. In the case of monochorionic twins (identical twins who share a single amniotic sac), some other options are available (ask your doctor). This procedure is performed only in a few centers throughout the country and is usually done by a maternal-fetal medicine specialist.

Having Another Baby

Doctors and parents haven't come to a consensus on the optimal time to get pregnant again. Probably the most important consideration is your overall health. If you are able to get back to your prepregnancy or ideal body weight quickly after you deliver, and if you are able to replenish any lost nutrients and vitamins (particularly iron and calcium) from your last pregnancy, then you can probably consider getting pregnant again fairly soon — about six months to a year. However, if you have had a complicated pregnancy, a difficult delivery, or excessive loss of blood, you should wait until you are in better shape before trying again.

Also ask yourself what you consider to be the ideal age difference in your children. Naturally, the answer varies according to each family's preference. Some people feel that it is better to have children close in age, so that the older child doesn't have so many years to settle into the role of *only child* and therefore may not feel so jealous when the new baby comes. Others feel that spacing the children further apart, so that the older child is mature enough to handle the introduction of a new sibling, is better. Most important is how you and your partner feel and how ready you are to take on another child. The decision may involve emotional and financial issues as well as physical ones. Ask yourself whether you can handle the pressure and the expense and can do the work that having another child takes.

How each pregnancy may be different

Naturally, any mother compares her second pregnancy with her first. The truth is that every pregnancy is different. If your last pregnancy went smoothly, you may think that any little thing that happens out of the ordinary in the next pregnancy is a signal that things are not going well. By the same token, if your first pregnancy was difficult, you needn't assume that the same complications are going to happen again.

One of the most common misconceptions is that things happening differently the second time around is a sign that the second baby is of a different sex. Many women believe that if they were nauseated in one pregnancy and had a girl, not feeling nauseated in the next pregnancy means that they are having a boy. Forget about it.

These are some of the ways in which you may experience pregnancy differently the second (or third or fourth) time around:

 ✔ Many women feel that they are showing sooner or are at least more bloated and distended. This condition may be due to the fact that their abdominal muscles have been stretched by their previous pregnancy and are now more lax.

✔ Many women find that nausea is not as severe as it was the first time around, and others find that it is even worse.

✔ You can usually identify fetal movement earlier.

✔ Labor is usually shorter, and delivery is easier.

✔ Many women find that they feel Braxton-Hicks contractions earlier and more frequently than with their first child.

✔ Most women are less anxious the second time around.

One thing that remains the same: As hard as it is to believe, you will love your second child as much as your first.

In their third pregnancy, many women commonly experience a special kind of worry: They feel that because their first two pregnancies were healthy and problem-free, the third one's bound to have complications. Many feel that they were lucky twice in a row, and that going for a third time is pushing their luck. If this is how you feel, believe us, you are not alone. Keep in mind that the chances of trouble are not inherently greater in a third pregnancy, even if the first two went smoothly.

Birth after a prior cesarean delivery

If you have had a cesarean delivery and you get pregnant again, the question arises as to whether you can deliver vaginally this time or need another cesarean. To some extent, the answer depends on the kind of cesarean you had. Most are done through what's called a *low transverse* incision (that is, across the floor in the lower part of the uterus). (See Figure 13-4a.) Women who have this kind of incision are usually able to deliver vaginally in a subsequent pregnancy — as long as they have no other complicating factors.

If, on the other hand, you have what's known as a *classical* cesarean, in which a vertical incision is made in the upper portion of the uterus (see Figure 13-4b), you should not try to have a vaginal delivery in a subsequent pregnancy, because this type of incision is more likely to rupture. Vertical incisions are sometimes performed in cases of very preterm birth or placenta previa (see Chapter 14), or when the mother's uterus is a very abnormal shape or has large fibroids.

A third type of cesarean incision is called a *low vertical* incision (see Figure 13-4 c). This method is performed less frequently than a low transverse incision, but it does enable the mother to attempt labor and delivery in a subsequent pregnancy.

The incision made on your skin does *not* reflect the type of incision on your uterus. In other words, you may have a transverse incision on your skin (a *bikini cut*) but still have a vertical incision on your uterus.

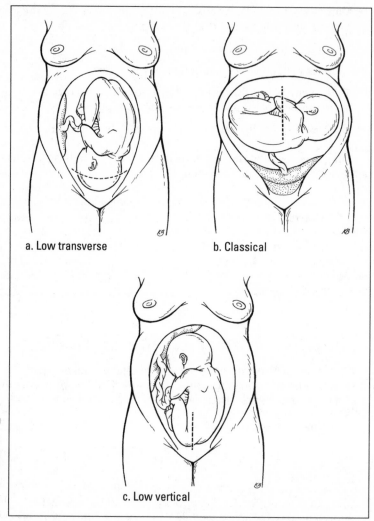

a. Low transverse   b. Classical

c. Low vertical

Figure 13-4:
Various
kinds of
uterine
incisions.

Doctors used to think that after a woman had a cesarean delivery, all her babies would have to be delivered the same way. Trying a vaginal delivery, it was thought, meant risking that the uterus would rupture through the old cesarean scar. But studies have demonstrated that the risk of such a rupture is actually quite low — less than half a percent. Other recent studies show that 70 percent of the time, women can successfully deliver a baby vaginally after they've had a cesarean. Of course, the likelihood of success depends to some extent on why a cesarean was performed in the first place. If it was done simply because the baby was breech, the chance that the next baby can be

Risks and benefits of attempted vaginal delivery after a cesarean birth

Benefits:

✔ Shorter recovery

✔ A lower risk of the kind of complications associated with abdominal surgery: anesthesia problems, infection, inadvertent injury to adjacent organs, possible blood clots from being immobile for a longer period of time

✔ For some women, a psychological benefit from experiencing a vaginal birth

✔ Shorter hospital stay

✔ For most patients, less pain following delivery

✔ The possibility, indicated by some studies, that the baby clears his or her secretions more efficiently if born vaginally

Risks:

✔ Rupture of the uterus in the area of the old scar

✔ Longer recovery if you are not successful, possibly longer than if you had elected to have a repeat cesarean

delivered vaginally is nearly 90 percent. If the cesarean was performed because the baby was too large to fit through the mother's pelvis, the chance of a future vaginal delivery falls to 50 to 60 percent.

Why would you want to deliver your next baby vaginally? The main benefit is that if you are successful, your recovery is much shorter. However, if you try labor and then end up with another cesarean, studies show that the complication rate is higher than if you went straight to a repeat cesarean without labor. Another potential benefit from a vaginal birth is that it is often associated with less postpartum pain. However, although most patients find the pain associated with vaginal birth to be less than that associated with cesarean delivery, some vaginal births have painful complications of their own. See Chapter 9 for more information.

Single Moms and Nontraditional Families

Single women and lesbian couples bearing children are becoming more and more common. If you fall into one of these categories, discussing your situation with your practitioner is important. You should not be worried that you will be judged or subject to ridicule. Practitioners are trained to be sensitive to *all* patients' needs, and you are no different. If your practitioner does seem to have a problem accepting your choice, move on to someone who's more understanding — the sooner the better.

In many single-mother and lesbian pregnancies, the father of the baby is not present. Still, try to have information about the father's family history and ethnicity so that you and your practitioner can go over any genetic implications. (See Chapter 5.)

If the father isn't going to be around for the whole process, you need to build your own support network. If you're a single mom, you may choose one or more people (family members or close friends) to share your pregnancy, labor, and delivery. If you are part of a lesbian couple, the nonpregnant partner can assume the primary support role. In either case, having your support people accompany you to any prenatal visits or prenatal classes and having them around for the labor and delivery process is completely appropriate.

Preparing Your Child (or Children) for a New Arrival

Many parents look forward to having a second child specifically because they want to provide a sibling for the first one. But this reasoning may not be easily understandable to that first child. He or she may feel completely content about being the only child, and it may take months or years before the first one appreciates the value of having the second one. For those of you who are having your second child — or third or fourth (or more!) — the following sections offer a few ideas about how to help prepare the older one(s) for the new arrival.

Explaining pregnancy

The ease or difficulty you may have introducing a new baby sister or brother depends quite a bit on how old the elder sibling is. Explaining a new baby to a 15-year-old is easy; getting the concept across to a 15-month-old can be tricky. And the challenge begins at the time you tell the first child that you're pregnant. A 2-year-old has little concept of time and may not understand that Mom is pregnant for months before the baby comes. He or she may be frustrated that the baby can't come immediately. So it may be a good idea to delay telling a very young child about your pregnancy until the second or third trimester.

If your child is old enough — at least 2 or 3 years old — you may want to bring him or her along to prenatal doctor visits, ultrasound examinations, or when you're shopping for baby items. (While you're doing that shopping, consider getting a small present for your child so that he or she doesn't feel neglected.) A child who is old enough may also like to join in discussions about what to name the new baby.

If you anticipate moving your child to a new room or having him or her graduate from a crib to a bed, make the change *before* the baby is born. This allows your older child to have a chance to acclimate and doesn't associate the new situation directly with the new baby's arrival.

As you near the end of your pregnancy, don't be surprised if your child starts to act up or becomes unusually clingy and dependent. Many children get a sense that things are about to change when they see their mother getting physically bigger or when they overhear conversations about the impending arrival. During this time, be supportive and loving. Include your child in the preparations as much as possible. And remember that although having a new sibling affects almost all children in certain predictable ways, each child is unique, and how yours reacts depends in large part on his or her personality.

Making baby-sitting arrangements for your delivery

Obviously, you need to make arrangements to have someone take care of your child when you and your partner go to deliver the new baby. If your delivery is scheduled (that is, you're having a planned cesarean or an elective induction), scheduling is relatively easy. But most women don't know exactly when the big moment will arrive. And you still need to be ready beforehand. If you go into labor spontaneously in the middle of the night, you want your child to be prepared in advance for what will happen and who will show up to take care of him or her while you're gone. Reassure your child that you will be okay and that he or she can come to see you and the new baby in the hospital very soon. If possible, phone your child at home while you are in the hospital to tell him or her that you are doing well, especially if your labor is unusually long. Many hospitals now have special sibling visiting hours, and you may want to check out the details ahead of time.

Pack a couple of gifts to take with you to the hospital — one for your child to give to the new baby and one for the baby to give to the child.

Coming home

During the first few days that the new siblings live together, you may be amazed at how well adjusted, happy, and excited your older child is. Part of this attitude is genuine enthusiasm. But keep in mind that part of it may also be your older child's attempt to share the limelight with the new baby. Some children have a short period of difficulty coping; others do fine at first but develop longer-lasting sibling rivalry. Don't be surprised if your child begins to regress in terms of some developmental milestones. A previously potty-trained child may resort to bedwetting, for example. Or a child may resume thumb-sucking or have difficulty sleeping. You may notice that your older child gets especially jealous while you are breast-feeding. During this period, understand that your child may need extra reassurance that you still love him and that the new baby hasn't replaced him in your heart at all.

Explain that your heart is big enough to love more than one child. If possible, allow her to participate in helping to care for the baby. How much "help" your child is capable of providing depends upon her age, but even small children can fetch a diaper if you need one or help give the baby a bath. Don't be surprised if at times your child expresses aggression toward you or the baby. Usually, these acts of aggression are harmless, but during this early stage of adjustment, you shouldn't leave your child alone with the baby unsupervised. She may not realize that certain ways of handling the baby may be harmful.

Several months may pass before your older child feels secure, but eventually most children do deal with the change successfully. Quite often the new baby is showered with gifts from friends, neighbors, and family. Again, having a stash of inexpensive new toys for your older child to prevent excessive jealousy may be a good idea. With extra love and understanding, you can help your child through what can be a difficult period.

Chapter 14

When Things Get Complicated

- -

In This Chapter

▶ Going into labor too soon

▶ Understanding problems with blood pressure

▶ Monitoring placental conditions and amniotic fluid levels

▶ Keeping track of the baby's growth

▶ Understanding the Rh factor

▶ Waiting for baby: When labor doesn't start on time

- -

*T*he vast majority of pregnancies are smooth, uncomplicated affairs — perfectly well managed by Mother Nature alone. Sometimes, though, things can get a little complicated. Even when they do, ultimately both baby and mother are healthy in most cases. If your pregnancy is uncomplicated and if you have no major medical problems going into pregnancy, you may just as well skip this chapter. If, on the other hand, you're the type of person who wants to know about every possibility, and it doesn't drive you nuts to do so, you may find this chapter interesting. Just do yourself a favor: Don't take it too much to heart. We have had many patients who, after reading other books about pregnancy, call us frantically, assuming that they are experiencing every complication the books describe. The information in this chapter is meant to reassure you that your pregnancy is safe — or if you do have some particular problem, it provides useful information to help you understand the problem better.

In many places in this chapter, you may find that practitioners disagree about certain strategies to combat complications. In obstetrical medicine, as in all areas of medicine, there is often some disagreement about which way of dealing with a problem is best, because the evidence for and against any one strategy may be inconclusive and therefore open to individual interpretation. Someone else's practitioner handling a situation differently than yours doesn't necessarily mean that either one of them is wrong. In this chapter we indicate our professional bias and mention the other options as well.

We're trying to avoid writing still another textbook in maternal-fetal medicine. To that end, we cover some conditions only briefly and omit some less common problems entirely. But our hope is that the following information gives you some familiarity with the kinds of complications that can occur, so that if you develop any problem, you know how to proceed.

Dealing with Preterm Labor

Normally, during the second half of pregnancy, the uterus contracts intermittently. As the end approaches, these contractions grow more frequent. Finally, they become regular and cause the cervix to dilate. When contractions and dilation occur before 37 weeks gestation, labor is considered *preterm*. Some women notice periods of regular contractions prior to 37 weeks. If the cervix doesn't dilate or efface, however, the condition is *not* considered preterm labor.

Of course, the earlier preterm labor occurs, the more troublesome it can be. The problems that a premature baby has if he or she is born after about 34 weeks are usually much less to worry about than those he or she would face if born at only 24 weeks. Prior to about 32 weeks, the main problem is that the baby's lungs may still be immature, but there can be other complications as well. Nevertheless, the majority of babies born at 26 to 32 weeks can be fine and healthy, especially if they have access to modern neonatal intensive care. Premature babies stand a higher risk of contracting some infection, they may experience problems with the gastrointestinal tract (stomach and intestines), or they may experience an *intraventricular hemorrhage,* which is bleeding into an area within the brain.

The following are signs and symptoms of preterm labor:

- ✔ Menstrual-like cramps
- ✔ Persistent lower-back pain
- ✔ An increase in mucous-like vaginal discharge
- ✔ Intense and persistent pressure in the pelvis or vaginal area
- ✔ Regular contractions that don't stop with rest or decreased activity
- ✔ A constant leakage of thin fluid from the vagina

Nobody knows for sure what causes premature labor, but clearly, some patients are at higher risk for developing it. If you fall into one of the high-risk categories, your practitioner probably wants to follow you more closely than usual. You may be asked to come to the office more frequently or to undergo certain tests. The following are some factors that put you at risk for preterm delivery:

✔ Prior preterm delivery

✔ Twins or more

✔ Abnormally shaped uterus

✔ Smoking

✔ Bleeding during pregnancy, especially during the second half (***Note:*** This does *not* include occasional spotting during the first trimester.)

✔ Some infections

✔ Abuse of certain illicit drugs

Checking for signs of preterm labor

Practitioners have various ways to try to detect preterm labor, but the techniques are not always effective. The most common way is for your practitioner to perform an internal exam to check the cervix and to monitor you for contractions.

Some practitioners look for symptoms of preterm labor using *transvaginal ultrasound* (a small ultrasound probe is placed into the vagina next to the cervix), which creates an image of the cervix. The cervix is measured to determine whether it is dilating or effacing (see Chapter 8 for more on labor). This may alert doctors that a patient is at a higher risk for preterm labor because her cervix is very short, effaced, or becoming funnel-shaped. More studies are needed so that doctors can find out how best to use transvaginal ultrasound.

What about monitoring from home?

Many patients ask us about the use of *home contraction monitoring*. This is a controversial technology because studies have not definitely proven its benefit. You are given a device that you strap to your abdomen for a period of half an hour or an hour each day (or sometimes twice a day), whatever your practitioner decides. This device can sense contractions that you may not be able to feel. The information that the device receives is then transmitted through a telephone modem to a nursing station. If it appears that you are contracting more frequently than you should be, your doctor is alerted. In this way, you may pick up preterm labor at an early stage. However, recent studies suggest that this kind of monitoring is no more useful than having the patient keep in close contact with nurses or teaching her to be aware of the symptoms of preterm labor.

Two relatively new tests involve checking a pregnant woman's secretions for substances that can indicate whether preterm delivery is likely to occur. One of these tests, called *fetal fibronectin,* involves swabbing the back of the vagina. A negative result on this test is a very good indicator that preterm delivery is unlikely within the next few weeks. A positive result, however, is a less strong indicator of whether a premature delivery will occur in the near future. Another test, called *salivary estriol,* involves swabbing the inside of the cheek and checking the saliva for signs that preterm delivery is likely. The effectiveness of this test is still under investigation.

Stopping preterm labor

Depending on how far along you are when you develop preterm labor, your doctor may attempt to stop your contractions (if he or she believes in the whole concept of trying to do so), and you may be admitted to the hospital. Several medications (called *tocolytics*) can be used to block preterm labor. Doctors have never come to widespread agreement that these medications are useful in the long run, though they have been shown to be helpful for a few days to a week. Most tocolytics have side effects on the mother. *Terbutaline,* for example, may cause an increase in heart rate or a jittery feeling. *Magnesium sulfate* may cause nausea, flushing, or drowsiness. However, they are thought to be safe for the baby.

If your doctor thinks that your preterm labor may lead to premature delivery prior to 34 weeks, he or she will probably recommend that you receive an injection of *corticosteroids,* which have been shown to decrease the risk of respiratory problems and other complications in the premature newborn. The risks to the mother of taking these drugs are negligible. And large studies have shown that the steroids are beneficial to the baby for about a week. Until more studies are done, however, doctors do not know for certain whether steroids should be repeated on a weekly basis if you remain at risk for preterm delivery.

Delivering the baby early

Sometimes it makes sense to deliver a baby early. When a woman experiences preterm labor at 35 or 36 weeks, for example, it's usually wise to just let her go ahead and deliver, because the outlook for the baby is so good and there's no reason to subject the mother to the side effects of medications to forestall labor. Regardless of the gestational age, premature delivery may also be the best option in some cases where the baby has a condition that doctors can't treat inside the uterus or when the mother has a condition that is worsening, such as preeclampsia (discussed next), and continuing the pregnancy would be risky.

Preeclampsia

Also known as *toxemia,* or *pregnancy-induced hypertension* (PIH), *preeclampsia* results when a woman experiences both elevated blood pressure and either fluid retention and/or protein spillage in the urine. This condition is not all that uncommon, occurring in about 7 percent of pregnancies. Women having their first child are especially susceptible.

Most often, preeclampsia occurs late in pregnancy, but it can develop in the late second or early third trimester. The condition goes away after delivery.

Doctors have different criteria for diagnosing the condition, but, in general, blood pressure that stays above 140/90 is considered elevated, if you have no history of blood pressure problems prior to pregnancy.

Following is a list of the signs and symptoms of preeclampsia:

- ✔ Sudden swelling of the hands, face, or legs

- ✔ Severe headache that won't go away even if you take pain medication

- ✔ Blurry vision or seeing spots in front of your eyes

- ✔ Pain in the upper-right part of your abdomen, near your liver

- ✔ Sudden weight gain (5 pounds in one week)

- ✔ Abnormalities in certain blood tests (decreased platelets, important in clotting) and elevations in liver tests

- ✔ Sudden onset of seizures

- ✔ Nausea, vomiting, and pain in the upper mid-abdominal area

A word of caution about the preceding list of symptoms. Most of the symptoms can occur harmlessly during any pregnancy. Unless they happen in combination with elevated blood pressure or protein spillage in the urine, they are quite normal. If one day you have a headache, or if for a second you see spots in front of your eyes, don't jump to the conclusion that you have preeclampsia. If the symptoms persist, let your doctor know.

No one knows exactly what causes preeclampsia. But doctors know that some women are at a higher risk for developing it than others. The following are risk factors for preeclampsia:

- ✔ History of preeclampsia in a prior pregnancy

- ✔ Existing chronic hypertension

- ✔ Long-standing diabetes

- ✔ Significant obesity

- ✔ Triplets or more (twins, also, but to a much lesser extent)

- ✔ First pregnancy

- ✔ Mother older than 40

- ✔ Some medical problems, such as serious kidney or liver disease, lupus, or other vascular diseases

Despite extensive ongoing medical research on preeclampsia, no one yet knows exactly how to prevent it. In the past several years, many treatment trials have been performed with low-dose aspirin, calcium supplementation, and fish oil, but none of these substances has proved to be a panacea.

The only real treatment for preeclampsia is delivering the baby. The decision on when you should deliver depends on how severe the condition is and how far along you are in your pregnancy. If you're close to your due date, induced delivery may be the wisest approach. If you're only 28 weeks along, on the other hand, your doctor may want to try bed rest and close observation, either at home or in the hospital. It's a matter of weighing the risks to the mother's health against the risks the baby runs from preterm delivery.

Placental Conditions

Two different problems with the baby's placenta can sometimes occur in the latter part of pregnancy: placenta previa and placental abruption. In this section, we describe both.

Placenta previa

Placenta previa is when the placenta partially or completely covers the cervix, as shown in Figure 14-1. Many patients are diagnosed with placenta previa when they have a routine ultrasound exam, but sometimes women find out about the problem only when they begin bleeding late in the second or early in the third trimester.

In early pregnancy, having the placenta positioned near the cervix or even partially covering it is common and usually poses no danger to the mother or the baby. In fact, this condition can happen in as many as one out of five pregnancies. In the vast majority of women (95 percent), the placenta rises as the uterus enlarges with the growing baby, which is why you have no reason to worry about the placenta covering the cervix early in pregnancy.

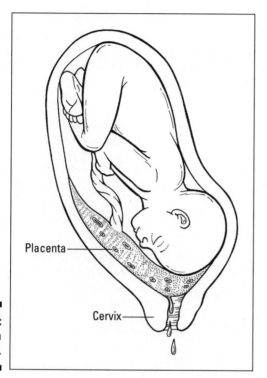

Placenta

Cervix

Figure 14-1:
Placenta
previa.

Even if the situation persists through the late second trimester and into the third, it can still be harmless. Many women who have placenta previa never bleed at all. However, the main concern with placenta previa is that heavy bleeding may occur. If bleeding is severe enough, the baby may have to be delivered just for this reason. Sometimes bleeding leads to preterm labor. In this case, an attempt is made to try to stop the contractions, which often stops the bleeding.

If you are in your third trimester and you have placenta previa, your practitioner may want you to have regular ultrasound examinations to see whether the placenta eventually moves out of the way. He or she may tell you to avoid intercourse and internal examinations in order to lower the risk of any bleeding. If the previa persists until 36 weeks, your doctor most likely recommends a cesarean delivery, because the baby can't come through the birth canal without disrupting the placenta, and that could lead to heavy bleeding.

Placental abruption

In some women, the placenta separates from the uterine wall before pregnancy is over. This condition is called *placental abruption* (sometimes also called *abruptio placentae* or *placental separation*). Figure 14-2 shows you what it looks like.

Placental abruption is a common cause of third trimester bleeding. Because blood is an irritant to the uterine muscle, it can also cause premature labor and abdominal pain. An abruption is difficult to see on an ultrasound exam unless it is quite large. So in many cases, doctors can make the diagnosis only after they rule out every other possible cause of bleeding. Rarely, a placental abruption occurs suddenly, and if the separation is large enough, it may necessitate rapid delivery. See Chapter 7 for other causes of third trimester bleeding.

If you experience a small placental abruption, your practitioner may recommend that you try bed rest. He or she will also start to observe your pregnancy more closely to make sure that the problem has no harmful side effects on the fetus.

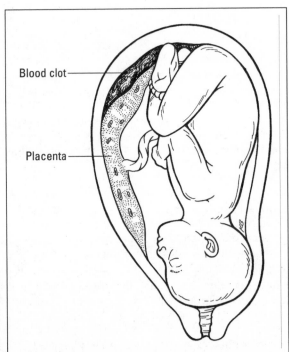

Figure 14-2:
Placental
abruption.

Problems with the Amniotic Fluid and Sac

As you know, the fetus grows within a bag of water known as the *amniotic sac*, which contains the *amniotic fluid*. This fluid increases in volume throughout the first part of pregnancy and reaches its maximum level at 34 weeks. After that, the volume gradually declines. Medical science has not yet discovered exactly what mechanism regulates the volume of amniotic fluid, although we do know that the fetus plays some role in how much fluid the sac contains. During the second half of pregnancy, the amniotic fluid is made up mainly of fetal urine. The fetus urinates into the sac and then also swallows the fluid.

Some of the fluid circulates around the fetal lungs, which aids in lung development. Sometimes, a practitioner may suspect that the amount of amniotic fluid is either above or below average, and he or she may do an ultrasound examination to see what's up. Minor increases or decreases in the amount of amniotic fluid are usually no big problem. But large variations in amniotic fluid volume may be a symptom of some other problem.

Too much amniotic fluid

The medical term for too much fluid is *polyhydramnios* or *hydramnios*. This situation occurs quite frequently, in about 1 to 10 percent of pregnancies. Often the increase in volume is small. Doctors don't always know what causes it, but it is known that a small increase is usually not a problem. Larger increases may be associated with some medical condition in the mother — diabetes or certain viral illnesses, for example. And in some rare cases, the excess fluid may be due to certain fetal problems. The fetus may be having difficulty swallowing the fluid, for example, so more of it accumulates inside the sac.

Too little amniotic fluid

A woman who has too little amniotic fluid has *oligohydramnios*. As we mention earlier, amniotic fluid volume normally decreases after 34 to 36 weeks. If yours starts to fall below a specific range, however, your practitioner may want to observe the fetus more closely by performing certain tests (see Chapter 7 and later in this chapter). One common cause of low amniotic fluid is a rupture of the membranes, which allows fluid to leak out.

A fluid level that drops significantly prior to 34 weeks may indicate a problem either with the mother or the baby. For example, some women with

hypertension or lupus may have less blood flow to the uterus and, consequently, less blood flow to the placenta and the baby. When the baby
receives less blood, the baby's kidneys make less urine, and that results in
lower levels of amniotic fluid.

If the reduction in fluid is mild or moderate, the baby is watched carefully
and undergoes tests of fetal well-being. Sometimes, oligohydramnios is a sign
that the baby's growth is restricted (see "Problems with Fetal Growth" later
in this chapter) or, rarely, that there are abnormalities in the baby's urinary
tract. Sometimes it is a sign that the placenta is not functioning optimally.

If you are found to have decreased amniotic fluid, your doctor may suggest
that you get more rest and try to stay off your feet. By doing so, you may promote more blood flow to the uterus and placenta and thus increase the
baby's urine output.

Rupture of the amniotic sac

Premature rupture of the membranes or amniotic sac (sometimes called
PROM) is when a woman's "water breaks" sometime before labor starts. It
can happen close to the due date *(term PROM)* or sometimes earlier than 37
weeks *(preterm PROM)*. If you experience term PROM, your practitioner may
simply wait until you go into labor on your own. Or he or she may induce
labor in order to avoid the risk that an infection may develop inside the
uterus. If you experience preterm PROM, you may or may not go into labor,
depending on how far along you are. If you are very far from your due date
and don't appear to have an infection in your uterus, your doctor may use
some medications (antibiotics, tocolytics, and steroids) to prolong the pregnancy as long as possible. If preterm PROM happens to you, your doctor will
probably perform frequent ultrasound exams and do fetal heart rate monitoring to ensure that the baby is managing okay.

Our patients want to know . . .

Q: "Is the amount of amniotic fluid determined
to any extent by the amount of water I drink?"

A: No. The mother's fluid intake has little to do
with it. Some recent studies suggest that a
mother can cause small increases in the
amount of amniotic fluid by drinking plenty of liquids, but the effect is not that great.
Nevertheless, it is always advisable to stay well
hydrated.

If you think your membranes may have ruptured and you are preterm, let your practitioner know right away. Tests can be performed to definitively let you know whether or not this has occurred.

Problems with Fetal Growth

One of the main reasons to get prenatal care is to assure that your baby is growing well. A practitioner typically gauges growth by measuring the fundal height (see Chapter 3). As a general rule (in a singleton pregnancy), the measurement in centimeters from the top of the pubic bone to the top of the uterus roughly equals the number of weeks gestation. If your practitioner finds that this measurement is greater or less than expected, he or she may recommend that you have an ultrasound exam to more precisely assess the baby's growth. During the exam, the technician measures various fetal body parts to come up with an approximate fetal weight. That estimate is then compared with the average weight for fetuses at the same gestational age and assigned to a certain percentile. The 50th percentile is average. But because fetuses (like babies, toddlers, children, teenagers, and grown-ups) come in different sizes, there is a range of normal weights. Anything between the 10th and the 90th percentile is considered normal (see Chapter 7 for more information about fetal weight).

These upper and lower limits are somewhat arbitrary. They do imply that 10 percent of the population is larger than normal and that 10 percent is smaller, but this statement is not exactly true. Most fetuses below the 10th percentile or above the 90th percentile are *completely* normal. On the other hand, some of them may not be growing normally and may need extra surveillance.

A fetus whose estimated weight falls below the 10th percentile may have *intrauterine growth restriction* (IUGR). IUGR can lead to the birth of a baby who is small-for-gestational-age (SGA). IUGR has many possible causes, including the following:

- ✔ **The baby is measuring small, but is otherwise normal.**

- ✔ **Genetic factors.** Some genetic factors cause the fetus to grow less than average.

- ✔ **Chromosomal abnormalities.** This cause is most common with early-onset IUGR, which occurs in the second trimester.

- ✔ **Infection such as cytomegalovirus (CMV), rubella, and toxoplasmosis.** Chapter 15 provides more information.

- ✔ **Heart and circulatory abnormalities in the fetus.**

- ✔ **Multiple gestation.** Fifteen to 25 percent of twins have IUGR, and even more triplets. Twins grow at the same rate as singletons until 28 to 32 weeks, when the twin growth curve drops off.

- ✔ **Inadequate nutrition for the mother.** Proper nutrition is especially important in the third trimester.

- ✔ **Placenta factors and uterine-placental problems.** Because the placenta provides nutrition and oxygen to the fetus, if it's functioning poorly or if the blood isn't flowing smoothly from the uterus to the placenta, the fetus may not grow properly. Women with *antiphospholipid antibody syndrome* (a blood clotting problem), recurrent bleeding, vascular diseases, or chronic hypertension are at risk for IUGR because those conditions cause poor placental function. Preeclampsia may also impair placental function and lead to IUGR.

- ✔ **Environmental toxins.** Cigarette smoking causes a decrease in birthweight between one-fourth and one-half of a pound, on average. Chronic alcohol consumption (of at least one to two drinks a day) and cocaine use also can cause low birthweight.

The way your practitioner responds to IUGR depends on the particulars of the situation. Fetuses with mild IUGR, normal chromosomes, and no evidence of infection are likely to be fine. Sometimes early delivery is warranted, however, because the fetus may grow better in the nursery than inside the uterus. The way your practitioner responds to signs of IUGR depends on both the cause of the problem and the gestational age at which it is diagnosed. He or she may recommend more frequent office visits, bed rest, periodic ultrasound examinations, fetal heart rate exams (known as NSTs — see Chapter 7), or other tests. If the problem is severe but the pregnancy is far enough along, your doctor may recommend delivery.

In many cases, SGA babies turn out to be perfectly normal. Unfortunately, though, severe cases have been associated with learning difficulties later in life and even fetal death, which is why it is important that your practitioner conduct some form of fetal surveillance.

A baby whose estimated weight is above the 90th percentile may have *macrosomia* ("big body") and end up being large-for-gestational-age, or LGA. There are many different reasons why a woman might have an exceptionally large baby, including the following:

- ✔ The pregnancy lasts longer than 40 weeks.

- ✔ Poorly controlled diabetes in the mother.

- ✔ Obesity in the mother.

- ✔ Excessive maternal weight gain during pregnancy.

- ✔ Delivery of a previous large baby.

- ✔ One parent was born very large — or both of them were.

The main risk to the mother, naturally, is that the delivery is more difficult. If she delivers vaginally, she may suffer increased trauma to the birth canal. And she has an increased chance of needing a cesarean delivery. The main

Our patients want to know . . .

Q: "If I eat more, will my baby grow into the normal range?"

A: Unfortunately, the answer is no. Eating more does not correct the problem unless you're significantly malnourished.

risk to the baby, likewise, is injury during delivery. Birth injury is more likely when a large baby is delivered vaginally, but it can also occur during a cesarean delivery. Most commonly, birth injury involves excessive stretching of the nerves in the baby's upper arm and neck resulting from a *shoulder dystocia* (see Chapter 9) during delivery.

If your practitioner thinks that your baby may be exceptionally large, based on either an ultrasound estimate of fetal weight or an abdominal exam, and it appears that your pelvic bones may make for a tight fit, he or she will discuss your delivery options with you.

Blood Incompatibilities

If a baby's parents have two different blood types, the baby's blood type can be different from the mother's. Usually this situation creates absolutely no problem for the mother or the baby. In some rare cases, these blood-type mismatches warrant special consideration. Even then, however, there is hardly ever a significant problem.

The Rh factor

The blood mismatch that most people have heard of is *Rh incompatibility*, which has to do with the *Rh factor*. The majority of people are Rh-positive, which means that they carry the Rh factor on their red blood cells. Those who don't carry the Rh factor are considered Rh-negative. If an Rh-positive man and an Rh-negative woman conceive, the fetus may be Rh-positive, thereby creating a mismatch between baby and mother. (The baby is Rh-positive if the father passes on an Rh-positive gene. If the father has two Rh-positive genes, he certainly passes one on. If he has one Rh-positive gene and one Rh-negative gene, chances are 50-50 that he passes on the Rh-positive one.)

This kind of mismatch is usually not a problem and is almost never a problem in a first pregnancy. If, however, any of the baby's blood leaks into the mother's circulation, her immune system may form antibodies to the Rh factor. And if any such antibodies reach a significant level in a future pregnancy, they can cross through the placenta into the baby's circulation and begin to destroy the baby's red blood cells. It sounds scary, we know. But the problem isn't insurmountable. In order to prevent it, the doctor usually gives the mother an injection of *Anti-D immune globulin* (also called *Rhogam*) at certain times to prevent the formation of antibodies. The following are times at which your doctor may recommend Rhogam if the baby's father is Rh-positive and you're Rh-negative:

- Within 72 hours of delivery (either vaginal or cesarean). The injection is given *after* delivery in order to prevent problems in future pregnancies.

- Routinely at about 28 weeks gestation (as a precaution, just in case any passage of blood across the placenta has already occurred) and again 12 to 13 weeks later, if you haven't already delivered.

- After amniocentesis (see Chapter 6), CVS (see Chapter 5), or any invasive procedure.

- After a miscarriage, abortion, or ectopic pregnancy (see Chapter 5 for more on ectopic pregnancy).

- After significant trauma to your abdomen during pregnancy, if your doctor thinks that some of the baby's blood may have leaked into your circulation.

- After significant bleeding during pregnancy.

In unusual circumstances — either when Rhogam was inadvertently not given (very rare) or when it did not work effectively (exceedingly rare) — a mother produces antibodies to the Rh factor. Then, if she ever becomes pregnant again, an Rh-positive fetus may be at risk of developing *anemia* (not enough red blood cells), depending on the levels of antibodies in the mother's blood and how they interact with the baby's blood. The anemia may be mild, requiring only that the baby be placed under special lights in the nursery to clear any extra *bilirubin* (a pigment that is released from red blood cells that are destroyed). In moderate cases, frequent ultrasound exams and a series of amniocenteses may be necessary to assess the severity of the situation. If the mother is close to her due date, her practitioner may recommend an early delivery. In the most severe cases, the baby may need to have a blood transfusion while he or she is still inside the uterus. The procedure is called a *fetal blood transfusion* (see Chapter 6), and it is performed by a maternal-fetal medicine specialist. A transfusion is the worst-case scenario, but even if things become this severe, a baby who has transfusions in a timely fashion can be born healthy. However, this procedure is associated with some small risks.

Other blood mismatches

Other kinds of blood mismatches are possible. *Kell, Duffy,* and *Kidd* are a few examples of blood factors that can differ between mother and baby. Fortunately, all of these factors are very rare. No Rhogam-like medications are available to treat these mismatches. But in the very few cases where a problem does occur, the babies can be taken care of in the other ways we describe previously for Rh incompatibility (special lights, early delivery, or blood transfusion). And these babies, too, are usually born healthy. Finally, some blood group antibodies — *Le, Lu,* and *P,* for example — can be mismatched but have no harmful effects on the fetus. Usually, no special action is needed.

Post-Date Pregnancy

The average pregnancy lasts about 40 weeks (or 280 days) after the last menstrual period, but only about 5 percent of women deliver on their due date. Some deliver a couple of weeks earlier and some a couple of weeks later, and all are considered to be "at term." You are not considered to have a *post-date pregnancy,* according to the medical definition, until you go beyond 42 weeks. Only a small number of pregnancies last longer than 42 weeks, and no one knows why they do.

Why should you or your practitioner care whether you go past your due date? Because the chance of certain complications rises as time goes on. From 40 to 42 weeks, the increases are small, but after 42 weeks, they climb into a range that is more worrisome. The worst complication, of course, is perinatal death (also called *perinatal mortality*). The chances of perinatal death start to go up after 41 to 42 weeks and double by 43 weeks.

This situation isn't as scary as it may sound, though, because the actual number of deaths is so low. The vast majority of late babies are born healthy. Even at 44 weeks, the point at which perinatal mortality rates quadruple, 95 percent of babies are fine if the appropriate testing is done.

Several factors are involved in the increase in mortality rates in post-date pregnancies:

> ✔ The placenta, an amazing organ that supplies the developing baby with oxygen and nutrients, can function efficiently for only a finite length of time. It is designed to last about 40 weeks, long enough for the average pregnancy. Fortunately, most placentas have some amount of "reserve," and they still work beyond 40 weeks. But some rare ones don't last as well. If a placenta can't get enough nutrients to the baby, he or she may actually lose some weight by remaining inside the uterus.

✔ In a post-date pregnancy, the volume of amniotic fluid may decrease. As we mentioned earlier in this chapter, amniotic fluid volume peaks at about 34 to 36 weeks gestation and starts to slowly drop after that. Most of the time, adequate fluid is left after 40 weeks. Sometimes, however, the fluid level drops into a range that doctors consider too low. In this situation, the umbilical cord has a chance of becoming compressed, and doctors may recommend that labor be induced.

✔ Babies can sometimes pass their first bowel movement while they are still inside the uterus, and the longer a pregnancy lasts, the more likely it is that this happens. In rare instances, the baby may breathe in this thick meconium, either before or during birth, which can cause problems with breathing in the first few days or weeks after birth (for more information, see Chapter 8).

✔ In a post-date pregnancy in which the placenta continues to function normally, the baby keeps growing. Therefore, late babies are more likely to be very large (*macrosomic;* see "Problems with Fetal Growth," earlier in this chapter), or large-for-gestational-age. So they may be at risk for all the problems that come with being extra large.

Practitioners use various strategies to manage post-date pregnancies, none of which is inherently better than another. Some want to be sure that all babies are delivered as soon after 40 weeks as feasible and induce labor to ensure that they are. Others are willing to wait longer for spontaneous labor. The argument for the first approach is that you don't have to worry about any of the aforementioned complications. With the second approach, on the other hand, you may have less chance of needing a cesarean delivery.

All sorts of other factors work into the equation of whether to induce labor or wait for spontaneous labor. For example, take the issue of the cervix. A cervix is said to be *ripe* if it is ready for labor and delivery — that is, soft, somewhat *effaced* (shortened), and a little dilated. If a cervix is ripe, the likelihood of being able to successfully induce labor and have a vaginal delivery is much greater. If it is *unripe* — hard, long, and closed — it is likely to take longer to induce labor, and the mother is more likely to end up with a cesarean delivery. See Chapter 8 for more information on induction of labor.

If you have a post-date pregnancy, discuss all the options with your practitioner and come up with a plan that is best for you, taking into account the baby's size, the amount of amniotic fluid, and the condition of the cervix. If your practitioner advises you to wait for spontaneous labor, you may undergo tests that assess the baby's well-being. These tests usually begin at about 40 or 41 weeks and continue until you deliver. They may include a non-stress test, a biophysical profile, a contraction stress test, an amniotic fluid check, or a combination of any of these (see Chapter 7). If the tests are reassuring, your chances of having a normal, healthy baby are excellent. You only need to get past the frustration of having to wait!

Chapter 15

Pregnancy in Sickness and in Health

*P*regnancy may give you a "maternal glow" and make you feel as if something magical is happening to your body. But face it: Pregnancy doesn't make you superhuman. You're still susceptible to all the illnesses and other health problems that can affect anyone who's not expecting a baby. When illnesses arise during pregnancy, they can have special consequences. In this chapter, we talk about how a variety of medical conditions affect pregnant women.

Getting an Infection during Pregnancy

Try as you might, avoiding every person who's carrying an infection during the time that you're pregnant may be impossible. Keep in mind that most infections don't hurt the baby at all; they just make life more uncomfortable for you for a while. In this section, we go over the most common infections and some of the more unusual ones.

Bladder and kidney infections

Bladder infections come in two basic types: those that have symptoms and those that do not. The "silent" (symptom-free) ones are common, occurring in about 6 percent of pregnant women. The other kind — what is called *cystitis* — comes with symptoms that include pain with urination, going to the bathroom more frequently than usual, discomfort above your pubic bone (where the bladder is), and the constant feeling that you need to urinate. If you develop either type of bladder infection, your doctor treats it with antibiotics.

If left untreated, a bladder infection can progress into a kidney infection, also known as _pyelonephritis_. A kidney infection produces the same symptoms described for cystitis, plus high fevers and _flank pain_ — pain over one or both kidneys (see Figure 15-1). Flank pain also can occur in someone who has kidney stones. The difference is that a kidney infection causes a constant pain, whereas kidney stones produce more severe, but intermittent, pain. Also, kidney stones are more often accompanied by small quantities of blood in the urine.

If your practitioner diagnoses you with pyelonephritis, he or she may want to admit you to the hospital for a few days so that you can get intravenous antibiotics. Because kidney infections tend to recur during pregnancy, your practitioner may also want to keep you on a daily antibiotic for the remainder of your pregnancy.

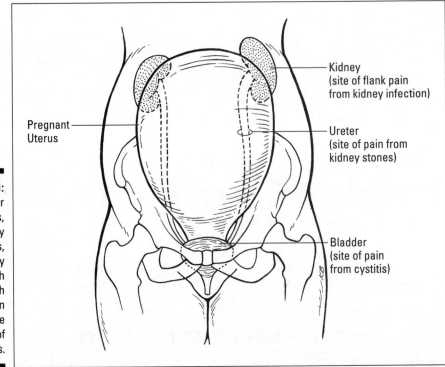

Figure 15-1: Bladder infections, kidney infections, and kidney stones each come with their own unique set of symptoms.

Kidney (site of flank pain from kidney infection)

Pregnant Uterus

Ureter (site of pain from kidney stones)

Bladder (site of pain from cystitis)

Chicken pox

Chicken pox is caused by the *varicella zoster* virus. The first time someone comes down with an infection caused by this virus, usually in childhood, he or she gets chicken pox. Chicken pox is pretty rare in adults, and pregnant women stand no greater risk of contracting this virus than nonpregnant people do.

If you have already had chicken pox, you are not likely to get it again, because your body has made antibodies that make you immune. Even if you've never had chicken pox, you have a good chance of having these protective antibodies in your blood, probably because you had some exposure to the virus in the past that didn't produce any illness. However, if you know that you have never been exposed to chicken pox, and you have not recently been vaccinated (a vaccine against this virus was just recently developed), or if you are unsure about your prior exposure, you should have your blood checked to see whether you are immune.

Because the chicken pox vaccine is so new, we have very little information about how safe it is for pregnant women, which is why the manufacturer of the vaccine recommends that pregnant women not have it. The recommendation is that women wait three months after receiving the vaccine before they get pregnant. If you get the vaccine and then suddenly find out you were pregnant at the time, let your doctor know. The little experience that pregnant women have had with the vaccine suggests that it probably does not increase the chances of birth defects. Nor has it led to any cases of *congenital varicella syndrome* (see the bulleted list that follows) in the baby.

Chicken pox can cause three potential problems during pregnancy:

- ✔ It can make the mother ill with flu-like symptoms, plus the famous skin rash (lots of little red blemishes). In rare circumstances, pneumonia may develop shortly (two to six days) after the rash appears. If you have chicken pox, and you develop symptoms like shortness of breath or a dry cough, let your doctor know right away.

- ✔ If you contract chicken pox during the first four months of pregnancy, the fetus has a small chance of developing the infection, too, leading to *congenital varicella syndrome*. With this syndrome, the fetus can have scarring (the same kinds of scars that little kids get on their bodies from chicken pox), some abnormal development of the limbs, problems with growth, and developmental delays.

Fortunately, congenital varicella syndrome is very rare (it happens in less than 1 percent of cases in which the infection occurs in the first trimester, 2 percent if in the early second trimester).

> ✔ If you contract chicken pox within the interval from five days before to five days after giving birth, the baby is at risk for developing a serious varicella infection in the newborn period. The chances of this are greatly reduced by giving the baby VZIG (explained next).

If you are not immune to chicken pox and you are exposed to someone with the infection, let your practitioner know as soon as possible so that you can receive an injection known as VZIG (varicella zoster immune globulin), which may reduce the risk of infection to you and the baby. Get this injection within three days of exposure, if possible. If you contract chicken pox within several days of giving birth (before or after) your baby should be given VZIG.

The same varicella zoster virus that causes chicken pox can also produce a recurrent form of the infection called *shingles* or *herpes zoster*. Most babies born to pregnant women who develop shingles are completely normal. Because shingles is much less common than chicken pox in pregnancy, it is not exactly known how common birth defects are after a pregnant woman develops this condition, although the incidence is thought to be less than the 1 to 2 percent seen with chicken pox.

If you know that you are susceptible to chicken pox, avoid direct contact with anyone who has herpes zoster, because their lesions contain the varicella zoster virus and can cause a chicken pox infection in susceptible women.

Colds and flu

Most people get a cold about once a year, so the fact that most women get one during pregnancy is not surprising. Nothing about pregnancy makes you more vulnerable to a cold virus, but the fatigue and congestion that go along with pregnancy can make a cold seem worse. In any case, the common cold is perfectly harmless to the developing fetus. As we all know, there is no cure, so the only option is to treat the symptoms. Contrary to popular belief, most cold medications — antihistamines, cough suppressants, and the like — are safe for pregnant women when taken in the recommended doses. (See the nearby sidebar for more information.)

Our patients want to know . . .

Q: "Is getting the flu vaccine safe while I'm pregnant?"

A: Yes: The vaccine is completely safe. So if you are likely to be around many people who are ill or if your local public health officials are predicting a particularly bad flu season, you may want to consider getting one. Remember, the vaccine does not protect against *all* flu viruses, only the ones that are thought to be common in your area.

Following are a few suggestions for dealing with cold and flu symptoms:

- ✔ **Fluids, fluids, and more fluids.** All viral illnesses promote dehydration, and being pregnant only makes the problem more extreme. Make sure that you drink plenty of water, juice, or soda when you have a cold or the flu.

- ✔ **Take a fever reducer.** It's okay to take acetaminophen (Tylenol) in the recommended doses to help bring a fever down. This action alone helps some people feel better. If your fever persists for more than a few days, however, call your doctor.

- ✔ **Take a decongestant.** Pseudoephedrine (Sudafed) is the decongestant of choice during pregnancy. There is no evidence that Sudafed taken in normal doses after the first trimester has any harmful effects. This statement is probably true for the first trimester, too, but few studies have been done on it.

- ✔ **Try nasal spray if you want, but keep it short-term.** Nasal spray decongestants are okay if you use them only short-term (the same is true for people who aren't pregnant). Used intermittently, decongestant sprays may allow you to breathe more comfortably. Used day after day, they may only make the problem last longer. The saline nasal sprays are fine long-term, but they are often not as effective in reducing congestion.

- ✔ **Eat some comfort food.** Last, but certainly not least, there's chicken soup. Scientific studies have shown that chicken soup has properties that help cold sufferers feel better, even though no one knows exactly what those properties are. (See Joanne's mother's recipe in the nearby sidebar.)

The same treatments for the common cold can also be used for influenza infections. If you get the flu while you're pregnant, you're likely to have the same experience as when you're not pregnant.

Many of our patients ask about the use of *echinacea* during pregnancy. This herb has been used for centuries in Asia to fight inflammation and the common cold. Typically, people use a preparation or supplement containing echinacea when they feel the first signs of a cold coming on. There is no evidence from the Asian countries where it has been used that echinacea causes a problem during pregnancy. The only study we could find was one that included only a small number of patients. Although no adverse effects were found, drawing any conclusions from such a limited study is difficult.

If your fever persists for more than a few days, or if you develop a cough with greenish or yellow phlegm or have difficulty breathing, call your doctor to make sure that you're not developing pneumonia.

Mother Regina's chicken soup recipe

4 quarts water

1 chicken, cut in large pieces

3 onions, peeled and quartered

4 parsnips, peeled and halved

6 celery stalks, halved

6 carrots, peeled and halved

4 tablespoons fresh parsley

4 tablespoons fresh dill

salt and pepper to taste

2 to 4 chicken bouillon cubes

1. Put water and chicken in a large stockpot and bring to a boil. Skim off froth.

2. Add onions, parsnips, celery, carrots, and salt and pepper.

3. Cover and simmer for 2 hours.

4. Add bouillon cubes (2 to 4, to taste).

5. Add parsley and dill.

6. Simmer for another hour.

7. Strain broth into another container, reserving the chicken and discarding the vegetables.

8. When cool enough to handle, cut up the chicken meat and use for chicken salad or whatever you want.

9. Either eat right way or, if possible, refrigerate overnight and then strain off the solidified fat that accumulates on top of the broth.

Tip: You can add cooked noodles to make chicken noodle soup.

Cytomegalovirus (CMV) infections

Cytomegalovirus (CMV) is a viral illness that's common among preschool-age children. The symptoms are very similar to the ones you get with the flu — fatigue, malaise, and aches. In most cases, though, an infection produces no symptoms at all. By the time they're old enough to have children, more than half of women have already had a CMV infection at some time in their lives, as evidenced by antibodies present in their blood.

The importance of CMV infection during pregnancy is that the virus can pass to the fetus and cause a congenital infection. Actually, congenital CMV is the most common cause of an infection inside the uterus, and it occurs in 0.5 to 2.5 percent of all newborns. However, most of the time, babies born with this infection are healthy at birth.

If you do develop CMV during pregnancy (and only 2 percent of susceptible pregnant women do), only about one-third of the time is the infection transmitted to the fetus. Even in those babies who contract CMV, 90 percent have no symptoms of this infection at birth (although a small percentage experience symptoms later in life — such as hearing loss or developmental problems).

Our patients want to know . . .

Q: "How can I tell if I've ever had a CMV infection?"

A: The way to tell is by checking to see whether your blood contains CMV antibodies. Most practitioners don't perform this test routinely because of the very small chance that a woman would acquire the infection during pregnancy. Also, the fact that the infection doesn't usually cause any symptoms means that a woman would have to be repeatedly tested to see whether she develops the infection during the course of the pregnancy. However, it is useful to check for susceptibility to the infection (that is, to check for antibodies) in women who are at higher risk — for example, women in close contact with preschool-age children. These women should minimize contact with young children's urine and saliva, wash their hands frequently, and practice very good hygiene.

Q: "If I am diagnosed with CMV during the first or second trimester, what should I do?"

A. The first thing to do, of course, is talk to your doctor and perhaps to a specialist in maternal-fetal medicine. Options for diagnosing the fetal infection include undergoing amniocentesis to check for evidence of infection in the amniotic fluid and ultrasound exams to look for any physical signs of the infection.

The chance that a baby who contracts CMV while in utero will have serious problems is influenced by the gestational age at which the infection occurs, and by whether the mother came down with CMV for the first time during pregnancy (a primary infection) or whether she ever had it in the past (a recurrent infection). If the mother came down with the infection after the second trimester or if it was a recurrent infection, the chance of serious problems in the newborn is much less.

Severe symptomatic congenital CMV is rare and occurs in only about 1 in 10,000 to 20,000 newborns. It can lead to hearing impairment, visual problems, and even some mental deficiencies. Because CMV is a virus, antibiotics don't help.

Hepatitis

Various types of hepatitis affect the mother and baby in different ways:

> ✔ **Hepatitis A** is transmitted by person-to-person contact or by exposure to contaminated food and water. Serious complications from hepatitis A in pregnancy are rare. The virus is not passed to the developing baby. If you are incidentally exposed during pregnancy, you should take *immune globulin* within two weeks after exposure.

✔ **Hepatitis B** virus is transmitted through sexual contact, intravenous drug use, or through a blood transfusion. A small percentage of women with hepatitis B infection have a chronic condition, which can lead to liver damage. While not that common, hepatitis B infection can be transmitted to the fetus. If you are found to be positive for hepatitis B infection, the baby's pediatrician should be informed after delivery, so that the baby can receive the appropriate immunizations.

✔ **Hepatitis C** is transmitted in the same way as hepatitis B. Less than 10 percent of hepatitis C positive women transmit the infection to their baby. If you are positive for this virus, you should not breast-feed.

✔ **Hepatitis D, E, and G** are much less common. Ask your practitioner if you want more information.

German measles (rubella)

German measles are caused by the rubella virus. These measles are the only kind that have any significant impact on pregnancy. If you contract rubella within the first trimester, the baby has about a 20 percent chance of developing *congenital rubella syndrome*. The chance of this, however, varies even within the first trimester from the first month to the third month. Fortunately, acute rubella infection during pregnancy is extremely uncommon.

Herpes infections

Herpes is a common virus that infects the mouth, the throat, the skin, and the genital tract. If you have a history of herpes, rest assured that the infection poses no risk to the developing fetus. The main concern is that you may have an active genital herpes lesion when you go into labor or when your water breaks. If you do, there is a small risk that you transmit the infection to the baby as he or she passes through the birth canal. If it is your first herpes infection, the chance that the fetus contracts the virus is greater, because you have no antibodies to the virus.

If you have active genital herpes lesions at the time of labor or ruptured membranes, let your practitioner know. He or she is likely to perform a cesarean delivery to avoid infecting the baby. If you see no lesions, but you feel as if you may be developing them, also tell your doctor. In this case, having a cesarean may also be advisable.

HIV

Over the past few years, studies have shown that some of the medications used to treat HIV infection can dramatically reduce the chance that the virus is transmitted from a mother to her baby. For this reason, doctors recommend that women undergo HIV testing prior to or during pregnancy, and that if a woman is HIV-positive, she receive these medications during pregnancy as well as during labor itself.

In order to decrease the chance that a baby becomes infected with HIV, invasive procedures that can cause bleeding, such as amniocentesis or CVS, should be avoided unless they're absolutely required. If they are done, doctors recommend that the mother receive intravenous doses of antiviral medications immediately beforehand to minimize the chance of infecting the fetus.

Breast-feeding is not recommended for women infected with HIV because of the risk that the virus may be transmitted to the baby. Whatever form of birth control you choose, the use of condoms, in addition, is absolutely necessary.

If you are HIV-positive, we strongly advise you to maintain close contact with HIV specialists so that you may benefit from the ever-improving treatments.

Lyme disease

Lyme disease is an infection transmitted through the bite of a deer tick. Pregnancy does not predispose you to getting Lyme disease or make it any worse if you get it. The great news is that Lyme disease is not thought to cause any harm to the fetus. The main problem is that it may make you sick.

If you think you have been bitten by a deer tick, let your practitioner know. He or she may want to draw blood to see whether you have contracted Lyme disease and possibly start you on antibiotics to prevent long-term effects.

Parvovirus infection (Fifth disease)

Parvovirus is a common childhood infection that comes with a fever and a characteristic "slapped cheek" rash. In adults, the infection can bring on flu-like symptoms — fever, aches, sore throat, runny nose, and joint pain. Or it may come without any symptoms whatsoever. Three-fourths of all pregnant women are immune to parvovirus, so even if they are exposed to someone who has it, no problems come of it.

If you are not immune to parvovirus or don't know whether you are, and you have come in contact with an infected person, let your practitioner know so that you can be tested. Pregnant women who spend a great deal of time around school-age children (teachers or day-care workers, for example) may undergo routine testing before pregnancy or in the early first trimester.

Even if you contract this illness, chances are very good that your baby will be born healthy. Parvovirus is not known to cause any birth defects. However, in rare cases, it can increase the risk of early miscarriage or the development of anemia in the fetus. For this reason, your practitioner may recommend that you have periodic ultrasound exams to look for signs of fetal anemia. If anemia does occur, doctors can perform a fetal blood transfusion (see Chapter 6) while the baby is still inside you or suggest that the baby be delivered, if you are toward the end of pregnancy,

The ultimate good news: Recent studies show that babies infected with parvovirus during pregnancy, even if they develop anemia, are likely to be born as healthy as any other baby if they are adequately treated.

Stomach viruses (Gastroenteritis)

A bout of stomach flu can occur any time, whether or not you are pregnant. Symptoms include stomach cramps, fever, diarrhea, and nausea, with or without vomiting, and they last anywhere from 24 to 72 hours. The viruses that cause gastroenteritis usually have no harmful effects on the baby.

Don't worry that the baby will not get adequate nutrition if you can't eat for a few days. Fetuses do just fine even when their mothers miss a few meals.

If you get a stomach virus, make sure that you drink plenty of liquids. Dehydration can lead to premature contractions, and it also can contribute to fatigue and dizziness. Try the chicken soup we mention earlier, as well as other liquids — water, ginger ale, tea, or broth. Basically take care of yourself in the same way you would if you weren't pregnant. If your symptoms persist for more than 72 hours, give your doctor a call.

Toxoplasmosis

Toxoplasmosis is an infection caused by a parasite that lives in raw meat and in cat feces. If the parasite enters a person's bloodstream, it may lead to flu-like symptoms or, in some cases, no symptoms at all. This type of infection is very rare in the United States, and infections in pregnant women are rarer still, occurring in only 2 out of every 1,000 women, whereas in France, it is more common. If a pregnant woman is infected, the chance that she will transmit the infection to her baby, and the possible effects it may have, depend largely on *when* she contracts it. If it is during the first trimester, the chance that the baby becomes infected is less than 2 percent. If it's later on in pregnancy, the chance that the baby is infected is greater, but the effects of infection are less severe. In a fetus, early toxoplasmosis infection can cause abnormalities of the central nervous system and in vision.

Some practitioners routinely screen, early in pregnancy, for evidence of a current or past toxoplasmosis infection. Because the rate of infection is so low in the U.S., however, many practitioners do not consider routine testing worthwhile. If you are found to have had the infection in the past and therefore have antibodies in your blood, it is highly unlikely that you get the infection again. If a screening indicates that you may have been recently infected, your practitioner is likely to have your blood tested by a special laboratory to confirm that the positive test result was real. (Many initial tests produce false positives.) If the result still comes back positive, and it appears that you contracted the infection after you became pregnant, your practitioner can give you special antibiotics to reduce the chance that the fetus also gets infected. Then, in the second trimester, your practitioner probably performs an amniocentesis to find out whether the fetus has been infected. In that case, taking additional antibiotics for the rest of the pregnancy is necessary.

You may be advised to consult a maternal-fetal medicine specialist to discuss all your options. If you get toxoplasmosis, keep in mind that recent studies from France, where toxoplasmosis is far more common, indicate that the vast majority of fetuses infected with the parasite who are treated with appropriate antibiotics have an excellent prognosis.

There is no vaccine to prevent toxoplasmosis. The best way to avoid the disease is to minimize your exposure to raw or undercooked meat. Skip the carpaccio. Order your steaks cooked at least medium. Also avoid cat feces. If you have an outdoor cat, ask someone else to change the litter. If no one else can do it, wear rubber gloves when you change the litter. Also wear gloves if you work in a garden and any cats live nearby and play in the garden.

Our patients want to know . . .

Q: "My cat is an indoor cat. Do I need to worry about toxoplasmosis?"

A: Not if your cat has never been outdoors and never comes in contact with mice or rats.

Vaginal infections

Bacteria and other organisms, when given half a chance, readily make themselves at home in a vagina, where the conditions — warm and moist — are perfect for them to grow and reproduce. A woman can get an infection at any time, even when she's pregnant.

Bacterial vaginosis

Bacterial vaginosis (BV) is a common vaginal infection. Symptoms include a whitish-yellow, odorous discharge that gets worse after sexual intercourse. BV has been linked to a slightly higher risk for premature delivery, which is why some practitioners screen for BV in patients known to be at risk for preterm delivery (if they've delivered early before, for example). Treatment includes oral antibiotics or antibiotic creams to use in the vagina.

Chlamydia

Chlamydia is one of the more common sexually transmitted diseases. It often comes with no symptoms. Some practitioners routinely perform a culture from the cervix to check for chlamydia at the same time they do a Pap smear. Some evidence indicates that if a pregnant woman has a chlamydia infection, she may be at higher risk for preterm delivery, and there may be a greater likelihood that the baby is of low birthweight. However, not all practitioners believe that this is the case because scientific studies on the question are inconclusive. If a newborn contracts chlamydia as he or she passes through the birth canal, the baby has a chance of developing *conjunctivitis* (an eye infection) or, less likely, pneumonia. Most hospitals routinely place an ointment in a newborn's eyes shortly after delivery to prevent conjunctivitis, whether or not the mother is infected with chlamydia.

Yeast infections

Yeast infections are very common in pregnancy. Many women who have never had one before get one or more when they're pregnant. The large amounts of estrogen that circulate in the bloodstream during pregnancy promote the growth of yeast in the vagina. Symptoms of an infection are vaginal itching and a thick, whitish-yellow discharge. However, many women get infections without any symptoms.

Often the only treatment needed is a short course of vaginal suppositories or creams. For stubborn infections, oral medications prescribed by your doctor may be helpful.

Yeast infections usually do not cause problems for the fetus or newborn.

Handling Prepregnancy Conditions

The following sections detail conditions that you may have before you get pregnant and how those conditions may affect your pregnancy and vice versa.

Asthma

Predicting how pregnancy will affect a woman's asthma is difficult. Some women find that their condition improves when they're expecting. Some find it gets worse, and about half notice no difference at all.

The main concern that women with asthma have is whether they can safely continue taking their medications during pregnancy. It is most important to realize, however, that the biggest problem with asthma is not the medications themselves but the possibility that pregnant women with asthma under-treat themselves. If you're having trouble breathing, you may not be getting enough oxygen to the baby. Most commonly used asthma treatments are quite safe for the baby, including the following:

- Beta-agonists (albuterol, metaproterenol, terbutaline, Proventil, Allupent)
- Corticosteroids (Prednisone)
- Cromolyn sodium
- Theophylline (Theodur)
- Inhaled steroids (Vanceril, Beclavent, Asmacort, and so on)

Preventative measures can be taken to try to control acute attacks. It's useful for patients with asthma to predict attacks by monitoring themselves with *peak expiratory flow rates* (most asthma patients know what these are, or if they don't, they should ask their lung specialist). Naturally, it helps to avoid situations that trigger attacks.

Chronic hypertension

Chronic hypertension refers to high blood pressure that occurs independently of pregnancy. Although many women who have this condition are aware that they have it before they conceive, doctors occasionally diagnose it during pregnancy. If you have mild or moderate chronic hypertension, chances are good that you have an uneventful pregnancy. However, your doctor will be on the lookout for certain conditions that can affect you or the baby.

Our patients want to know . . .

Q: "Are blood pressure medications safe?"

A: Most medications are safe, but many have not been well studied during pregnancy (as is the case with so many medications). Discuss this important question with your doctor. Certain medications, however, should be avoided. Angiotensin converting enzyme inhibitors (known as ACE inhibitors) pose some risk for kidney problems in the fetus. Beta-blockers, although considered quite safe, pose a very small risk of IUGR (intrauterine growth restriction). Also, diuretics are better avoided, unless this is the only way of treating the high blood pressure.

Women with chronic hypertension stand an increased risk of developing preeclampsia, so your doctor looks for any signs that you are developing this condition. The main risk for the baby is intrauterine growth restriction (IUGR) or placental abruption. Your doctor may suggest that you have repeated sonograms to check on the baby's growth and to make sure that you have adequate amniotic fluid. He or she may also suggest that you undergo some tests for fetal well-being, such as non-stress tests, in the latter part of your pregnancy. The overall management of your pregnancy, of course, depends on how well controlled your blood pressure is, your overall health, and how the baby grows. (For more information on all the complications discussed in this section, see Chapter 14.)

Deep vein thrombosis/pulmonary embolus

A *deep-vein thrombosis* (DVT) is a blood clot that develops within a deep vein, most commonly in the leg, but it can be anywhere. A *pulmonary embolus* is a blood clot within the lung, which is often a clot that has dislodged from one of the deep veins of the leg and made its way to the lung. Both of these conditions are rare, affecting far less than 1 percent of pregnant women.

Symptoms of a DVT include pain, swelling, and tenderness, usually in the calf, and a rope-like hardness running down the back of the lower leg. It is important to diagnose DVT before it has the chance to lead to a pulmonary embolus.

Keep in mind that muscle pain, cramping, and swelling are common symptoms of a normal pregnancy, and a DVT is quite unusual. Therefore, although it is important to let your doctor know when you are experiencing the sudden onset of these symptoms, don't panic about them.

Pulmonary embolisms are even rarer than DVTs, but they are also more serious. Symptoms include sudden shortness of breath, chest pain, increased heart rate, coughing up blood, and very rapid breathing. Let your doctor know immediately if you experience these symptoms.

Diabetes

Diabetes comes up as a problem in pregnancy in two ways: Either you already have the condition before you become pregnant, or you develop what's called *gestational diabetes,* which is unique to pregnancy and which usually goes away after pregnancy. Gestational diabetes is one of the most common medical complications in pregnancy, occurring in 2 to 3 percent of all pregnant women.

Gestational diabetes

The way your practitioner can diagnose gestational diabetes is by giving you a special blood test. (See Chapter 6 for more information about this test.)

You may wonder why you should bother to go through all this testing. If you have gestational diabetes and your glucose levels are not well controlled, the baby may be at higher risk for certain problems. If your blood sugar levels are high, for example, the fetus's are, too. And high blood sugar levels cause the fetus to produce certain hormones that stimulate fetal growth. This may cause him or her to grow too large (to become *macrosomic;* see Chapter 14). What's more, if the fetus has high blood sugar levels while still in the uterus, there is a chance that, after birth, he or she may have temporary problems with sugar regulation. If the mother's (and fetus's) glucose levels are well controlled during pregnancy, the risk of these complications drops dramatically.

You need to control your sugar levels if you have gestational diabetes. Most of the time, it's enough merely to alter your diet. (Most women have a consultation with a nurse and/or a nutritionist to come up with a specific diet plan.) Exercise also helps. Only in rare cases do women need to resort to taking medication — insulin — to keep their sugar level under control. If you develop gestational diabetes, your doctor may ask you to check your sugar level several times during the day or on a weekly basis. You do this by pricking your finger (called a *fingerstick*) and placing the drop of blood into a little portable machine that gives immediate results.

Diabetes before pregnancy

If you have a history of diabetes, it is important that you talk to your doctor about it before you get pregnant. If you have your blood sugar level under good control before you conceive, your pregnancy is more likely to proceed smoothly. Women with pregestational diabetes stand a higher-than-average risk of having a fetus with certain birth defects, but this risk can be brought down to the normal range if the mothers achieve excellent glucose control.

Our patients want to know . . .

Q: "If I develop gestational diabetes, will I recover when my pregnancy ends?"

A: Most women do recover completely, but a minority remain diabetic. In these cases, pregnancy itself didn't cause the diabetes. Instead, the women were already at risk for developing the condition. This is why, if you develop what is thought to be gestational diabetes, being tested for diabetes within a few months after you deliver is important. Also, keep in mind that your risk for developing diabetes at some point later in your life is increased.

Some doctors suggest that you have a blood test called a *hemoglobin A1C* to check how well your sugar has been controlled over the past few months. Your doctor may also suggest that you have a special sonogram, called a *fetal echocardiogram,* to make sure that the baby's heart is okay. If you take an oral medication to control your blood sugar, your practitioner probably tells you to switch to insulin injections for better control. Some women with diabetes suffer kidney complications, but this kind of problem is not likely to be made worse by pregnancy. Other women who have eye problems related to diabetes *(proliferative retinopathy)* need to have their eyes monitored closely and possibly treated during pregnancy.

The vast majority of women with diabetes proceed through pregnancy without a hitch. However, the dose of insulin often needs to be adjusted. Your doctor also follows the baby's growth with periodic ultrasound exams and is on the lookout to see that you do not develop high blood pressure. In the third trimester, your doctor probably begins to monitor the fetus closely, performing certain tests for fetal well-being (periodic NSTs, for example — see Chapter 7).

When you're in labor, your doctor keeps a close eye on your glucose level and may give you insulin while you are in labor. With optimal glucose control and close monitoring of the baby and mother-to-be, most women with diabetes have an excellent outlook for pregnancy.

Fibroids

Fibroids (also called *uterine myomas*) are benign growths of the muscle cells that make up the uterus. They are extremely common and are often diagnosed during pregnancy during routine sonograms. The high levels of estrogen in a pregnant woman's bloodstream can encourage fibroids to grow larger. Yet predicting whether any woman's fibroids grow, stay the same, or shrink during pregnancy is difficult. Most of the time, fibroids cause no problems for a pregnancy.

In extreme cases, fibroids can cause difficulties:

- Fibroids may grow so fast that they outgrow their blood supply and begin to degenerate, which sometimes causes pain, uterine contractions, and even preterm labor. Symptoms of degeneration include pain and tenderness directly over the fibroid (in the lower abdomen). Short-term treatment with anti-inflammatory medications (Motrin or Indocin, for example) may help.

- Very, very large fibroids in the lower portion of the uterus or near the cervix may interfere with the baby's ability to make its way through the birth canal. Thus, they may increase the risk for cesarean delivery, although this situation is quite unusual.

- Large fibroids within the uterus can sometimes increase the likelihood that the baby will be in the breech or transverse position. But this possibility, too, is rare. Most commonly, fibroids cause no problem at all. And most often, they shrink in size after delivery.

Immunological problems

Immunological problems are conditions in which a person's immune system produces atypical antibodies, which can lead to a variety of problems. In most cases, women who have immunological problems already know they have them before they become pregnant. If you are one of those women, discuss your problem with your doctor before you become pregnant or as early in your pregnancy as possible.

Antiphospholipid antibodies

Antiphospholipid antibodies are a class of antibodies that circulate in the blood of some women. The two most common kinds are *lupus anticoagulant* and *anticardiolipin antibodies*. They may be found in some women with collagen vascular diseases (such as lupus), in women who have had blood clots, and in some women with no known medical problems. They are significant in pregnancy because they have been associated with recurrent miscarriages, unexplained fetal death, early onset of preeclampsia, and intrauterine growth restriction. Doctors do not routinely screen for these antibodies because many women who have them experience no resulting problems. But if you have one of the following conditions, your doctor will probably want to test you:

- Lupus (or other collagen vascular disease)
- A history of spontaneous blood clots in the legs or lungs

✔ A history of stroke or *transient ischemic attacks* (a "temporary" kind of stroke)

✔ A false positive test for syphilis

✔ Autoimmune platelet conditions

Your doctor may also want to test you if you have had any of the following obstetrical problems in the past:

✔ Recurrent miscarriages

✔ Unexplained stillbirth or fetal death

✔ Early-onset preeclampsia

✔ Problems with fetal growth (intrauterine growth restriction)

Antiphospholipid antibody syndrome is diagnosed when a woman has antiphospholipid antibodies in her bloodstream *plus* one of the listed risk factors. If you have the syndrome, depending on its severity, your doctor may recommend that you take baby aspirin, heparin, oral steroids, or some combination of these medications. He or she probably will also recommend that you have periodic ultrasound exams, to make sure that the baby is growing appropriately, and that you undergo tests for fetal well-being (see Chapter 7).

We realize that this syndrome may sound scary, but the good news is that most women who receive adequate medical care have normal pregnancies and healthy babies.

Lupus

Systemic lupus erythematosus (SLE, or *lupus*) is one of several so-called *collagen vascular diseases*. Pregnancy doesn't make the disease worse, but some women do experience more flare-ups during pregnancy.

On the other hand, lupus can affect pregnancy in some cases, depending on the severity of the problem going into pregnancy. If you have a mild form of lupus, chances are it has little effect on your pregnancy. Some women with more severe lupus stand an increased risk of miscarriage, problems with fetal growth, and preeclampsia (see Chapter 14). Depending on your specific medical history, your doctor may recommend certain medications — such as heparin, baby aspirin, or oral steroids. He or she may also recommend more frequent sonograms and other measures of fetal well-being. As is so often the case with chronic medical conditions, the best way to increase your chance for a successful pregnancy is to have the disorder under control as much as possible before you become pregnant.

Inflammatory bowel disease

The two kinds of inflammatory bowel disease are *Crohn's disease* and *ulcerative colitis*. Fortunately, pregnancy does nothing to exacerbate either condition. If you have inflammatory bowel disease, but your symptoms were minor or nonexistent during the months before you became pregnant, chances are good that they remain at bay during your pregnancy. Doctors often recommend that women whose symptoms are frequent and severe postpone pregnancy until the disease abates or is brought under control.

The best news is that most doctors believe that inflammatory bowel disease doesn't cause significant problems for a pregnancy. What's more, most medications used to treat inflammatory bowel disease are considered to be safe and effective during pregnancy. In fact, most doctors think that if medication is needed to control disease activity, it is better to continue taking the medication during pregnancy than to stop taking it and risk the possibility that the disease gets worse.

Seizure disorders (Epilepsy)

Most women who have epilepsy can have an uneventful pregnancy and give birth to a perfectly healthy baby. However, epilepsy does require that a woman's obstetrician and her neurologist work together to come up with the right strategy for controlling seizures. If you have epilepsy, make an effort *before* you get pregnant to control your seizures with the lowest possible dose of medication. Studies show that women whose seizures are well controlled on a minimal dose of a single medication before they get pregnant have the best pregnancy outcomes. So by all means, consult your neurologist before you get pregnant. If your seizures can't be controlled on a single medication, there's still no need to worry. Simply try to get on the lowest doses of the medications you must take. Never stop taking your medications unless your doctor advises you to.

All medications used to treat seizures pose some risk of birth defects. The problems they can cause vary, depending on the particular medication, but they include facial abnormalities, cleft lip and cleft palate, congenital heart defects, and neural tube defects. For this reason, women who take seizure medications need to have an ultrasound to evaluate fetal anatomy and a fetal echocardiogram (see Chapter 6) to look for abnormalities in the baby's heart.

Women with seizure disorders should begin taking extra folic acid about three months before trying to conceive, because some seizure medications can affect folic acid levels.

Do *not* adjust your medications on your own, especially after you become pregnant. Your seizure activity could increase, which would probably be worse for the developing baby than the medications themselves.

Thyroid problems

Problems with thyroid function are relatively common in women of reproductive age, which is why we see many women with overactive or underactive thyroids during pregnancy. Although these conditions require extra testing, they usually do not cause significant problems for pregnancy.

Hyperthyroidism (overactive thyroid)

There are many different causes of hyperthyroidism, but the most common by far is Grave's disease, which is associated with its own special set of antibodies (*thyroid stimulating immunoglobulins,* or TSIs) in the blood. These antibodies cause the thyroid to make too much hormone. Women with an overactive thyroid must receive adequate treatment during pregnancy (ideally, beginning *before* conception) in order to reduce their risk of such complications as miscarriage, preterm delivery, and low birthweight. If you have an overactive thyroid, unless your condition is extremely mild, your doctor most likely recommends that you take certain medications to lower the amount of thyroid hormone circulating in your blood. Some of these medications may cross the placenta, so your doctor watches the fetus closely, usually by performing regular sonograms, to look for any evidence that the medications are lowering the baby's thyroid levels too much. Specifically, he or she monitors the baby's growth and heart rate to see that they are normal and checks for any evidence that the fetus has developed a *goiter* (an enlarged thyroid).

Your doctor probably also monitors the levels of thyroid-stimulating antibodies in your blood because these antibodies may, in some rare cases, cross the placenta and stimulate the baby's thyroid as well. After delivery, your baby's pediatrician watches the baby carefully for any evidence of thyroid problems.

Hypothyroidism (underactive thyroid)

A woman with an underactive thyroid (hypothyroidism) can have a healthy pregnancy as long as her condition is adequately treated. If it is not, she stands a higher risk of developing certain complications, such as having a low birthweight baby. The condition is treated with a thyroid replacement hormone (Synthroid, for example). This medication is safe for the baby, because very little of it crosses the placenta. If you have an underactive thyroid, your doctor may want to periodically check your hormone levels to see whether your medication needs to be adjusted.

Chapter 16

When the Unexpected Happens

● ●

In This Chapter

▶ Dealing with multiple miscarriages

▶ Suffering a loss late in pregnancy

▶ Making a decision when the baby develops an abnormality

▶ Finding help

▶ Trying again

● ●

*W*e wish we had no reason to include this chapter. We wish every pregnant couple could end up delivering a healthy baby. Most do, but not everyone is so fortunate. And so there are times when couples need to know what happens and how to respond when things go wrong. If you are experiencing any of the problems we cover in this chapter, we hope that you find some of this information helpful.

Perhaps you are drawn to this chapter because you have had an unsuccessful pregnancy in the past. If so, you may be anxious about your current pregnancy. That's entirely normal. We take care of many women who have had poor outcomes in the past, and we realize that the only thing that can truly alleviate their anxiety is to hold a healthy baby. This is especially true for women who have no other children.

 One way to at least minimize your worry is to sit down with your doctor and discuss the situation. Ask him or her to map out a plan for your current pregnancy that maximizes your chances for a favorable outcome. When you feel certain that you are doing everything you possibly can do to avoid a recurring problem, you may rest a little easier. Your worry probably won't entirely disappear, but remember that although a certain part of the process is in Mother Nature's hands, you can take medical steps to maximize your chances of having a healthy baby.

Surviving Recurrent Miscarriages

Unfortunately, first trimester miscarriage is a fairly common occurrence. Doctors estimate that about 15 to 20 percent of recognized pregnancies — those that have yielded a positive pregnancy test — end up in miscarriage. Still more early embryos (also called *conceptuses*) are lost before they are actually known to exist — that is, before a pregnancy test is taken. About half the time, the cause of first trimester miscarriage is the presence of some chromosomal abnormality in the embryo or fetus. Another 20 percent of early miscarriages are due to structural abnormalities in the embryo.

Fortunately, 80 to 90 percent of women who experience a single early miscarriage subsequently deliver a normal baby.

Recurrent miscarriage — technically, the loss of three consecutive pregnancies — is far less common. This problem occurs in only ½ to 1 percent of women. A variety of causes contribute to recurrent miscarriage, including the following:

- ✔ Genetic causes

- ✔ Uterine abnormalities

- ✔ Immunologic causes (though not all physicians agree that this is a factor)

- ✔ Possibly, inadequate progesterone secretion

- ✔ Possibly, certain infections (though this cause is also controversial)

- ✔ Antiphospholipid antibody syndrome (see Chapter 15)

- ✔ Rarely, certain environmental toxins or drugs (such as antimalarials and some anesthetic agents)

Most doctors suggest that women undergo certain tests after having three miscarriages; some begin testing even sooner. Because chromosomal abnormalities are the most common cause of miscarriage, an important first diagnostic step is to run tests on the chromosomes of the fetal tissue.

There are various strategies for treating recurrent miscarriage, but doctors may disagree about which one, if any, is best. Choosing a strategy is easier if you know what the problem is. An abnormally shaped uterus may be repaired surgically, for example. If doctors can't find a cause for recurrent miscarriage, knowing which treatment is best may be difficult. Note, however, that even if no treatment is attempted, women who have had three consecutive miscarriages still have a 50 percent or higher chance of having a normal, successful pregnancy.

Coping with Late-Pregnancy Loss

Late-pregnancy loss refers to a fetal death, stillbirth, or death of an infant in the immediate newborn period. Fortunately, these losses are infrequent and rarely occur more than once. Some causes of late losses include

- Chromosomal abnormalities

- Other genetic syndromes

- Structural defects

- A massive placental abruption (see Chapter 14)

- Antiphospholipid antibodies (see Chapter 15)

- Umbilical cord compression

- Unexplained reason, which is, unfortunately, very common

Women who suffer a loss of pregnancy often ask, "Did I do something to cause this?" The answer is almost always no. So you have no reason to add to your grief by mixing in guilt. Many patients find it helpful, after the initial hurt has begun to subside, to gather all their pregnancy records, including any pathology reports, and consult with their doctor or a specialist. Sometimes a cause can be identified, and sometimes not. Either way, most patients benefit from sitting down with their doctor and mapping out a strategy for preventing a loss in future pregnancies. Having a plan to focus on makes many patients feel less helpless. Support groups are also very helpful and should not be overlooked (see "Finding Help" later in this chapter).

In subsequent pregnancies, your doctor may recommend that you undergo blood tests to check for certain abnormalities that have been associated with fetal loss. Often, if you have experienced a prior late-pregnancy loss, doctors follow your progress with regular ultrasound examinations and tests of fetal well-being. Your doctor may recommend that you deliver somewhat early, before you go into labor. You're likely to feel anxious in subsequent pregnancies, which is completely normal. But keep in mind, it is quite unlikely that you will suffer a pregnancy loss a second time — that lightning will strike twice in the same place.

Dealing with Fetal Abnormalities

All prospective parents wonder whether their baby will be "normal." And for most, the answer is yes. Still, 2 to 3 percent of babies end up having a significant abnormality. Some of these abnormalities can be repaired and have very little impact on the baby's overall quality of life. Occasionally, however, the condition can be significant, whether it is a structural, chromosomal, or genetic abnormality.

When an abnormality occurs, the first question many women ask us is, "Is this my fault?" And the answer, most often, is no. From what is known about fetal abnormalities, most are what are called *sporadic,* meaning that they occur randomly and have no identifiable cause. If there is no known cause, chances are unlikely that the same kind of abnormality will recur in a subsequent pregnancy. (If the cause is genetic, there may be some chance that the abnormality could occur again.)

If your fetus is diagnosed with an abnormality, by ultrasound or some other test, your doctor may recommend that you have additional tests to look for other things that have been associated with that particular abnormality. He or she may recommend that you see a genetic counselor to discuss the implications of the abnormality. If the abnormality is a defect that can be surgically repaired or treated, you doctor may recommend that you meet with the specialist who will treat the baby after he or she is born. These discussions help you prepare for what lies ahead during the newborn period and also later on in the child's life.

Nobody wants to get the news that they have a fetus with an abnormality, but having this information is helpful for several reasons:

- ✔ It is important to diagnose some disorders because doctors can treat some of them.
- ✔ The knowledge helps to prepare you for what happens after the baby is born.
- ✔ This information helps you manage your pregnancy and consider all possible options.
- ✔ The information can give you important insights into the management of future pregnancies.

Finding Help

If your pregnancy did not turn out as you had hoped, the first and most obvious place to look for support is from your partner. Family members, friends, and clergy can also be very helpful. Professional advice or treatment from a psychotherapist or social worker may be useful for many couples. Support groups also can provide understanding and expert insight into your problem. If you have a computer and are online, you can find hundreds of support groups on the Internet. Dozens of helpful books are also available, including:

✔ *How to Go on Living After the Death of a Baby,* by Larry G. Peppers and Ronald J. Knapp (Peachtree Publishers, 1985).

✔ *When Mourning Breaks: Coping with Miscarriage,* by Melissa Sexson Hanson (Morehouse Publishing Co., 1998).

✔ *Loss During Pregnancy or in the Newborn Period,* by James Woods and Jennifer Woods (Jannetti Publications, Inc., 1997).

✔ *Roses in December,* by Marilyn Willett Heavilin (Harvest House Publishers, 1998).

Beginning to Heal

Couples naturally feel a strong emotional attachment to their unborn child, beginning as early as the first trimester. So it's no wonder that many couples experience the same grief after the loss of a fetus as they would after the loss of a family member or close friend. The loss of a fetus is no less significant than the loss of a child. Parents who decide to terminate a pregnancy because of an abnormality also go through tremendous grief.

Both parents should acknowledge their need — and their right — to grieve after a pregnancy loss. The emotional response takes time and typically goes through a number of stages, beginning with shock and denial, progressing to anger, and eventually reaching acceptance and the ability to carry on with life.

Our patients want to know . . .

Q: "After a loss, when should we start trying again?"

A: If you have gone through the stages of grief and feel that you are physically and emotionally strong, then you are probably ready. In some couples, one person progresses through the grieving process faster than the other. Make sure that both of you are ready before you begin trying to get pregnant again. And remember that a successful pregnancy, while joyful, does not replace a lost one — so the grieving process is necessary. From a medical perspective, make sure that you finish looking into possible causes for the loss and have a plan of action for the next pregnancy. Realize that your next pregnancy will be somewhat stressful and that you will need extra attention and compassion from your family, friends, and health care professionals.

Part V
The Part of Tens

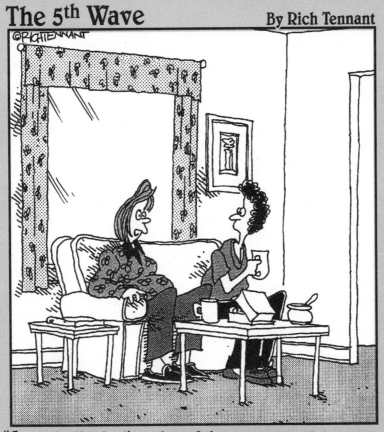

The 5th Wave   By Rich Tennant

"I really think it's a boy. Why else would I turn off 'Masterpiece Theater' to hog the remote through a two-hour 'Wrestlemania'?"

In this part . . .

*H*ere's the part where we get to put things in a nutshell. We describe how the baby grows over the
course of pregnancy and how your practitioner can
observe that growth and development via ultrasound. We
also tell you ten things that pregnant women don't often
hear from their friends and family or even their doctors.
And in keeping with our repeated advice that you not get
bogged down with needless worry while you're pregnant,
we expose ten old wives' tales about pregnancy and ten
myths about predicting your baby's sex.

Chapter 17

Ten Things Nobody Tells You

*I*t isn't as if some conspiracy is keeping you from knowing all there is to know about pregnancy. But your friends, sisters, cousins — whoever tells you what it's going to be like — often forget the little details, especially the more unpleasant ones. Other books, too, often gloss over this stuff, perhaps in the interest of decorum. Well, at the risk of being indecorous, we're going to give it to you straight.

Pregnancy Lasts Longer than Nine Months

Patients always ask, "How many months along am I?" and we have trouble giving them a precise answer. Pregnancy is said to last nine months, but that number isn't exactly accurate. The average pregnancy lasts 280 days, or 40 weeks, starting from the date of the mother's last menstrual period. If a month is four weeks, then that calculation comes out to ten months. On the calendar, however, most months contain four weeks plus two or three days, so nine calendar months often do contain close to 40 weeks. Practitioners speak in terms of weeks when measuring gestational age because it's more accurate and less confusing.

Other People Can Drive You Crazy

Friends, relatives, acquaintances, and strangers alike give you unsolicited opinions and advice and want to share with you every pregnancy horror story they've ever heard. They may tell you that your rear looks big, that you are too fat (or too thin), or that you shouldn't be eating whatever you're putting in your mouth.

We realize that these people usually have only good intentions when they tell you how their sister's pregnancy ended badly, or about the trouble a friend of a friend had. They don't realize that they're increasing your anxiety. Do your best to not pay attention. Try to politely smile and ignore them. Tell them you really don't want to hear this story right now. If you have any real problems or concerns, talk them over with your practitioner.

You Feel Exhausted in the First Trimester

You may already have heard that you're going to feel tired during the first trimester, but until you go through it yourself, you really have no idea how overwhelming the fatigue can be. You may find yourself looking for every possible opportunity to catch a few winks — on the bus, the train, at work, or even on the exam table waiting for your practitioner to come into the room. Rest assured that this fatigue does go away, usually by the end of the first trimester (at about 13 weeks), and you do get your usual energy back. Look out, though. Around 30 to 34 weeks, the physical stress of pregnancy may overwhelm you again, and you may go back to feeling pretty washed out for several weeks.

Round Ligament Pain Really Hurts

The round ligaments run from the top of the uterus down into the labia. As the uterus grows, these ligaments stretch, and many women feel discomfort or pain on one or both sides of the groin area, especially at about 16 to 22 weeks. Practitioners tell you that this symptom is only round ligament pain and that it's nothing to worry about. And they're right — you shouldn't worry. But you deserve some sympathy (you have ours), because this pain can be fairly intense.

You can probably ease round ligament pain a bit by getting off your feet, thereby taking the pressure off the ligaments. The good news is that round ligament pain usually diminishes by about 24 weeks.

Your Belly Becomes a Hand Magnet

After your stomach protrudes noticeably with pregnancy, you're likely to find that suddenly everyone presumes it's okay to touch it — not only your friends, family members, and the people you work with, but also the mailman, the cashier at the supermarket, and people you've never even met. Although some women appreciate the extra attention, many find it an invasion of privacy. You can either grin and bear it or learn to say, "Hey, hands off!"

Hemorrhoids Are a Royal Pain in the Butt

Your best friend may say that she's told you everything about her own pregnancy. But has she remembered her hemorrhoids? Believe us, hemorrhoids happen pretty often, and when they do, you're in for some very noticeable pain and discomfort. *Hemorrhoids* are dilated veins near the rectum that become engorged because of the pressure on that part of the body or because of pushing during delivery. Some women notice hemorrhoids during pregnancy, others don't have any problem with them until after delivery, and some very lucky women never have hemorrhoids at all.

If your hemorrhoids are significant, be prepared for some discomfort after vaginal delivery (see Chapter 11). Most hemorrhoids go away within a few weeks. If you are fortunate enough not to have them, realize how lucky you are — and have sympathy for all the other new mothers who do have them.

Sometimes Women Poop While Pushing

Our patients frequently ask us about having a bowel movement during labor, so although it may not be the most genteel subject to bring up, we're going to anyway. Pooping while pushing doesn't happen every time, but it isn't that uncommon. In all likelihood, you and your partner are not even aware of it happening, because your nurse quickly wipes away any mess and keeps you clean throughout the pushing process. If it does happen, don't give it a thought. No one — neither your doctor nor your partner — is going to be grossed out.

Don't Weigh Yourself the Day After You Deliver

Most women can't wait to weigh themselves after delivering 10 pounds or so of baby, placenta, and fluid. But contain yourself. Wait at least a week. After delivery, many women swell up like dumplings, especially their hands and feet. This extra water retention adds pounds. If you step on the scale right away, you may be very disappointed at the number that comes up. The swelling generally takes about a week or two to go away.

Bring a Box of Modern Pads to the Hospital

At most hospitals, the nurses offer you sanitary napkins from the 1920s — and a cute little elastic belt to hang them on. If you're a time traveler or if for some other reason you prefer this kind, great. But if you want something a little more contemporary, bring your own box of large-size pads with side tabs (along with some fairly sturdy underwear — no thongs).

Breast Engorgement Really Sucks

Of course you know that your breasts fill up with milk after you deliver your baby. But what you may not have heard is how painful and cumbersome this engorgement can be if you are not breast-feeding, or when you decide to stop breast-feeding. Your breasts may become rock hard, tender, and warm, and they sometimes seem to grow to the size of blimps. Fortunately, the discomfort is temporary; this intense period of engorgement lasts only a couple of days.

Chapter 18

Ten Myths about Predicting Your Baby's Sex

In This Chapter

▶ Ultrasound can't always tell

▶ Blowing holes through superstitions

F rom time immemorial, women have been curious to know ahead of time whether they're carrying a boy or a girl. How else do you explain why there are so many superstitious ways of making the prediction? These days, amniocentesis and chorionic villus sampling can give a definitive answer (see Chapters 5 and 6). And in many cases, ultrasound can let you know. But if anyone mentions Drano, look out. In this chapter, we tell you ten gender indicators that don't work.

If we could, we'd put one giant Myth icon on this entire chapter. Remember, the headings are false!

Ultrasound Can Always Tell the Baby's Sex

Often, by about 18 to 20 weeks gestation, it's possible to see the genitalia of a fetus on ultrasound. But being able tell the sex of the baby depends on whether the baby is in position to give you a good view. Sometimes the sonographer can't see between the baby's legs and therefore can't determine the sex. Sometimes, too, the sonographer may be wrong, especially if the ultrasound is done very early in the pregnancy. So even though you can find out the sex of the baby through ultrasound in most cases, it's not 100 percent guaranteed.

The Only Way to Tell the Sex by Ultrasound Is to See the Penis

If you had to see the penis to determine the sex of the baby, then the only way to know that the baby is a girl is if you *don't* see a penis. But that isn't true. A skilled sonographer can see either a penis or labia, if the fetus is in an advantageous position.

If the Woman Initiates the Sex That Leads to Conception, the Baby Is a Girl

A related myth: If the woman's on top when the baby is conceived, it's a boy. But think about it. You know how babies are conceived. (If you don't, see Chapter 1.) How could either scenario possibly make a difference?

If a Pregnant Woman Gains Weight in Her Face, the Baby Is a Girl

And the corollary myth says that if a woman gains weight in her butt, the baby is a boy. Neither statement is true, obviously enough. The baby's sex has no influence whatsoever on the way the mother stores fat.

Another seemingly related myth is that if the mother's nose begins to grow and widen, the baby is a girl. The so-called reasoning here is that a daughter always steals her mother's beauty. Strange concept — and quite untrue.

If a Pregnant Woman's Belly Is Round, the Baby Is a Girl

And if it's more bullet-like, it's a boy. Forget about it. Belly shape differs from woman to woman, but the sex of the child has nothing to do with it.

If a Woman Is Moody during Pregnancy, the Baby Is a Girl

This superstition sounds as if it's based on the old stereotype of the hysterical female. It's total nonsense.

If the Fetal Heart Rate Is Fast, the Baby Is a Girl

And if the heart rate is slow, the baby is a boy. Medical researchers actually looked into this myth. They did find a very slight difference between the average heart rate of boys and that of girls, but it was not significant enough to make heart rate an accurate predictor of sex.

If the Locket Swings Back and Forth, the Baby Is a Boy

Dangle a locket on a chain (or a pencil on a string, or your wedding ring on a chain . . .) over a pregnant woman's abdomen. If it swings back and forth, the baby is a boy. If it swings in a circle, the baby is a girl. Or is it the other way around?

The Old Spoon-and-Fork Myth

Here are the instructions for this one: Place a spoon under one cushion of a sofa and a fork under another. Then invite a pregnant woman to come in and sit down. If she sits on the cushion over the spoon, she's carrying a girl. If she sits over the fork, the baby is a boy. We don't think so.

The Great Drano Hoax

This one is our favorite. Pour a tablespoon of Drano into the toilet bowl and then have the pregnant woman urinate into it. If the water turns pink, she is carrying — you guessed it — a girl. If it turns blue, the baby is a boy. At least if you act on this superstition, your drain will be clog-free.

This "test" can cause noxious fumes — and possibly splatters.

Chapter 19

Ten Old Wives' Tales

. . . .

In This Chapter

▶ Nonproblems you don't have to worry about

▶ Weird notions you don't even have to think about

▶ Strange beliefs you can only shake your head in wonder about

. . . .

Pregnancy has a certain mystique. Millions of women have been through it, yet predicting in detail what any one woman's experience is going to be like is difficult. Perhaps that's why so many myths have formed (and survived) over the centuries, most of which are designed to foresee the unknowable future. Here are ten tales that, alas, are really just so much nonsense.

The Old Heartburn Myth

The oldest one in the book: If a pregnant woman frequently experiences heartburn, her baby will have a full head of hair. Simply not true.

The You-Can't-Be-Too-Careful Myth

If a pregnant woman lifts her hands above her head or steps over a rope, she will choke the baby. Give us a break.

The Curse Myth

Anyone who denies a pregnant woman the food that she craves will get a sty in his or her eye. Nope. (Good thing no one kept Joanne from her pickles and ketchup!)

The Ugly Stick Myth

If a pregnant woman sees something ugly or horrible, she will have an ugly baby. How could this possibly be true? There's no such thing as an ugly baby!

The Java Myth

If a baby is born with *cafe au lait spots* (light-brown birthmarks), the mother drank too much coffee or had unfulfilled cravings during her pregnancy. Nope.

The Myth of International Cuisine

Many people still believe that eating spicy food brings on labor. It doesn't, so go ahead and enjoy your dinner.

The Great Sex Myth

Having passionate sex brings on labor. It doesn't, but go ahead and try it (if you feel like it when you're nine months pregnant). It's likely to be worth the effort.

The Moon Maid Myth

This one holds that more women go into labor during a full moon. Although many labor and delivery personnel insist that the labor floor is busier during a full moon (police say their precinct houses are livelier then, too), the scientific data just doesn't support the idea.

No Good Pregnancy Books

Who says there are no good books about pregnancy? (There's one now!)

Pregnancy Is for Dummies

We realize that your picking up this book doesn't mean that you actually think of yourself as a "dummy" in the negative sense of the word. In fact, we hope that you're reading it to find accurate, up-to-date information and advice from practicing obstetricians. You can go through a pregnancy without knowing much about the process, and things probably turn out fine. But there is so much to know that having the correct information may lessen your anxiety about pregnancy. Knowledge is liberating. A well-informed pregnant woman and her partner know enough not to sweat minor discomforts, inaccurate advice from friends and strangers, and old wives' tales.

Chapter 20

Ten Landmarks in Fetal Development

In This Chapter
▶ Finding out how pregnancy begins
▶ Knowing when the baby takes shape
▶ Recognizing when the baby starts calling attention to him- or herself

*P*regnant women are naturally curious to know how their babies grow. On any given day during pregnancy, they want to know which body parts have developed, which organs are working, and, later on in pregnancy, whether the baby has matured to the point where he or she would be able to thrive outside the uterus. In this chapter, we describe ten major landmarks in fetal development. The sections of this chapter show you the basic scenario for how a fetus develops before birth.

The Baby Is Conceived

The essential first moment of pregnancy occurs when the father's sperm penetrates or fertilizes the mother's egg. Conception occurs, on average, about 14 days after the first day of the mother's last menstrual period (assuming she has a typical 28-day cycle). The average pregnancy lasts 40 weeks after the last menstrual period (38 weeks after conception). See Chapter 2 for more information on the difference between measuring pregnancy in terms of weeks or months.

The Embryo Implants Itself

Implantation usually occurs about seven days after conception. The embryo (or *zygote,* as it's known in the very early stages) spends the first week traveling down the fallopian tube. It reaches the inside of the uterus on about day 5 and begins to implant on about day 6 or 7. The zygote takes several days to implant in the lining of the uterus.

The Heart Begins Beating

The first organ system to start operating in a developing fetus is the cardiovascular system. The embryonic heart starts beating only three weeks after conception. The motion of the beating heart is often one of the first signs of a viable pregnancy that practitioners can detect on ultrasound. In fact, you can sometimes see the beating heart on the ultrasound screen before you can see the embryo itself.

The Neural Tube Closes

The neural tube is the beginning of the central nervous system — the brain and spinal cord. It starts as a flat plate of cells that rolls up into a tube during development. After the ends of this tube close, the primitive nervous system begins the long process of maturing, which continues after the baby is born. The neural tube is normally closed on both ends by day 28 after conception.

The Face Develops

Although fetal facial features mature throughout gestation, the critical period for face development is from five to eight weeks after conception.

The Embryonic Period Ends

The rudiments of all the organs and structures of a normal baby are formed during the so-called *embryonic period,* the first eight weeks of gestation. The *fetal period* that follows is characterized by further maturation of these primitive organs until a happy, healthy, crying baby is born.

The Sexual Organs Appear

Although your baby's sex was determined at the time of conception, the very early embryo appears the same whether it is a male or female. Only after about 12 weeks gestation do either the penis and scrotum or the clitoris and vagina become apparent.

Quickening Occurs

Quickening refers to the mother's first perception of fetal movement. It typically occurs at about 18 to 20 weeks gestation. Although you can see fetal movements on ultrasound much earlier than this, quickening is the first sign of life that the expectant mom can feel.

The Lungs Reach Maturity

The foundations of the fetal respiratory system are present and functioning by 26 to 28 weeks gestation. Some babies born at this time can breathe on their own, but many need the help of a mechanical ventilator. Some babies' lungs mature earlier than others do, but the overwhelming majority of babies have well-developed lungs by 36 to 37 weeks gestation.

A Baby Is Born

This one needs no (further) explanation.

Chapter 21

Ten Key Things You Can See on Ultrasound

If you've ever had a parent-to-be show you an ultrasound picture of the baby, you know it's not always easy to tell what you're looking at. Detecting a family resemblance is out of the question! But ultrasound pictures can be amazingly clear and useful — if you know what you're looking for. In this chapter, we show you the kinds of things that doctors and sonographers try to pick out on ultrasound to find out whether the baby is growing and developing well.

Reproducing ultrasound images in a book like this one is unprecedented. But we think that doing so is worth a try because no other pregnancy book has ultrasound images, and so many of our patients ask questions about what they see.

Measurement of Crown-Rump Length

The crown-rump length is also referred to by its acronym, CRL. This measurement, shown in Figure 21-1, is made from the top of the fetus's head (crown) to the buttocks (rump) during the first trimester. It is the most precise sonographic measurement that your practitioner can use to estimate gestational age.

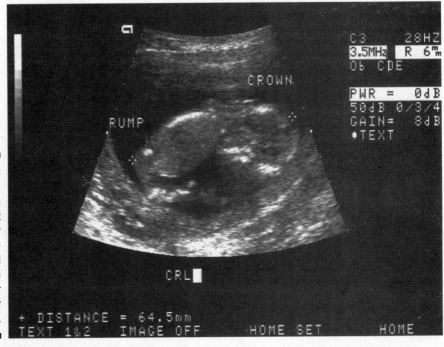

Figure 21-1:
The crown-rump length is a first trimester measurement used to determine how far along your pregnancy is.

The Face

Many people think that the view of the fetus in Figure 21-2, taken during the second trimester, is sort of ghoulish. Some say that the baby looks like ET. But keep in mind that it's not a traditional photograph of the baby's face. The ultrasound beam passes *through* the fetus wherever it is directed and renders a picture of a "section" of the inside of the baby, not the surface.

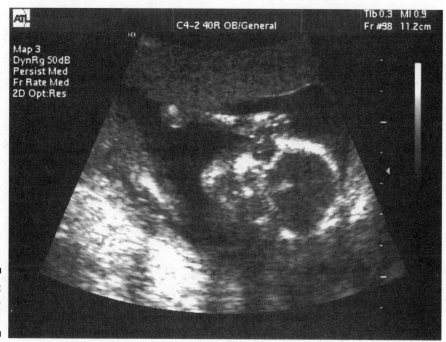

Figure 21-2:
Smile for the camera!

The Spine

The spine is one thing that even most novices at ultrasound can easily find. Take a look at it in Figure 21-3. In the second trimester, imaging the entire spine is important in order to rule out neural tube defects (see Chapter 6).

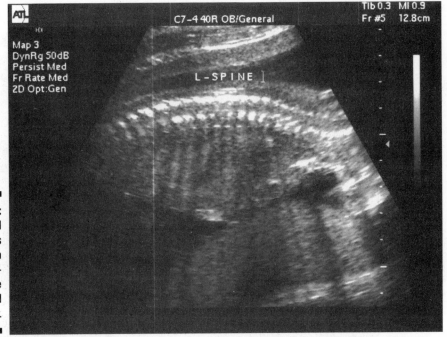

Figure 21-3: The fetal spine is easily seen on ultrasound in the second trimester.

The Heart

The image in Figure 21-4 is the classic four-chamber view of the fetal heart that your practitioner looks for on ultrasound in the second trimester. You can clearly see two *atria* and two *ventricles*. A normal four-chamber view rules out the most major heart abnormalities. During an actual ultrasound, you can see the heart beating and the valves moving.

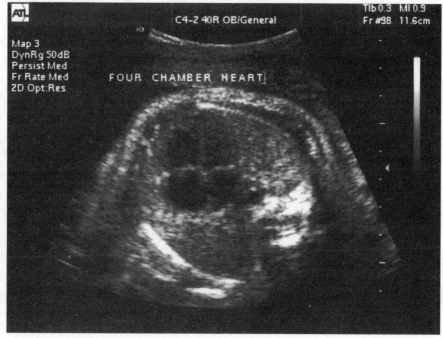

Figure 21-4:
In this picture, you can see the four chambers of the fetal heart. During the actual exam, you also see the heart beating.

The Hands

In the second trimester, counting fetal fingers and toes is a challenge because the fetus moves constantly. But in Figure 21-5, we captured them all in the picture at the same time. You can see five fingers in the lower hand and five in the upper (that's just the tip of the upper hand's thumb you see).

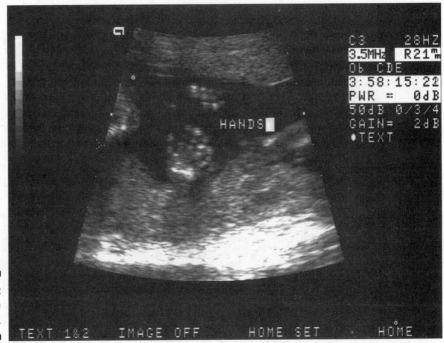

Figure 21-5:
All five
fingers . . .

The Foot

Although you can't predict shoe size yet, you can see five toes on the foot in Figure 21-6, caught on ultrasound in the second trimester.

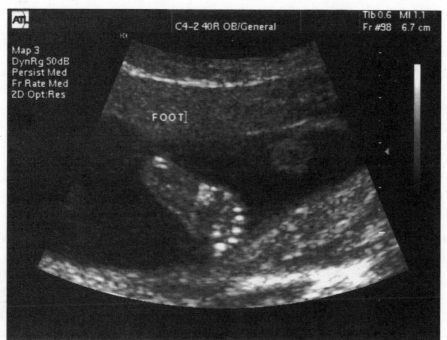

Figure 21-6:
... and all
five toes.

The Fetal Profile

In Figure 21-7, you can see a fetus in the second trimester taking a rest from his or her busy play schedule.

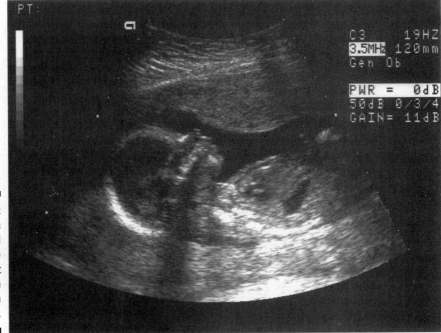

Figure 21-7:
In this ultrasound image, the fetus is at rest and can be seen in clear profile.

The Stomach

Anything that is fluid-filled shows up dark on ultrasound. Because the baby is constantly swallowing amniotic fluid, the stomach shows up as a dark "bubble." (This fetus in Figure 21-8 is also second-trimester.)

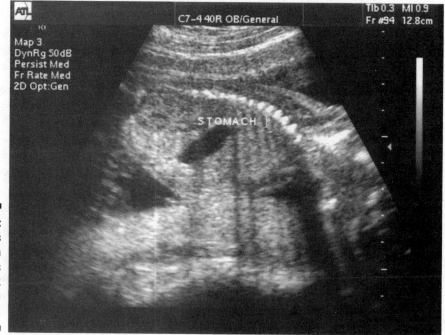

Figure 21-8:
The fetus's
stomach
shows up as
a dark
bubble on
ultrasound.

It's a Boy!

As you can see in Figure 21-9, it's often possible to get a very clear view of the developing penis.

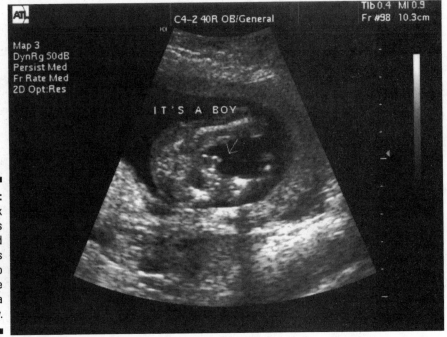

Figure 21-9:
One look at this ultrasound image is enough to tell that the baby is a boy.

It's a Girl!

Figure 21-10 shows an easily recognizable image of the labia.

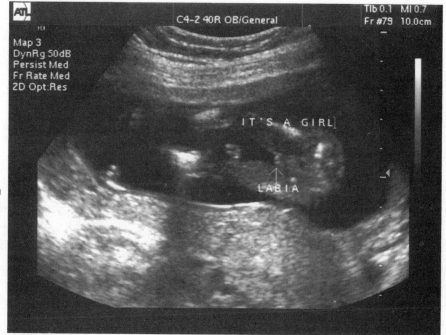

Figure 21-10: This baby, the ultrasound image clearly shows, is a girl.

The Pregnant Man: Having a Baby from a Dad's Perspective

• •

*B*iologically speaking, a woman's role in pregnancy is undoubtedly pivotal. But she can't do it alone. Your part is vital, too, right from the start. The DNA from your sperm provides half the baby's total DNA. And it's your share that determines the baby's sex. If you donate an X chromosome, it's a girl; if you hand in a Y, it's a boy. (A woman's egg always contains an X chromosome.)

Sperm, of course, is only the first contribution you make to the project. The support you provide the mother during pregnancy in some ways is at least as important. Just as pregnancy is a time of tremendous change in a woman's body, so is it a time of tremendous emotional change for both the father and mother, and it is a time of transition for you as a couple — a transition to parenthood. Recognizing this fact can make it easier for you to become comfortable with the whole process and play your role as well as possible. You can do a great deal to make things easier for both of you. Studies clearly show that pregnancy, labor, and delivery are associated with fewer complications when the father is involved and supportive.

Reacting to the news

"Honey, I think I'm pregnant!" You hear the words that millions of other men before you have heard — and you feel pure joy and excitement. Well, not really. You probably also feel some concern, even fear for the future. No matter what you feel, rest assured that it's completely normal. You may be concerned about how parenthood will change your relationship with your partner. You may be concerned about how parenthood will change your life in general. You may worry that you and your partner won't be able to support a family financially, or that you won't be a good father. Just keep in mind that your partner's feelings about having a baby aren't all that simple, either. She's probably having a few worries of her own. So talk to her about what you're both feeling.

Everything every dad wants to know about sex

One of the most common questions that dads ask is about sex during pregnancy. Your desire for sex — like that of your partner — may increase or decrease. Many men worry that inserting the penis into the vagina, next to the cervix, may injure the baby or lead to preterm delivery. But in an uncomplicated pregnancy, you have nothing to worry about at all in this regard. Another common worry is that you may crush the baby by lying on top of your partner. Again, if the pregnancy is normal (especially during the first months), being on top isn't a problem. The baby is surrounded by a cushion of amniotic fluid. Later on in pregnancy, the size of the mother's abdomen may make the missionary position awkward, or your partner may find it uncomfortable. If she is willing, take the time to find alternative positions that are comfortable for her. Also, remember that libido can wax and wane during pregnancy, or it may

wane only (see Chapter 4). For some women, pregnancy is just a sexual turnoff. So try to be understanding if your partner is not interested in sex.

In some cases, intercourse during pregnancy may not be a good idea. If the mother goes into preterm labor, for example, and her cervix is open significantly, refraining may be wise. In the case of placenta previa (see Chapter 14) with bleeding and in some cases of incompetent cervix (see Chapter 6), foregoing intercourse also makes sense. If your partner has one of these problems, and if you are unsure about your partner's situation, talk to her practitioner. And keep in mind that intercourse is not the only way that you and your partner can express your sexual feelings for each other. Often, embracing, cuddling, or fondling can be just as satisfying.

Dad's first trimester

After both of you get over the initial surprise, you are faced with the realities of pregnancy during the first trimester. Your partner is likely to feel exceptionally tired and may need to urinate with remarkable frequency. Chances are she also has morning sickness (see Chapter 2). You are the one who can help most, by assuming more of the day-to-day responsibilities of running the household. Give her the extra time she needs to rest. And be aware of what a drag it can be to be nauseated all the time. Don't get too upset if she can't stand to be around steak (your favorite) or some other food. Be as supportive as you can. If she asks you to run out for more pickles and ketchup (Joanne's favorite first-trimester snack), just smile and ask, "Whole or slices?" "Dill or gherkins?" Try to make room in your schedule to accompany your partner to her first prenatal visit to her practitioner. Your participation is important not only because it telegraphs your support, but also because you may need to answer questions about your family medical history. In addition, you probably have questions to ask the practitioner.

Watching mom grow — the second trimester

"Honey, do you think I'm fat and ugly now?" You may start to hear this question during the second trimester when the mother's body *really* begins to change. Here's a tip: It's not a multiple-choice question. There's only one answer, and you may as well commit it to memory so that you can answer without hesitation: "Absolutely not, honey. You're the most beautiful woman I've ever laid eyes on."

Enjoy the second trimester. Often, it's the most fun part of pregnancy for both parents. Morning sickness fades away, fatigue subsides, and your partner begins to feel the baby move around inside her. Often, you, too, can feel the baby move by placing your hand on the mom's abdomen. During this trimester, many mothers get an ultrasound exam to check the baby's anatomy.

Try to go along to see the ultrasound exam (see Chapter 21); it's one of the most enjoyable prenatal tests. You get to see the baby's hands, feet, and face, and you get to watch the baby move around. For the first time, you see the living, moving, growing little human inside, and suddenly the whole enterprise seems so much more real!

By the end of the second trimester, it may be time to begin prenatal classes. You should go; they are designed for both father and mother. During this time, you can find out how to be useful during labor and delivery. And you can also ask questions about what to anticipate — to relieve some of your own anxiety.

Down to the wire — the third trimester

"I can't sleep." "I look like a beached whale." "I've lost my ankles." The third trimester has arrived. Your partner may begin to feel uncomfortable because of all the changes in her body — and because of her sheer size. Many women do have trouble sleeping late in pregnancy, which only makes it harder for her to tolerate her discomfort. As you did during the first trimester, take on more of the day-to-day household duties and give her the time she needs to rest. Consider treating her to a "day of beauty" at her favorite salon, or send her out for a massage or something else that makes her feel special. She deserves to feel good about herself and the changes her body is going through. And things will go easier for both of you if you can find a way to help her accept her pregnant body, relax, and take things a little easier.

Later in the third trimester, naturally, both of you start to focus on labor and delivery. Your mind may be filled with a million questions: Will the baby be okay? Do I really want to be in the delivery room? How will my partner tolerate labor? How will I tolerate labor? Will I get queasy during the delivery? Psychologically, childbirth can be a real challenge for the father. You care about the course of events very much, but you're clearly not in the driver's seat, and this situation may make you feel anxious.

At the same time, you are faced with truly imminent fatherhood. And the onset of this new responsibility may cause still more anxiety and more questions: Will I be able to provide for my family? Will I be a good father? Can I learn to change a diaper? How will I know how to handle a fragile newborn? These questions are all normal. Again, they are probably very similar to the questions running through your partner's head. Communication is everything. Most couples find that they can talk each other through their respective panic attacks.

Dad in the delivery room

If you plan to join your partner in the delivery room (and we wholeheartedly encourage you to do so!), remember that after you arrive on the labor floor, all attention is focused on Mom, not you. Your primary role is to support your partner. Play that role to the hilt. Help her breathe and focus during her painful contractions. Hold her hands. Fetch ice chips. Encourage her gently when she gets frustrated. If she occasionally snaps at you, don't be surprised, and don't think it means that she wishes you weren't there. After it's all over, she will appreciate your presence. If decisions need to be made about pain management — about whether to have an epidural, for example — help her make them, without being judgmental. She has to make the final decision; after all, it's her body, her pain.

Some fathers may prefer not to watch the actual delivery. Some mothers prefer that their partner not see all the blood involved, the feces that may come out during pushes, or the baby's head emerging from and greatly distending the vagina. Some men opt to avoid the whole scene, too, not wanting to view their partner's genitalia in such a different light. (Indeed, some men who do observe childbirth suffer some sexual dysfunction for a period of time afterward.)

In any case, after the baby is born — and, really, it goes without saying — congratulate your partner on a job well done.

Home at last — with the new family

If pregnancy, labor, and delivery weren't enough to jolt you into the realization that your life is changing forever, getting home from the hospital with your new family certainly does. You and your partner now have a new set of responsibilities. Long gone are the days when it was normal for men to assume that the mother would take them on all by herself. It goes without saying that men can help change diapers (they even have changing tables in men's restrooms these days), feed the baby, shop, and do household chores. Even if the mother is breast-feeding, you can sometimes feed the baby breast milk she has pumped and put into a bottle. In fact, you may want to ask her to prepare bottles this way for you regularly, because feeding the baby is an important and highly satisfying way to bond with him or her.

Your partner is going to need *at least* six weeks to get back to prepregnancy shape, and probably longer. During the first couple of months, she may be exhausted. She's recovering from labor and delivery, after all. And chances are good that both you and she are somewhat sleep deprived. Conditions like these make it easy for anyone to lose his patience from time to time or to lose her temper more often than usual. Simply being aware of the fact that you're operating under special circumstances for a while is helpful. See that your partner has time for rest — and make the effort to take naps yourself when you can.

In a somewhat stressful (even if very joyful) situation such as having a new baby, sex may not be a huge priority. Give yourself and your partner the time you both need to adjust your sex drives to your new life. Even after your partner's practitioner has given her the go-ahead to resume sex (usually about six weeks after delivery) and you are both ready, take things slow and easy at first. The tissue around your partner's vagina and perineum (the area between her vagina and rectum) may still be a little sore. And the fact that it has been some number of weeks or months since the two of you have had intercourse may add to the discomfort. Many couples find it useful to use a lubricant (K-Y jelly, vegetable oil, whatever) for the first few times.

Finally, don't be surprised if you feel unprepared for parenthood, lacking in the skills and understanding it takes to do a good job. Unlike cats, dogs, or jungle animals, humans are not born with sure-fire instincts about how to be perfect parents. Both you *and* your partner need time to develop the skills it takes to handle babies — and children, and teenagers. . . . Along the way, you often work by trial and error. Just realize and accept this situation. Talk about it with each other — often. And fasten your seat belts. You're in for an incredible adventure.

Index

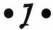

FREE

american baby

for expectant mothers!

To receive your FREE subscription to the #1 prenatal magazine, simply fill out this mail-in coupon. Each issue is filled with information and advice to help you through the exciting months ahead.

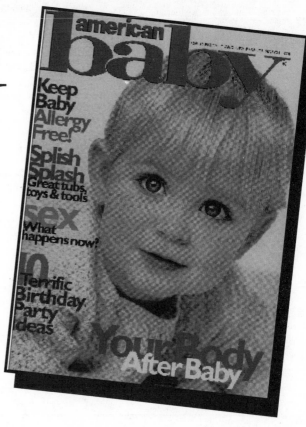

For myself

☐ **Yes**, I wish to receive **American Baby Free!**
☐ No

Name _____ (Please print)

Address _____ Apt.#

City _____ State ___ Zip

Due date ____/____ First Child? ☐ Yes
Month Year

Signature _____ Date ___ WPDA

For my friend

☐ **Yes**, I wish to receive **American Baby Free!**
☐ No

Name _____ (Please print)

Address _____ Apt.#

City _____ State ___ Zip

Due date ____/____ First Child? ☐ Yes
Month Year

Signature _____ Date ___ WPDB

Send now for **FREE subscription** to :
American Baby P.O. Box 53093
Boulder, CO 80322-3093
or for fastest service fax to 212-462-4690.
Available only in the U.S.

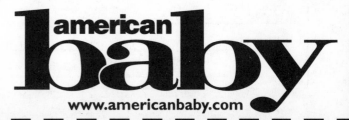

www.americanbaby.com

Notes